Cardiac Surgery Essentials

Cardiac Surgery Essentials

Edited by Evie Brooks

hayle medical

New York

Hayle Medical,
750 Third Avenue, 9th Floor,
New York, NY 10017, USA

Visit us on the World Wide Web at:
www.haylemedical.com

ISBN: 978-1-63241-920-0

Cataloging-in-publication Data

Cardiac surgery essentials / edited by Evie Brooks.
    p. cm.
Includes bibliographical references and index.
ISBN 978-1-63241-920-0
1. Heart--Surgery. 2. Heart--Diseases--Nursing. 3. Surgical emergencies.
4. Cardiology. I. Brooks, Evie.
RD598 .C37 2020
617.412--dc23

Table of Contents

Permissions

List of Contributors

Index

Preface

Cardiac surgery, also known as cardiovascular surgery, is the surgery which is performed either on the heart or the great vessels. It is performed to treat various conditions such as congenital heart disease, valvular heart disease and ischemic heart disease. There are numerous types of cardiac surgeries like open-heart surgery, coronary artery bypass grafting, minimally invasive surgery and heart transplantation. Postoperative care is vital after a cardiac surgery had been performed. This is to ensure that complications and infections do not occur, and scarring is kept to a minimum. After surgery, the patient is closely monitored in an intensive care unit for heart rate, oxygen levels and blood pressure. Stroke, postperfusion syndrome and skumin syndrome are some complications that can occur in patients after surgery. This book elucidates new procedures of cardiac surgery in a comprehensive manner. It will also provide interesting topics for research which interested readers can take up. This book, with its detailed analyses and data, will prove immensely beneficial to professionals and students involved in this area at various levels.

After months of intensive research and writing, this book is the end result of all who devoted their time and efforts in the initiation and progress of this book. It will surely be a source of reference in enhancing the required knowledge of the new developments in the area. During the course of developing this book, certain measures such as accuracy, authenticity and research focused analytical studies were given preference in order to produce a comprehensive book in the area of study.

This book would not have been possible without the efforts of the authors and the publisher. I extend my sincere thanks to them. Secondly, I express my gratitude to my family and well-wishers. And most importantly, I thank my students for constantly expressing their willingness and curiosity in enhancing their knowledge in the field, which encourages me to take up further research projects for the advancement of the area.

Editor

Cardiac tamponade and para-aortic hematoma post elective surgical myocardial revascularization on a beating heart – a possible complication of the Lima-stitch and sequential venous anastomosis

Anna Marcinkiewicz[1*], Ryszard Jaszewski[1], Katarzyna Piestrzeniewicz[2] and Radosław Zwoliński[1]

Abstract

Background: Off-pump coronary artery bypass (OPCAB) surgery can be associated with some intrinsic, but relatively rare complications. A pericardial effusion is a common finding after cardiac surgeries, but the prevalence of a cardiac tamponade does not exceed 2% and is less frequent after myocardial revascularization.

Authors believe that in our patient an injury of a nutritional pericardial or descending aorta vessel caused by the Lima stitch resulted in oozing bleeding, which gradually leaded to cardiac tamponade. The bleeding increased after introduction of double antiplatelet therapy and caused life-threatening hemodynamic destabilization. According to our knowledge it is the first report of such a complication after OPCAB.

Case presentation: We present a case of a 61-year old man, who underwent elective surgical myocardial revascularization on a beating heart. On the 11th postoperative day the patient was readmitted emergently to the intensive care unit for severe chest pain, dyspnoea and hypotension. Coronary angiographic control showed a patency of the bypass grafts and significant narrowing of circumflex artery, treated with angioplasty and stenting. The symptoms and hemodynamic instability exacerbated. A suspicion of dissection of the ascending aorta and para-aortic hematoma was stated on 16-slice cardiac computed tomography. The patient was referred to the Cardiovascular Surgery Clinic. Transthoracic echocardiography revealed cardiac tamponade. On transesophageal echocardiography there were no signs of the ascending aorta dissection, but a possible lesion of the descending aorta with para-aortic hematoma was visualized. Emergent rethoracotomy and cardiac tamponade decompression were performed. 12 days after intervention the control 64-slice computed tomography showed no lesions of the ascending or descending aorta. On one-year follow-up patient is in a good condition, the left ventricular function is preserved and there is no pathology in thoracic aorta on echocardiography.

Conclusions: Mechanical complications of surgical myocardial revascularization on a beating heart should be considered as a cause of the clinical and hemodynamic instability relatively early in the postoperative period. Echocardiographic examination must be the first step in diagnostics process in a patient after cardiac surgery.

Keywords: Lima-stitch, Cardiac tamponade, Aortic dissection

* Correspondence: annamar87@o2.pl
[1]Cardiac Surgery Clinic, Chair of Cardiology and Cardiac Surgery, Military Medical Academy University Teaching Hospital - Central Veterans' Hospital in Lodz, Sterling 1/3 St, Lodz 91-425, Poland
Full list of author information is available at the end of the article

Background

Avoiding extracorporeal circulation (ECC) results in a lower inflammatory response, less myocardial or kidney damage and blood–brain barrier injury. Elimination of the ECC decreased the sex-depending differences in the results of surgical revascularization [1]. Still, there is no consensus about the long-term results of the beating heart surgery. Off-pump coronary artery bypass (OPCAB) surgery is associated with some intrinsic, but relatively rare complications: mechanical damage of the cardiac walls by suction stabilizers, coronary arteries injury by vascular loops or shunts, acute aortic dissection, lesions of the pulmonary vein, descending aorta or esophagus, gaseous embolism, as well as some exceptional adverse events as vasoplegic syndrome [2,3]. The crucial issue during revascularization on a beating heart allowing to perform anastomoses on the posterior and lateral wall is insertion of the pericardial stitch (firstly performed by Ricardo Lima) [4].

We presented a case of a patient who developed cardiac tamponade on the 11th postoperative day. Authors believe that it was a result of an injury of a nutritional pericardial or descending aorta vessel caused by the Lima stitch. A double antiplatelet therapy aggravated the bleeding. Echocardiography performed on the readmission could have allowed to make a proper diagnosis. According to our knowledge it is the first report of such a complication after OPCAB.

Case presentation

A 61-year old man with a history of arterial hypertension with a 3-month history of unstable angina was admitted to hospital. Coronary angiography revealed significant bi-level stenosis of the left anterior descending artery (LAD) and 70% stenosis in the central segment of circumflex artery (Cx) with its further amputation. The patient was referred to elective myocardial surgical revascularization on a beating heart, without extracorporeal circulation. Left internal mammary artery (LIMA) was used to bypass the left anterior descending artery (LAD) and the sequential venous anastomosis to diagonal and marginal branches was performed. A pericardial deep stitch (Lima stich) allowed to perform anastomoses on the lateral cardiac wall. The surgery and the postoperative period was uneventful. Patient was extubated the same day and discharged in a good condition 7 days later. Early postoperative transthoracic echocardiography (TTE) revealed mild hypokinesis of the para-apical and central segments of the interventricular septum and basal segments of the infero-posterior wall with preserved ejection fraction (EF) - 54% and small pericardial effusion (0,9 cm).

On the 11th postoperative day the patient was readmitted to the intensive care unit in a local hospital for severe chest pain, dyspnoea NYHA IV functional class and hypotension. The blood pressure was 80/50 mmHg and the heart rate was 120/min. On electrocardiogram (ECG) nonspecific changes of ST-segment in left precordial leads were observed (1 mm downsloping depression, with flat/slight negative T waves in I, aVL, V4-V6). The diagnosis of an acute coronary syndrome without persistent ST-segment elevation was made. Mild elevation in cardiac enzymes was detected. The arterial pressure was maintained with catecholamines infusion. Coronary angiographic control showed patent LIMA and sequential venous grafts. Significant narrowing of circumflex artery which was treated with angioplasty and stenting with drug-eluting stent (DES) was also found. Consequently a double antiplatelet therapy was commenced. The symptoms and hemodynamic instability even exacerbated. 16-slice computed tomography (CT) disclosed effusion in the pericardial sac and around the ascending aorta what was suggestive for the dissection of the anterior wall of the ascending aorta. Patient in severe clinical condition was emergently referred to the Cardiovascular Surgery Clinic in Lodz where mechanical ventilation was applied for the cardiorespiratory insufficiency not controlled with catecholamines infusion. The blood tests showed increased level of troponin T (119,3 ng/L), leukocytes count (21.700 mc/L), platelets count (453.000 mc/L), C-reactive protein (201,3 mg/L), significantly increased liver enzymes and high creatinine level suggesting multiple organ dysfunction syndrome (MODS). Creatine kinase-MB was within normal limits (18 U/L). The clinical presentation together with TTE/TEE allowed to diagnose cardiac tamponade. There were no echocardiographic signs of dissection of the ascending aorta, but an increased distance between the probe and the aortic wall was suggestive for the para-aortic effusion (mediastinal hematoma) (Figure 1). A slight flow from the descending aorta towards the effusion was noticed suggesting either the ostial flow in the pericardial or esophageal aortic branch or the aortic rupture (Figure 2).

Patient was emergently transferred to the operating theatre, where rethoracotomy was performed. Blood from the pericardial sac was evacuated and cardiac tamponade decompressed with dramatic improvement in clinical status of the patient. Para-aortic hematoma was confirmed but there was no evidence of damage to the aorta. The drainage from pericardial sac was 270 ml during the following day.

12 days after intervention the control 64-slice CT showed no lesions of the ascending or descending aorta. On one-year follow-up patient is in a good condition, the left ventricular function is preserved and there is no pathology in thoracic aorta on TEE.

Discussion

The presented case requires differential diagnosis of several possible causes of the significant hemodynamic

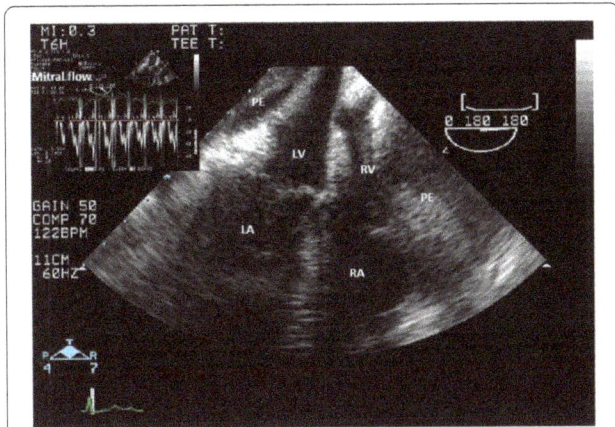

Figure 1 Transesophageal echocardiography. Cardiac tamponade. Pericardial effusion with collapse of left and right ventricles and significant respiratory variations of the transmitral flow velocities (left upper corner) – typical for cardiac tamponade. PE – pericardial effusion, LV - left ventricle, RV – right ventricle, LA - left atrium, RA – right atrium.

decompensation that occurred on the 11th postoperative day.

Early graft occlusion and myocardial infarction was one of the considered causes of patient's symptoms and hemodynamic instability. Prevalence of this complication is estimated on 3-12% for venous grafts and 1–2,5% for the internal thoracic artery [5]. Vascular loops and tourniquets passed under the coronary arteries may damage arterial walls and intraluminal shunts may cause lesions of the vascular endothelium. Although pericardial effusion is a common finding after cardiac surgeries, but the prevalence of a cardiac tamponade does not exceed 2% and is less frequent after myocardial revascularization [6]. The effusion or hematoma is usually not massive and is more likely regional than circumferential. That is

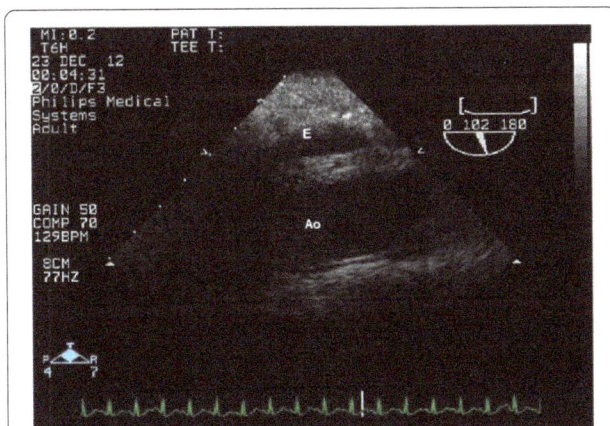

Figure 2 Transesophageal echocardiography. Descending aorta – long axis view. Increased distance between the probe and the aortic wall with the echo-free space suggestive for the para-aortic effusion. Ao – aorta, E - effusion.

why the role of fluid accumulated in pericardium that should be considered as a cause of severe clinical condition and cardiac tamponade is neglected. The final clinical outcome depends on the appropriate time of rethoracotomy [7].

Dressler's syndrome was considered but during rethoracotomy not a bloody effusion but hematoma and fresh blood filling the pericardial sac were found. It seemed apparent that bleeding was a cause of the cardiac tamponade.

Unfortunately TTE, that should be the first step of diagnostic process in this particular case and might have disclosed pericardial effusion was not performed on admission in the local hospital. At that time, mild elevation of troponin T level was not diagnostic for an acute coronary event, as blood levels of this marker may remain increased up to 2 weeks after surgical myocardial revascularization. Cardiac tamponade was another possible cause of the elevation of troponin level. In our opinion stenting of the circumflex artery was not appropriate as the marginal venous bypass graft was well functioning. Introduction of double antiplatelet therapy might have increased the oozing bleeding and caused further patient's destabilization.

Another possible complication after beating heart surgery is an intraoperative mechanical heart wall damage with suction devices. Mandke et al. [8] presented a case of subepicardial hematoma, which was evacuated intraoperatively, but early after the surgery dissecting intramural hematoma with tamponade occurred.

OPCAB procedure may lead to an acute ascending aorta dissection as a result of the partial clamping of the aorta for suturing the proximal anastomoses. Hagl and Griepp [9] suggested that in case of poor aortic wall quality the risk of dissection is even higher for OPCAB than procedures under ECC. Some authors emphasized underestimation of this complication, which prevalence is 3-5%, especially in cases of sudden postoperative deaths with ventricular tachyarrhythmias [10]. Iatrogenic ascending aorta dissection can occur at any time after the operation. It often presents as acute neurological deficits, rapidly arising mediastinal hematoma and finally aortic rupture. Such cases must be aggressively treated. However iatrogenic dissection can be clinically silent and found incidentally with conservative treatment as a solution [10]. In our patient neither the clinical presentation nor the dynamics of arising effusion indicated dissection. The diagnosis of our experienced echocardiographist based on TEE excluded the presence of aortic dissection and was definitively confirmed during re-exploration of the mediastinum.

The most interesting issue in this case are the confusing results of imaging examinations. The firstly performed 16-slice CT, considered as diagnostic tool of relatively low sensitivity and specificity, revealed limited dissection of the ascending aorta at the area of the proximal bypass graft anastomosis, which was not confirmed on subsequent TEE. Thinking of the possible explanation of this diagnostic discrepancy we considered iatrogenic aortic dissection as a result of proximal bypass graft anastomosis or at the time of coronary artery bypass angiography, self-healed within following hours. Garg P et al. [11] described spontaneous recovery of aortic dissection in several hours.

Salerno et al. [12] reported a fatal case of descending aorta injury. Fukui et al. [13] described a case of a lesion in the pulmonary vein with retrocardiac hematoma formation.

The presented case is an example of a rare but extremely dangerous complication of beating heart revascularization. The authors believe that a lesion of a pericardial or aortic nutritional vessel caused by Lima-stitch resulted in the life-threatening complication. Echocardiographic examination remains the first step in diagnostic process in a patient after cardiac surgery.

Conclusions
Mechanical complications of surgical myocardial revascularization on a beating heart should be considered as a cause of the clinical and hemodynamic instability relatively early in the postoperative period.

Consent
Written informed consent was obtained from the patient for publication of this Case report and any accompanying images. A copy of the written consent is available for review by the Editor of this journal.

Abbreviations
DES: Drug-eluting stent; CT: Computed tomography; TTE: Transthoracic echocardiography; TEE: Transesophageal echocardiography; ECC: Extracorporeal circulation; OPCAB: Off-pump coronary artery bypass; LAD: Left anterior descending artery; Cx: Circumflex artery; LIMA: Left internal mammary artery; EF: Ejection fraction; ECG: Electrocardiogram; MODS: Multiple organ dysfunction syndrome.

Competing interest
The authors declare that they have no competing interests.

Authors' contributions
AM made the conception and design of the paper, drafted the manuscript, was responsible for acquisition of the data, literature searching, interpretation of the data and its revision. RJ helped to revise it critically for important intellectual content, participated in its design and coordinated. KP prepared the echocardiograms, helped to draft the manuscript, helped to revise it critically for important intellectual content. RZ helped to draft the manuscript, helped to design it properly and choose appropriate literature, helped to revise it critically for important intellectual content. All authors were involved in the patient's treatment and made a substantial contribution to the manuscript preparation. All authors read and approved the final manuscript.

Author details
[1]Cardiac Surgery Clinic, Chair of Cardiology and Cardiac Surgery, Military Medical Academy University Teaching Hospital - Central Veterans' Hospital in Lodz, Sterling 1/3 St, Lodz 91-425, Poland. [2]Department of Cardiology, Chair of Cardiology and Cardiac Surgery, Military Medical Academy University Teaching Hospital - Central Veterans' Hospital in Lodz, Lodz, Poland.

References
1.   Puskas JD, Kilgo PD, Kutner M, Pusca SV, Lattouf O, Guyton RA: Off-pump techniques disproportionately benefit women and narrow the gender disparity in outcomes after coronary artery bypass surgery. *Circulation* 2007, 116(11):192–199.
2.   Mantovani V, Sala A: Off-pump coronary artery bypass surgery: surgical complications. *New Technologies in Surgery* 2009, 1(1):1–3.
3.   Raja SG, Dreyfus GD: Vasoplegic syndrome after off-pump coronary artery bypass surgery: an unusual complication. *Tex Heart Inst J* 2004, 31(4):421–424.
4.   Lima RC, Escobar MAS, Lobo Filho JG, Diniz R, Saraiva A, Césio A, Gesteira M, Vasconcelos F: Resultados cirúrgicos na revascularização do miocárdio sem circulação extracorpórea: análise de 3.410 pacientes. *Rev Bras Cir Cardiovasc* 2003, 18(3):261–267.
5.   Laflamme M, DeMey N, Bouchard D, Carrier M, Demers P, Pellerin M, Couture P, Perrault LP: Management of early postoperative coronary artery bypass graft failure. *Interact Cardiovasc Thorac Surg* 2012, 14(4):452–456.
6.   Pepi M, Muratori M, Barbier P, Doria E, Arena V, Berti M, Celeste F, Guazzi M, Tamborini G: Pericardial effusion after cardiac surgery: incidence, site, size, and haemodynamic consequences. *Br Heart J* 1994, 72(4):327–331.
7.   ten Tusscher BL, Groeneveld JAB, Otto K, Jansen EK, Albertus B, Gribes ARJ: Predicting outcome of rethoracotmy for suspected pericardial tamponade following cardio-thoracic surgery in the intensive care unit. *J Cardiothorac Surg* 2011, 6:79.
8.   Mandke NV, Nalladaru ZM, Chougule A, Mandke AN: Intra myocardial dissecting hematoma with epicardial rupture - an unusual complication of the Octopus 3 stabilizer. *Eur J Cardiothorac Surg* 2002, 21(3):566–567.
9.   Hagl C, Griepp RB: Aortocoronary bypass surgery and ascending aortic dissection: letter 1. *Ann Thorac Surg* 2001, 72(4):1444–1446.
10. Tabry IF, Costantini EM: Acute Aortic Dissection Early after Off-Pump Coronary Surgery True Frequency Underestimated? *Tex Heart Inst J* 2009, 36(5):462–467.
11. Garg P, Buckley O, Rybicki FJ, Resnic FS: Resolution of iatrogenic aortic dissection illustrated by computed tomography. *Circ Cardiovasc Interv* 2009, 2(3):261–263.
12. Salerno TA: A word of caution on deep pericardial sutures for off-pump coronary bypass procedures. *Ann Thorac Surg* 2003, 76(1):339.
13. Fukui T, Suehiro S, Shibata T, Hattori K, Hirai H: Retropericardial hematoma complicating off-pump coronary artery bypass surgery. *Ann Thorac Surg* 2002, 73(5):1629–1631.

Mediterranean dietary quality index and dietary phytochemical index among patients candidate for coronary artery bypass grafting (CABG) surgery

Mahdieh Abbasalizad Farhangi[1], Mahdi Najafi[2]*, Mohammad Asghari Jafarabadi[3] and Leila Jahangiry[4]

Abstract

Background: The aim of the present research was to evaluate the relationship between Mediterranean dietary quality index (Med-DQI) and dietary phytochemical index (DPI) with metabolic risk factors of cardiovascular disease in candidates for coronary artery bypass graft (CABG) surgery.

Methods: This was a cross-sectional study on 454 patients aged 35–80 years as candidates of CABG and hospitalized in Tehran Heart Center. Anthropometric and demographic characteristics were obtained from all participants and a 138-item semi-quantitative food frequency questionnaire (FFQ) was used to evaluate Med-DQI and DPI. Biochemical parameters including HbA1C, serum lipids, albumin, creatinine and C-reactive protein (CRP) were assessed by commercial laboratory methods.

Results: Patients with higher scores of "saturated fatty acids" had lower serum albumin concentrations ($P < 0.05$). High scores of "cholesterol" subgroup was also accompanied with higher serum Hb A1C percent ($P = 0.04$). Significantly higher concentrations of serum creatinine were also observed in categorizes with lower "fish" scores. Patients with lower phytochemical intakes had significantly higher Med-DQI scores.

Conclusion: According to our findings, high dietary intakes of saturated fatty acids and cholesterol were associated with low serum albumin and Hb A1C concentration. Further studies are needed to better clarify these associations and possible underlying mechanisms.

Keywords: Med-DQI, Mediterranean dietary style, Dietary phytochemical index, CABG

Backgrounds

Cardiovascular disease (CVD) is one of the most common causes of morbidity and mortality in different communities accounting for more than 31% or 17.5 million deaths worldwide; more that 75% of these deaths occur in low and middle income countries and nearly 50% of all deaths in Iran [1, 2]. Coronary artery bypass grafting (CABG) is the most common type of open-heart surgical interventions for the treatment of patients in the higher stages of coronary artery disease (CAD), where atherosclerosis of one or more of coronary arteries is severe enough to show at least 50% stenosis of arterial lumen in angiographic image. The number of CABG operations carried out to treat CAD has increased more than fivefold since 1980, and the general trend has been an almost steady rise in the number of operations performed each year [3]. Independent risk factors of CVD include a family history of premature coronary artery disease, cigarette smoking, diabetes mellitus, hypertension, dyslipidemia, sedentary life style, unhealthy food choices and poor eating habits [4].

The role of dietary factors and nutritional regimens in prevention of CVD and its progression has been extensively studied; numerous reports suggested the role of healthy dietary choices and improved life style with higher physical activity level [5] and higher intakes of

* Correspondence: najafik@sina.tums.ac.ir
[2]Department of Research, Tehran Heart Center, Tehran University of Medical Sciences, North Karegar Street, Tehran 1411713138, Iran
Full list of author information is available at the end of the article

healthy food choices including fruits and vegetables and dietary antioxidants in prevention and treatment of cardiovascular events [6].

The Mediterranean diet is considered as one of the healthiest dietary models, and numerous epidemiological and nutritional studies have shown that Mediterranean countries benefit from lower rates of morbidity from chronic disease and higher life expectancy [7]. The Mediterranean dietary pattern is characterized by a high intake of vegetables, legumes, fruits and nuts, cereals (that in the past were largely unrefined), a high intake of olive oil but a low intake of saturated lipids, a moderately high intake of fish, a low-to-moderate intake of dairy products (and then mostly in the form of cheese or yoghurt), a low intake of meat and poultry and a regular but moderate intake of alcohol [8]. The diet exerts most of its health-promoting effects via its bioactive compounds including phytochemicals. These phenolic ingredients mostly concentrated in olives, grapes and nuts protect against cardiovascular events, oxidative stress and vascular dysfunction [9, 10]. The Mediterranean diet is the best example of a phytochemical-rich diet; recently, two studies have reported that Mediterranean and phytochemicals-rich diets both reduce total cholesterol, LDL-C and non-HDL-C levels and has significant cardio-protective effects [11]. Dietary phytochemical content can be evaluated by dietary phytochemical index (DPI) first proposed by McCarty [12]. DPI, defined as the percent of dietary calories derived from foods rich in phytochemicals could be used as an index of total dietary phytochemical content; this index is a simple method for assessment of phytochemical intake that, despite its limitations, could provide important background for diet quality and may have high practical and clinical uses [12, 13].

Several previous studies suggested the protective role of Mediterranean dietary regimen in prevention of cardiovascular events [6] and other chronic disease like diabetes and metabolic syndrome [6, 14]. In a multicenter trial in Spain, a Mediterranean diet supplemented with extra-virgin olive oil and a Mediterranean diet supplemented with mixed nuts reduced the risk of major cardiovascular disease by 30% and 28% respectively [6]. In other study by Hoscan et al. in Turkish population, for each score of reduction in Mediterranean diet intake, in men, the risk of myocardial infarction, coronary bypass, coronary angioplasty, and any cardiovascular disease in men increased by 1.3 ($P = 0.02$), 1.4 ($P = 0.03$), 1.5 ($P = 0.01$), and 1.3 ($P = 0.02$) respectively, while in women, the risk of myocardial infarction and angioplasty increased by 1.3 ($P = 0.02$) and 1.5 ($P = 0.01$), respectively [15]. In a meta-analysis by Martinez-Gonzalez MA [16], an intervention with a Mediterranean diet was associated with a 38% relative reduction in the risk of CVD clinical events (pooled random-effects risk ratio: 0.62; 95% confidence interval, CI: 0.45–0.85). It has been suggested that there would be a synergy among the nutrient-rich foods included in the Mediterranean diet that fosters favorable changes in intermediate pathways of cardio-metabolic risk factors, like blood lipids, insulin sensitivity, resistance to oxidation, inflammation, and vaso-reactivity [17].

Almost all of the above-mentioned studies focused on evaluating the relations between Mediterranean dietary pattern and the risk of disease. However, findings based on dietary patterns that depend on the consumption characteristics of the sample under study cannot be generalized; In fact, based on real cultural heritage and traditions, a priori indices like Mediterranean dietary scores, used to evaluate adherence to the Mediterranean diet should consider classifying whole grains and refined grains olive oil and monounsaturated fats, and wine and alcohol differently [18]; Mediterranean dietary quality index (Med-DQI) first developed by Gerber et al. [19] is a useful tool to evaluate quality of diet highlighting two different sources of fat (saturated and olive oil) and two different sources of protein (meat and fish) with the opposite scores, one on the poor side and other on the good side respectively (Table 1). There are some studies assessing dietary quality in patients with myocardial infarction [20] or established CAD [21] in which a priori healthy diet pattern score was used. However, to our review of literature, no report was found evaluating the Mediterranean dietary quality index or dietary phytochemical index in patients undergoing CABG surgery in Iran. Therefore in the current study we aimed to investigate Med-DQI and DPI in CABG patients during 1 year pre-operation period, and looked for associations with some demographic factors and biochemical risk factors.

Methods
Subjects
Participants in the current cross-sectional study were candidates for isolated CABG with cardiopulmonary bypass and were recruited for Tehran Heart Center-

Table 1 Construction of the score for the Mediterranean Dietary Quality Index

Scoring	0	1	2
Saturated fatty acids (% energy)	<10	10–13	>13
Cholesterol (milligram)	<300	300–400	>400
Meats (gram)	<25	25–125	>125
Olive oil (milliliter)	>15	15–5	<5
Fish (gram)	>60	60–30	<30
Cereals (gram)	>300	300–100	<100
Vegetables + fruits (gram)	>700	700–400	<400

Table 2 General characteristics of study participants according to different categorizes of total Med-DQI and DPI scores

	Med-DQI score		$P^\dagger$ value	DPI tertiles			P value‡
	<6	> 6		1st	2nd	3rd	
Age (y)	58.99 ± 8.93	58.27 ± 3.80	0.95	58.45 ± 9.92	59.52 ± 8.61	59.04 ± 8.38	0.59
Male (%)	233 (77.2)	100 (65.8)	*0.004*	125 (83.9)	100 (67.6)	108 (68.8)	*0.016*
Body mass index (kg/m^2)							
<24.9	82 (27.7)	48 (32.2)	0.28	52 (35.6)	31 (21.2)	37 (30.7)	*0.02*
25–29.9	132 (44.6)	65 (43.6)		69 (47.3)	71 (48.6)	57 (37.3)	
≥ 30	82 (27.7)	36 (24.2)		25 (17.1)	44 (30.1)	49 (32.0)	
Educational level (%)							
Uneducated	148 (50.5)	93 (62.4)	*0.02*	77 (52.7)	88 (60.7)	76 (50.3)	0.34
< Diploma	96 (32.8)	39 (26.2)		51 (34.9)	36 (24.8)	48 (31.8)	
Diploma and higher	49 (16.7)	17 (11.4)		18 (12.3)	21 (14.5)	27 (17.9)	
Diabetes (%)	119 (39.4)	73 (48.0)	*0.04*	60 (40.3)	62 (41.9)	70 (44.6)	0.44
Hyperlipidemia (%)	219 (72.5)	104 (68.4)	0.21	104 (69.8)	109 (73.6)	110 (70.1)	0.69
Hypertension (%)	145 (48.2)	72 (47.4)	0.47	65 (43.6)	75 (50.7)	77 (49.4)	0.32

†P values from independent sample T-test, ‡P values from ANOVA analysis. The comparison of discrete variables is performed by χ^2 test. The significant P values are presented as italic

Coronary Outcome Measurement (THC-COM) study. The study was carried out between May–September 2006. Participants in this study were patients admitted to the cardiothoracic ward for CABG surgery at a large Heart Center in this time period (Tehran heart center, Iran). The sample size calculation has been explained before [22]; briefly, the sample size was calculated using the formula for comparing two proportions: n = [(Zα/2 + Zβ)2 × {(p$_1$ (1-p$_1$) + (p2 (1-p$_2$))}]/ (p$_1$ - p$_2$)^2 where p$_1$ is the proportion of the women with low quality Mediterranean regimen (0.3), p$_2$ is the proportion of the men with low quality Mediterranean regimen (0.25), α error = 0.05, and power = 80% (1-β). Accordingly, a 125-subject sample size was determined for the study (125 in each group). We also assumed 20% loss (125 + 25) and as men with CAD are twice as women (150 + 300), the final sample size of 450 was considered for the study [22, 23]. Reasons for drop-out or exclusion were incomplete dietary questionnaires (*n* = 1), and incomplete demographic questionnaires (*n* = 5). The final analytic sample in this study consisted of 454 patients aged 35–80 years who completed both the questionnaire and the medical examination. More details of study procedure and biochemical assays have been provided elsewhere [22]. Written informed consent was obtained from each participating subject. The study was approved by Tehran Heart Center, Tehran University of Medical Sciences.

Dietary assessment methods

A 138-item semi-quantitative food frequency questionnaire (FFQ) was used to assess the habitual dietary intakes of patients. The FFQ consisted of a list of foods with standard serving sizes commonly consumed by Iranians. Participants were asked to report how often they consumed each of the food items listed as the number of times per day, per week, per month or per year during the previous year. The reported frequency for each food item was then converted to a daily intake. Portion sizes of consumed foods were converted to grams by using household measures [24]. The questionnaire was previously validated for healthy Iranian population [25].

We calculated the diet score on the basis of Mediterranean diet quality index (Med-DQI) (Table 1). The index assigns a score of 0, 1 or 2 according to the daily intake of each of the seven components and then final score was reported as a summation of all nutrient scores ranged between 0 and 14. A lower score on this index denotes a better nutrition quality and higher adherence to Mediterranean dietary pattern [19].

The dietary phytochemical index (DPI) was defined as the percent of dietary calories derived from foods rich in phytochemicals. Calories derived from fruits, vegetables (except for potatoes), legumes, whole grains, nuts, seeds, fruit/vegetable juices, soy products, wine, beer, and cider are enumerated in this index. The higher score denotes the higher phytochemical content of diet [12].

Statistical analysis

Data analysis was performed by SPSS statistical software package version 16 (SPSS Inc., Chicago, IL, USA). Kolmogorov–Smirnov test was performed for normality of the distributions of variables. The comparison of discrete variables was performed by Chi- square test. Continuous variables between groups were compared by independents sample- *t* test or one way analysis of variance (ANOVA). Analysis of covariance (ANCOVA) was used to compare continuous variables between three groups adjusting for the confounding effects of age, gender and body mass index. General linear model was also applied for evaluating the association between total Med-DQI score and biochemical parameters adjusting for the mediating effects of dietary phytochemical score. P values less than 0.05 considered as significance level.

Results

As mentioned previously, higher MED-DQI scores denote higher adherence to Mediterranean dietary pattern and better nutrition quality. While higher DPI score indicates higher intake of dietary phytochemicals. Patients general information according to different categorizes of Med-DQI and DPI are presented in Table 2. Mean age and BMI were not significantly different between two categorizes of Med-DQI. However patients with lower Med-DQI score were more likely to be male and have higher educational attainment ($P < 0.05$). Additionally the prevalence of diabetes was lower in the higher scores of Med-DQI. Patients in higher tertiles of dietary phytochemical index had higher BMI and were most likely to be male ($P < 0.05$).

Table 3 presents the comparison of laboratory parameters according to components of Mediterranean dietary quality index in patients. As shown in this Table, patients with higher intakes of "saturated fatty acids" had lower serum albumin concentrations ($P < 0.05$). High scores of "cholesterol" subgroup was also accompanied with higher serum Hb A1C percent ($P = 0.04$) denoting the higher likelihood of diabetes by high intake of dietary cholesterol. Significantly higher concentration of serum creatinine was also observed in categorizes with higher "fish" intakes; while serum lipoprotein (Lp) (a) concentration was increased in top scores of "cereals". In other word, lower cereal intake was associated with higher serum Lp (a) concentrations ($P = 0.05$). In General linear model for evaluation of the association between total Med-DQI score and biochemical parameters adjusting for the mediating effects of DPI, total Med-DQI score was associated with serum CRP and creatinine concentrations and these associations remained significant even after adjusting for the mediating effects of DPI (Table 4). Moreover, patients with lower dietary phytochemical intake had significantly higher Med-DQI scores (Fig. 1, $P < 0.004$).

Discussion

Adherence to Mediterranean diet lowers the risk of coronary artery events and reduces the risk myocardial infarction, coronary bypass graft, percutaneous coronary intervention and coronary artery disease rates [15]; on the other hand, patients candidate for CABG, did not have an acceptable nutritional status before and after surgery and malnutrition is a common feature of CABG [26, 27]. Therefore, having a good nutritional status before surgery can be a useful strategy for prevention of CABG-induced malnutrition. Therefore it is very important to develop healthy dietary regiments for improving the patients' nutritional status and quality of life.

Numerous evidences suggested the protective role of Mediterranean dietary pattern against cardiovascular disease [28] and its associated risk factors including metabolic syndrome, diabetes and obesity [29, 30]. In fact, over the past decades, numerous dietary models have been proposed to protect against metabolic abnormalities and among them, only the Mediterranean diet demonstrated a beneficial effect [31].

In the current study we demonstrated that patients with lower Med-DQI scores had higher educational attainment compared with patients with higher scores. Moreover, patients with higher scores of "saturated fatty acids" and "cholesterol" had significantly lower serum albumin and creatinine concentrations and higher Hb A1C percent respectively.

In a sub-analysis of the EPIC study analyzed a cohort of 497,308 people showed that a higher adherence to the Mediterranean diet was associated with a significantly lower body mass index and waist circumference within 3 years [29]. Likewise, the beneficial role of Mediterranean dietary pattern in protecting against CVD risk factors has been supported by several studies. A two point increase of Mediterranean dietary score was associated with 33% reduced risk of mortality from cardiovascular causes (RR = 0.67, 95%, CI: 0.47–0.94) [28]. The role of Mediterranean dietary style in primary prevention of CVD in a sample of 7747 adults at high risk of CVD but without a manifest disease has been established in a large interventional study before [6].

The Mediterranean dietary quality index (Med-DQI) is a useful tool for predicting dietary quality and has been validated previously using nutritional biomarkers [19]. This index was based on the recommendations made by the National Research Council and American Heart Association regarding the diet and health [32]. These recommendations are based on consumption of 30% or less of the daily total energy from fat, 10% or less of the total energy from saturated fat, 30 mg/d or less from cholesterol, 55% of energy from complex carbohydrates and 5 servings or more from fruits and vegetables.

In the current study, for the first time, we evaluated the Med-DQI in patients undergoing CABG and according to our findings, higher scores of "saturated fatty acid" was associated with lower serum albumin concentrations ($P = 0.04$). Albumin is a main fatty acid transporter in the extracellular fluids and dietary factors influence its plasma concentrations [33]. Several animal studies observed the albumin- lowering effects of high fat diets. Andrson et al. [34] found that feeding high fat diet in mice induces a slight decrease in serum albumin

Table 3 Comparison of laboratory parameters according to components of Mediterranean dietary quality index in patients candidate for CABG

Characteristics	Hb A$_1$C (%)	TG(mg/dl)	TC(mg/dl)	HDL(mg/dl)	LDL(mg/dl)	CRP(mg/dl)	Albumin (g/dl)	Creatinine (mg/dl)	Lipoprotein (a) (mg/dl)
Saturated fatty acid (n)									
0 (216)	6.05 ± 1.72	172.48 ± 82.66	158.27 ± 43.66	40.19 ± 8.61	85.52 ± 40.88	6.84 ± 0.87	4.69 ± 0.36	1.33 ± 0.29	31.43 ± 24.76
1 (163)	6.20 ± 1.85	176.46 ± 99.20	162.85 ± 48.75	40.90 ± 9.14	88.05 ± 39.15	6.58 ± 0.25	4.63 ± 0.32	1.27 ± 0.27	34.18 ± 27.15
2 (63)	6.07 ± 1.57	179.28 ± 92.85	165.09 ± 44.94	40.53 ± 9.20	89.35 ± 38.88	6.89 ± 0.69	4.59 ± 0.25	1.26 ± 0.20	31.88 ± 29.37
P value*	0.73	0.83	0.45	0.74	0.72	0.87	*0.04*	0.08	0.58
Cholesterol (n)									
0 (318)	6.01 ± 1.65	173.03 ± 1.12	160.89 ± 43.89	40.42 ± 8.56	87.95 ± 40.74	6.64 ± 5.22	4.65 ± 0.32	1.28 ± 0.28	33.32 ± 26.85
1 (66)	6.14 ± 1.74	178.76 ± 80.16	163.33 ± 49.12	40.81 ± 10.22	87.74 ± 41.45	6.63 ± 3.40	4.62 ± 0.34	1.39 ± 0.29	30.21 ± 23.38
2 (58)	6.63 ± 2.15	181.18 ± 97.78	158.46 ± 52.26	40.61 ± 9.16	80.80 ± 32.82	7.51 ± 7.25	4.74 ± 0.35	1.28 ± 0.20	30.40 ± 26.67
P value*	*0.04*	0.76	0.83	0.94	0.45	0.51	0.11	0.68	0.57
Meats (n)									
0 (16)	6.03 ± 1.56	164.09 ± 80.62	171.49 ± 51.21	39.98 ± 7.93	89.53 ± 23.43	5.65 ± 2.06	4.65 ± 0.30	1.28 ± 0.21	22.28 ± 12.29
1 (313)	6.03 ± 1.62	171.88 ± 80.49	161.93 ± 45.14	40.84 ± 8.73	87.92 ± 39.62	6.55 ± 5.15	4.65 ± 0.34	1.29 ± 0.27	32.31 ± 25.63
2 (113)	6.33 ± 2.07	184.96 ± 114.19	156.58 ± 46.51	39.65 ± 9.43	84.10 ± 42.75	7.46 ± 5.93	4.67 ± 0.31	1.33 ± 0.28	34.63 ± 29.38
P value*	0.27	0.35	0.34	0.45	0.65	0.20	0.78	0.32	0.17
Olive oil (n)									
0 (52)	6.09 ± 1.53	164.07 ± 79.41	155.09 ± 40.85	41.88 ± 8.82	87.86 ± 58.85	5.57 ± 1.30	4.70 ± 0.36	1.30 ± 0.24	30.85 ± 24.81
1 (136)	6.03 ± 1.53	184.01 ± 104.87	160.25 ± 40.84	40.32 ± 8.79	84.19 ± 34.46	6.50 ± 3.49	4.66 ± 0.29	1.33 ± 0.31	32.82 ± 25.31
2 (254)	6.15 ± 1.89	172.33 ± 83.81	162.49 ± 49.07	40.32 ± 8.95	88.31 ± 37.93	7.13 ± 6.45	4.65 ± 0.34	1.28 ± 0.25	32.66 ± 27.23
P value*	0.82	0.31	0.55	0.48	0.61	0.12	0.53	0.15	0.88
Fish (n)									
0 (57)	6.20 ± 2.32	163.62 ± 80.35	158.86 ± 45.51	40.40 ± 8.22	91.34 ± 57.50	5.30 ± 0.69	4.64 ± 0.32	1.39 ± 0.34	32.49 ± 27.09
1 (91)	6.09 ± 1.56	188.57 ± 107.92	156.73 ± 36.06	39.72 ± 9.10	82.02 ± 27.85	4.29 ± 0.44	4.70 ± 0.32	1.30 ± 0.25	33.74 ± 29.66
2 (294)	6.09 ± 1.68	172.94 ± 86.01	162.62 ± 48.38	40.76 ± 8.95	87.69 ± 38.92	5.58 ± 0.34	4.64 ± 0.34	1.28 ± 0.26	32.12 ± 25.14
P value*	0.91	0.21	0.52	0.61	0.33	0.62	0.31	*0.02*	0.41
Cereal (n)									
0 (315)	6.11 ± 1.80	179.55 ± 95.83	159.84 ± 44.89	40.18 ± 8.73	6.39 ± 3.49	4.67 ± 0.32	1.31 ± 0.26	31.78 ± 24.57	39.61 ± 11.44
1 (119)	6.12 ± 1.62	162.60 ± 73.23	161.77 ± 46.83	41.17 ± 9.27	7.78 ± 8.42	4.64 ± 0.36	1.27 ± 0.31	35.51 ± 30.71	42.17 ± 13.74
2 (8)	5.66 ± 1.23	174.88 ± 88.19	192.62 ± 57.75	43.50 ± 8.83	5.73 ± 0.69	4.47 ± 0.26	1.32 ± 0.08	16.12 ± 14.61	45.62 ± 12.78
P value *	0.76	0.21	0.13	0.36	0.11	0.44	0.23	0.45	*0.059*
Fruits and vegetables (n)									
0 (369)	6.10 ± 1.73	175.64 ± 94.06	160.17 ± 43.46	40.62 ± 9.31	39.69 ± 2.04	6.65 ± 5.28	4.66 ± 0.33	1.31 ± 0.28	31.29 ± 25.22
1 (62)	6.16 ± 1.93	166.79 ± 64.37	162.13 ± 56.29	40.37 ± 6.48	40.79 ± 5.09	7.44 ± 5.84	4.62 ± 0.33	1.25 ± 0.22	39.89 ± 31.82
2 (11)	5.94 ± 1.35	197.82 ± 90.95	180.27 ± 54.44	37.18 ± 4.16	42.11 ± 12.69	6.55 ± 1.64	4.71 ± 0.17	1.14 ± 0.17	32.55 ± 25.00
P value*	0.92	0.53	0.34	0.44	0.33	0.55	0.58	0.09	0.06

*P values from ANCOVA adjusted for the confounding effects of age, gender and body mass index. The significant P values are presented as italic

concentrations. Since Albumin synthesis is sensitive to insulin, they speculated that reduced serum albumin concentrations and biosynthesis is a result of high fat diet- induced insulin resistance. In other study, female rats feeding high-fat diets had 25% lower serum albumin concentrations [35].

Interestingly, patients in the lower categorizes of "cholesterol" subgroup had significantly higher serum HbA$_1$C concentrations. Hb A1C is a better predictor of circulating lipids and better diagnostic marker of developing cardiovascular and micro-vascular complications [36, 37]. Previous studies observed a positive association between

Table 4 General Linear Model (GLM) for evaluating the association between total MED-DQI score and biochemical parameters with and without mediating effects of DPI

| | With DPI as co-variate | | Without DPI as co-variate | |
	F	P value*	F	P value*
Hb A₁C (%)	0.84	0.58	0.85	0.58
TG(mg/dl)	0.51	0.88	0.51	0.88
TC(mg/dl)	1.2	0.28	1.2	0.24
HDL (mg/dl)	1	0.44	0.99	0.44
LDL(mg/dl)	1.25	0.25	1.23	0.27
CRP(mg/dl)	1.72	*0.05*	1.71	*0.049*
Albumin(g/dl)	1.58	0.11	1.65	0.089
Creatinine (mg/dl)	2.46	*0.007*	2.29	*0.012*
Lipoprotein (a) (mg/dl)	1.37	0.19	1.36	0.19

P-values obtained from general linear model with and without mediating effects of DPI. The significant P values are presented as italic

dietary cholesterol intake and risk of type 2 diabetes mellitus [38, 39]. Since cholesterol is only present in products of animal origin, one can speculate that these associations could represent an adverse effect of a food pattern characterized by a high consumption of meat and eggs, or even an unidentified component of animal products [40]. However dietary cholesterol could have direct effects in incidence of type 2 diabetes via stimulating inflammatory pathways [41]. In animal models, dietary cholesterol per se produces an increase in serum amiloid A, a potent inflammatory mediator [42]. These inflammatory mediators can lead to incidence of type 2 diabetes mellitus [43]. Moreover, dietary cholesterol disrupts glucose metabolism and increases serum insulin concentrations [38].

Serum creatinine is a marker of muscle mass and also dietary protein intake [44]. High dietary protein can also significantly raise serum creatinine concentrations [45]. In our study, patients with higher fish intake had higher serum creatinine concentrations, although none of these

differences were out of normal range and these variations occurred in the physiologically normal range of serum creatinine. Previous studies also confirm our findings. In the study by Rasmussen et al. the higher dietary fish intake was associated with higher urinary creatinine excretion [46].

We also observed high serum Lp (a) concentrations in patient with low intakes of cereals. Accordingly, the beneficial effects of cereals on serum Lp (a) have been previously confirmed. In the study by Xiong et al. breakfast and bran cereals had potent positive effects on reduction of serum Lp (a) concentrations [47]. Lp (a) is essentially an LDL particle with an apoprotein (a) attached to it. Numerous evidences have revealed that high serum Lp (a) concentration is associated with a variety of CVD events, including peripheral vascular disease, cerebrovascular disease, premature coronary disease and vascular injury [48]. The impact of cereals in improving serum lipoproteins and lipids are attributed to their fiber content as previously confirmed [49].

Conclusions
The present study reported that patients with higher scores of "saturated fatty acids" and "cholesterol" had significantly lower serum albumin and higher Hb A1C percent respectively. Higher intake of "fish" was also associated with higher serum creatinine concentration. Further studies with interventional approaches are needed to better clarify the causal inference of these associations.

Abbreviations
ANCOVA: Analysis of co-variance; BMI: Body mass index; CABG: Coronary artery bypass grafting; CRP: C-reactive protein; CVD: Cardiovascular disease; FBS: Fasting blood sugar; FFQ: Food frequency questionnaire; HC: Hip circumference; HDL-C: High density lipoprotein cholesterol; LDL-C: Low density lipoprotein cholesterol; MED-DQI: Mediterranean dietary quality index; TC: Total cholesterol; TG: Triglyceride; THC-COM: Tehran heart center-coronary outcome measurement; WC: Waist circumference; WHR: Waist to hip ratio

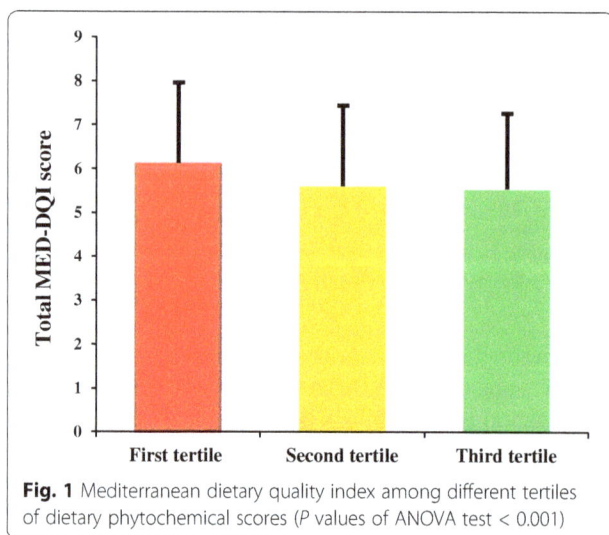
Fig. 1 Mediterranean dietary quality index among different tertiles of dietary phytochemical scores (P values of ANOVA test < 0.001)

Acknowledgement
We thank all of the study participants.

Funding
This research has been performed by a grant from Tehran University of Medical Sciences.

Authors' contributions
MAF wrote the manuscript and performed the statistical analysis, MN supervised the project and revised the manuscript, MAJ was involved in data analysis and LJ collected the data. All authors read and approved the final manuscript.

Competing interests
The authors declare that they have no competing of interests.

Author details
[1]Drug Applied Research Center, Nutrition Research Center, Faculty of Nutrition, Tabriz University of Medical Sciences, Tabriz, Iran. [2]Department of Research, Tehran Heart Center, Tehran University of Medical Sciences, North Karegar Street, Tehran 1411713138, Iran. [3]Road Traffic Injury Research Center, Tabriz University of Medical Sciences, Tabriz, Iran. [4]Tabriz Health Services Managment Research Center, Tabriz University of Medical Sciences, Tabriz, Iran.

References
1. Hatmi ZN, Tahvildari S, Motlag AG, Kashani AS. Prevalence of coronary artery disease risk factors in Iran: a population based survey. BMC Cardiovasc Disord. 2007;7:32–7.
2. WHO. New initiative launched to tackle cardiovascular disease, the world's number one killer. Global Hearts. 2016 [cited 2016; Available from: http://www.who.int/cardiovascular_diseases/global-hearts/Global_hearts_initiative/en/.
3. National Institute of Health. National Heart, Lung and Blood Institute. What is coronary artery bypass grafting? https://www.nhlbi.nih.gov/health/health-topics/topics/cabg. Accessed 23 Feb 2012.
4. Yusuf S, Reddy S, Ounpuu S, Anand S. Global burden of cardiovascular diseases: part I: general considerations, the epidemiologic transition, risk factors, and impact of urbanization. Circulation. 2001;104(22):2746–53.
5. Lichtenstein AH, Appel LJ, Brands M, Carnethon M, Daniels S, Franch HA, et al. Diet and lifestyle recommendations revision 2006 A scientific statement from the American Heart Association nutrition committee. Circulation. 2006;114(1):82–96.
6. Estruch R, Ros E, Salas-Salvadó J, Covas MI, Corella D, Aros F, et al. Primary prevention of cardiovascular disease with a Mediterranean diet. New Engl J Med. 2013;368(14):1279–90.
7. Mariscal-Arcas M, Rivas A, Velasco J, Ortega M, Caballero AM, Olea-Serrano F. Evaluation of the Mediterranean Diet Quality Index (KIDMED) in children and adolescents in Southern Spain. Pub Health Nutr. 2009;12(9):1408–12.
8. Tur JA, Romaguera D, Pons A. The Diet Quality Index-International (DQI-I): is it a useful tool to evaluate the quality of the Mediterranean diet? British J Nutr. 2005;93(3):369–76.
9. Carluccio MA, Siculella L, Ancora MA, Massaro M, Scoditti E, Storelli C, et al. Olive oil and red wine antioxidant polyphenols inhibit endothelial activation: antiatherogenic properties of mediterranean diet phytochemicals. Arterioscler Thromb Vasc Biol. 2003;23(4):622–9.
10. Mottaghi A, Bahadoran Z, Mirmiran P, Mirzaei S, Azizi F. Is dietary phytochemical index in association with the occurrence of hypertriglyceridemic waist phenotype and changes in lipid accumulation product index? A prospective approach in Tehran Lipid and Glucose Study. Int J Pharmacog & Phytochem Res. 2015;7(1):16–21.
11. Lukaczer D, Liska DJ, Lerman RH, Darland G, Schiltz B, Tripp M. Effect of a low glycemic index diet with soy protein and phytosterols on CVD risk factors in postmenopausal women. Nutrition. 2006;22(2):104–13.
12. McCarty MF. Proposal for a dietary "phytochemical index". Med Hypoth. 2004;63(5):813–7.
13. Vincent HK, Bourguignon CM, Taylor AG. Relationship of the dietary phytochemical index to weight gain, oxidative stress and inflammation in overweight young adults. J Hum Nutr Diet. 2010;23(1):20–9.
14. Fraser A, Abel R, Lawlor DA, Fraser D, Elhayany A. A modified Mediterranean diet is associated with the greatest reduction in alanine aminotransferase levels in obese type 2 diabetes patients: results of a quasi-randomised controlled trial. Diabetologia. 2008;51(9):1616–22.
15. Hoscan Y, Yigit F, Müderrisoglu H. Adherence to Mediterranean diet and its relation with cardiovascular diseases in Turkish population. Int J Clin Exp Med. 2015;8(2):2860–6.
16. Martinez-Gonzalez MA, Bes-Rastrollo M. Dietary patterns, Mediterranean diet, and cardiovascular disease. Curr Opin Lipidol. 2014;25(1):20–6.
17. Jacobs DR Jr, Gross MD, Tapsell LC. Food synergy: an operational concept for understanding nutrition. Am J Clin Nutr. 2009;89:1543S–8S.
18. D'Alessandro A, Pergola GD. Mediterranean diet and cardiovascular disease: A critical evaluation of a priori dietary indexes. Nutrients. 2015;7(9):7863–88.
19. Gerber M. The comprehensive approach to diet: a critical review. J Nutr. 2001;131(11):3051S–5S.
20. Lockheart MS, Steffen LM, Rebnord HM, Fimreite RL, Ringstad J, Thelle DS, et al. Dietary patterns, food groups and myocardial infarction: a case-control study. Br J Nutr. 2007;98(2):380–7.
21. Ma Y, Li W, Olendzki BC, Pagoto SL, Merriam PA, Chiriboga DE, et al. Dietary quality 1 year after diagnosis of coronary heart disease. J Am Diet Assoc. 2008;108(2):240–6.
22. Najafi M, Sheikhvatan M. Gender differences in coronary artery disease: correlational study on dietary pattern and known cardiovascular risk factors. Int Cardiovasc Res J. 2013;7(4):124–9.
23. Farhangi MA, Ataie-Jafari A, Najafi M, Foroushani GS, Tehrani MM, Jahangiry L. Gender differences in major dietary patterns and their relationship with cardio-metabolic risk factors in a year before coronary artery bypass grafting (CABG) surgery period. Arch Iran Med. 2016;19(7):470–9.
24. Ghaffarpour M, Houshiar-Rad A, Kianfar H. The manual for household measures, cooking yields factors and edible portion of foods (In Persian). Tehran: Keshaverzi Press; 1999.
25. Esmaillzadeh A, Mirmiran P, Azizi F. Whole-grain intake and the prevalence of hypertriglyceridemic waist phenotype in Tehranian adults. Am J Clin Nutr. 2005;81:55–63.
26. Ringaitiene D, Gineityte D, Vicka V, Žvirblis T, Šipylaite J, Irnius A, et al. Impact of malnutrition on postoperative delirium development after on pump coronary artery bypass grafting. J Cardiothorac Surg. 2015;10:74–81.
27. DiMaria-Ghalili RA. Changes in nutritional status and postoperative outcomes in elderly CABG patients. Biol Res Nurs. 2002;4(2):73–84.
28. Trichopoulou A, Costacou T, Bamia C, Trichopoulos D. Adherence to a Mediterranean diet and survival in a Greek population. N Engl J Med. 2003; 348:2599–608.
29. Romaguera D, Norat T, Mouw T, May AM, Bamia C, Slimani N, et al. Adherence to the Mediterranean diet is associated with lower abdominal adiposity in European men and women. J Nutr. 2009;139:1728–37.
30. Martínez-González MA, de la Fuente-Arrillaga C, Nunez-Cordoba JM, Basterra-Gortari FJ, Beunza JJ, Vazquez Z, et al. Adherence to Mediterranean diet and risk of developing diabetes: prospective cohort study. BMJ. 2008; 336:1348–51.
31. Sofi F, Casini A. Mediterranean diet and non-alcoholic fatty liver disease: New therapeutic option around the corner? World J Gastroentrol. 2014; 20(23):7339–46.
32. Gerber MJ, Scali JD, Michaud A, Durand MD, Astre CM, Dallongeville J, et al. Profiles of a healthful diet and its relationship to biomarkers in a population sample from Mediterranean southern France. J Am Diet Assoc. 2000;100(10): 1164–71.
33. Van der Vuees GJ. Albumin as fatty acid transporter. Drug Metab Pharmacokinet. 2009;24(4):300–7.
34. Anderson SR, Gilge DA, Steiber AL, Previs SF. Diet-induced obesity alters protein synthesis: tissue-specific effects in fasted versus fed mice. Metabolism. 2008;57(3):347–54.
35. Brito PD, Ramos CF, Passos MCF, Moura EG. Adaptive changes in thyroid function of female rats fed a high-fat and low-protein diet during gestation and lactation. Brazil J Med Biol Res. 2006;39(6):809–16.
36. Prabhavathi K, Kunikullaya KU, Goturu J. Glycosylated Haemoglobin (HbA1c) - A Marker of Circulating Lipids in Type 2 Diabetic Patients. J Clin Diagn Res. 2014;8(2):20–3.
37. Sacks DB. A1C versus glucose testing: A comparison. Diabetes Care. 2011; 34(2):518–23.
38. Lajous M, Bijon A, Fagherazzi G, Balkau B, Boutron-Ruaul MC, Clavel-Chapelon F. Egg and cholesterol intake and incident type 2 diabetes among French women. British J Nutr. 2015;114:1667–73.
39. Salmerón J, Hu FB, Manson JE, Stampfer MJ, Colditz GA, Rimm EB, et al. Dietary fat intake and risk of type 2 diabetes in women. Am J Clin Nutr. 2001;73:1019–26.

40. Kahn BB, Flier JS. Obesity and insulin resistance. J Clin Invest. 2000;106:473–81.
41. Bjorkbacka H, Kunjathoor VV, Moore KJ, Koehn S, Ordija CM, Lee MA, et al. Reduced atherosclerosis in MyD88-null mice links elevated serum cholesterol levels to activation of innate immunity signaling pathways. Nat Med. 2004;10:416–21.
42. Lewis KE, Kirk EA, Mcdonald TO, Wang S, Wight TN, O'Brien KD, et al. Increase in serum amyloid an evoked by dietary cholesterol is associated with increased atherosclerosis in mice. Circulation. 2004;110:540–5.
43. Gonzalez-Clemente JM, Carro O, Gallach I, Vioque J, Humanes A, Sauret C, et al. Increased cholesterol intake in women with gestational diabetes mellitus. Diab & Met. 2007;33(1):25–9.
44. Patel SS, Molnar MZ, Tayek JA, Ix JH, Noori N, Benner D, et al. Serum creatinine as a marker of muscle mass in chronic kidney disease: results of a cross-sectional study and review of literature. J Cachexia Sarcopenia Muscle. 2013;4(1):19–29.
45. Butani L, Polinsky MS, Kaiser BA, Baluarte HJ. Dietary protein intake significantly affects the serum creatinine concentration. Kidney Int. 2002;61(5):1907.
46. Rasmussen LG, Winning H, Savorani F, Toft H, Larsen TM, Dragsted LO, et al. Assessment of the effect of high or low protein diet on the human urine metabolome as measured by NMR. Nutrients. 2012;4(2):112–31.
47. Xiong ZW, Wahlqvist ML, Wattanapenpaiboon NT, Biegler BM, Balazs NDH, Xiong DW, et al. Factors contributing to variation in lipoprotein (a) in Melbourne Anglo-Celtic population. Eur J Clin Nutr. 2003;57:447–54.
48. Ritu M, Manika M. Blood homocystiene and lipoprotein (A) levels, stress and faulty diet as major risk factors for early cardiovascular diseases in Indians. J Cardiovasc Dis Diagn. 2014;2(4):1–6.
49. Hosseinpour-Niazi S, Azizi F, Mirmiran P. Nutritional Management of Disturbances in Lipoprotein Concentrations. Croatia: INTECH Open Access Publisher; 2012.

3

Outcomes following the implementation of a quality control campaign to decrease sternal wound infections after coronary artery by-pass grafting

Rickard P. F. Lindblom[1*], Birgitta Lytsy[2], Camilla Sandström[1], Nadjira Ligata[1], Beata Larsson[1], Ulrika Ransjö[2] and Christine Leo Swenne[1,3]

Abstract

Background: Coronary artery by-pass grafting (CABG) remains the optimal strategy in achieving complete revascularization in patients with complex coronary artery disease. However, sternal wound infections (SWI), especially deep SWI are potentially severe complications to the surgery. At the department of cardiothoracic surgery in Uppsala University Hospital a gradual increase in all types of SWI occurred, which peaked in 2009. This prompted an in-depth revision of the whole surgical process. To monitor the frequency of post-operative infections all patients receive a questionnaire that enquires whether any treatment for wound infection has been carried out.

Methods: All patients operated with isolated CABG between start of 2006 and end of 2012 were included in the study. 1515 of 1642 patients answered and returned the questionnaire (92.3 %). The study period is divided into the time before the intervention program was implemented (2006-early 2010) and the time after the intervention (early 2010- end 2012). To assess whether potential differences in frequency of SWI were a consequence of change in the characteristics of the patient population rather than an effect of the intervention a retrospective assessment of medical records was performed, where multiple of the most known risk factors for developing SWI were studied.

Results: We noticed a clear decrease in the frequency of SWI after the intervention. This was not a consequence of a healthier population.

Conclusions: Our results from implementing the intervention program are positive in that they reduce the number of SWI. As several changes in the perioperative care were introduced simultaneously we cannot deduce which is the most effective.

Keywords: CABG, Sternal wound infection, Quality control campaign

Background

Complete revascularization in patients with severe coronary artery disease is optimally achieved with coronary artery bypass-grafting (CABG) [1–3]. However, CABG is also vitiated with complications, out of which one of the most serious is sternal wound infection (SWI) [4]. SWI leads to both increased patient morbidity and mortality as well as augmented health care costs. Compared to a CABG operation without SWI the median cost of a single CABG procedure with SWI was $49.449 compared to $18.218 [5]. The incidence of reported SWI following CABG is highly variable due to differences in patient profiles and surgical techniques. There are also differences in classification of the SWI, where most studies have focused on the more severe, deep infections which typically occur in 1–2 % of CABG operations [4] others also report more superficial infections which are more common, with incidences between 5–12.0 % [6, 7].

* Correspondence: rickard.lindblom@ki.se

[1]Department of Cardiothoracic Surgery and Anesthesia, Uppsala University Hospital, 751 85 Uppsala, Sweden

Full list of author information is available at the end of the article

There are a number of known patient-related, pre- intra- and postoperative risk factors associated with increased risk of developing SWI after CABG which have been studied extensively [6, 8]. Accordingly, major attempts have been made to decrease the incidence of SWI. It is reasonable to believe that strict adherence to good hygienic routines in the perioperative period is beneficial, and there is documented evidence of the efficacy of hygiene interventions in the setting of cardiac surgery [9, 10]. However, these studies were small (less than 200 patients), spanned short periods of time (1–2 years) and included mixed patient groups, i.e. different kinds of open heart procedures. Also, there are multiple challenges to overcome when introducing changes in organizations [11]. In particular the leadership is challenged and methods of evaluating the performance of the clinic are of essence. Health care processes are complex and multivariate. It is therefore recommended to analyze the events when a patient is harmed or severely threatened to be so within the health care process using a standardized method, for instance a root cause analysis (The Swedish National board of Health and Welfare, http://www.socialstyrelsen.se/patientsakerhet/ledningssystem/analyserarisker). The focus of continuous event analysis should be on system aspects and organizational issues and complications identified related to the surgical care should be recorded continuously [11]. Furthermore, collaboration with support functions and other professions constitutes an important step in improving medical organizations [12].

During 2009 especially the number of deep, but also superficial, postoperative sternal wound infections within 30 days of surgery increased dramatically at the Department of Cardiothoracic Surgery and Anesthesia, Uppsala University Hospital. This was considered a serious problem and an extensive event analysis was performed. The aim of the current study was to assess how the semi-structured quality interventions that were implemented following the campaign impacted on the number of self-reported SWI 30 days after CABG.

Methods

Data collection

The study was performed at the department of Cardiothoracic Surgery and Anesthesia, Uppsala University Hospital, Sweden. The unit performs around 700 open heart surgeries annually out of which 250 to 300 are isolated CABG. During the period between the start 2006 and the end of 2012 1642 patients underwent isolated CABG. To evaluate the incidence of sternal wound infection 30 days after surgery a prospective, post-discharge patient registered evaluation was performed (Additional files 1 and 2). The infections were self-reported and the response rate was high throughout the study period; 1515 of 1642 patients (92.3 % response rate) answered the post-discharge

evaluation. Any kind of postoperative SWI (superficial, subcutaneous, to the sternum or deep/mediastinitis) that warranted active treatment with either/or antibiotics or surgical revision was included. 1334 (81.2) of the 1642 patients were men and 308 women (18.8 %). The mean age was 67 ± 9 years.

To perform a more detailed study of potential risk factors for SWI and better characterize the population a retrospective review of the medical records of every third patient, in chronological order of operation date, that had answered the post-discharge evaluation was selected and included in a separate cohort (Fig. 1). 503 of 1515 (33.2 %) patients were eligible for records review, the characteristics of this cohort were similar to the whole study population regarding age and sex (age 67 ± 9, M/F 410/93, 81.5/ 18.5 %). A chronological sampling, as opposed to stricter randomization, was chosen in order to reflect the seasonal fluctuations in operation volume and infection frequency [13].

The review of the 503 medical records included specific studies of patient-related risk factors such as age, gender, body mass index (kg/m^2), preoperative insulin-like growth factor 1 (IGF-1) levels, diabetes, preoperative hemoglobin

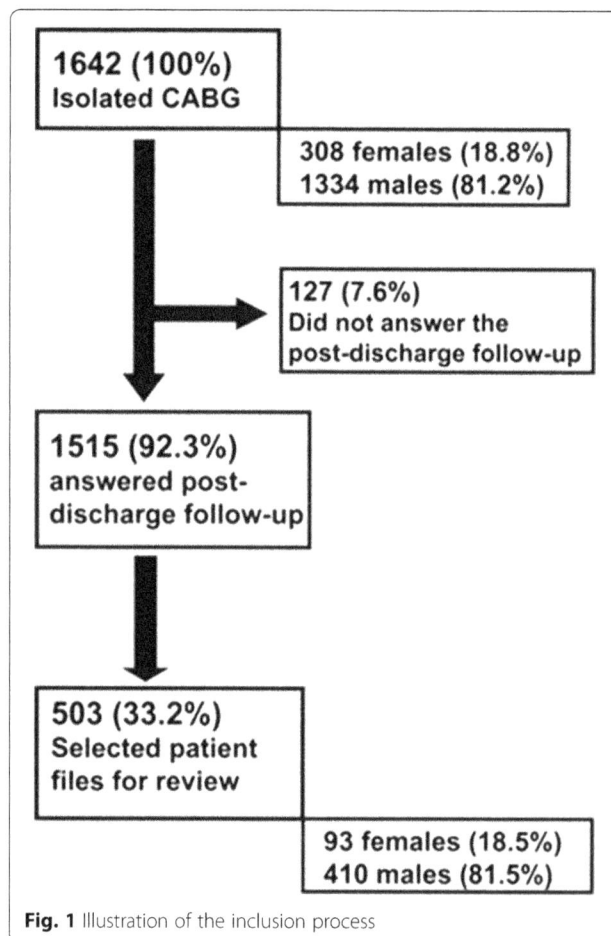

Fig. 1 Illustration of the inclusion process

concentrations, preoperative serum creatinine concentrations, chronic obstructive pulmonary disease (COPD), corticoid steroid treatment, current smoking status and preoperative ejection fraction (EF). The review of intraoperative risk factors included the number of saphenous vein grafts and internal mammary arteries used and the duration of cardiopulmonary by-pass and aortic cross clamp time. The review of postoperative risk factors included if erythrocyte transfusions had been given on day 0, 1 and 2 and also assessment of mean blood glucose concentration day 0, 1 and 2. The day of operation was denoted as day 0 and day 1 started 6 am in the morning after surgery.

Hygiene routines before intervention
Preoperatively
Elective and semi-urgent cases were normally admitted to the hospital the day before surgery, but sometimes earlier. The patients had one shower at home and one shower at the hospital. Hair removal on the leg and chest hair was done using a disposable clipping machine the night before surgery.

Intraoperatively
In the operating room, the skin was scrubbed with 0.5 % chlorhexidine in 70 % ethanol, which was allowed to air dry. The surgical procedures were performed in an operating room with ultra clean air with 10 cfu/m^3. The staff wore tightly woven scrub suits with cuffs and helmets tucked under the neckline of the shirt. Cloxacillin, 2 g, was administered intravenously three times a day for 2 days, starting in the morning of surgery.

Postoperatively
During the study period the policy of normalization of blood glucose concentrations in the immediate postoperative period changed; for patients without diabetes it was 5–7 mmol/l in 2006 to 2007 and 4–6 mmol/l from 2007 and onwards. For patients with diabetes the goal was 5–7 mmol/l in 2008 to 2011. Wound dressings were in the first period (2006–2010) allowed to stay in place for 4 days if dry.

Changes in hygiene routines after intervention
When the increase in SWI was detected an action plan was devised. Representatives from all personnel categories (surgeons, anaesthesiologists, nurses and nurses aids) from all three units (operation, intensive care unit and ward unit) of the department as well as from the departments of Clinical Microbiology and Infectious Medicine met at regular intervals during September 2009–April 2010 to perform a structured root cause analysis for infection according to The National board of Health and Welfare (http://www.socialstyrelsen.se/patientsakerhet/ledningssystem/

analyserarisker) and [14]. All elective operations ceased for 1 week. The changes in routines are summarized below.

Preoperatively
The preoperative washing routines were changed to two showers and scrubbing with a 4 % chlorhexidine detergent solution at the hospital. In the elective cases, care was taken to admit the patients to the ward only on the day before surgery, with a polyclinical meeting with a surgeon several days before admittance in order to spend as little time possible preoperatively in the hospital.

Intraoperatively
After the intervention the routine for antibiotic prophylaxis changed; Cloxacillin 2 g was instead administered four to five times all in the day of surgery, every four hours. The first dose started 30–60 min before the skin incision to achieve the maximum concentration in the blood at time of surgery.

A general policy of increased overall discipline in the operating theatre, which aimed at restricting the number of door-openings and minimizing the number of people in the operating theatre (maximum 11) was enforced. Regarding surgical technique, a standardized closure of the sternotomy with preferably eight single sternal wires that were not in figure-of-eights was introduced for all surgeons. There are no RCT's comparing closure techniques, although there is some evidence from biomechanical studies that supports the use of single wires as compared to the figure-of-eight configuration [15, 16]. All surgeons were urged to wear double gloves. Also, the WHO checklist for Safe surgery was introduced [17]. At the end of surgery the skin around the incision was scrubbed with 0.5 % chlorhexidine in 70 % ethanol before applying the wound dressing. Lastly, a revision of cleaning procedures for the operation theatre and of reusable materials was done with purchase of disinfectable keyboards and more disposable materials.

Postoperatively
In the second period (2010–2012) all sterile wound dressings were removed after 48 h and the wound inspected. No new dressing was added after this unless the wound was still open in which case a new dressing was placed after washing with sterile saline, the wound was then inspected the next day again and the procedure repeated if necessary. For patients with diabetes the blood glucose goal was changed to 6–8 mmol/l from 2011 and onwards

General attitudes
In general, a higher level of alertness and adherence to general and basic hand hygiene routines was enforced after the intervention as well as the introduction of disposable

plastic aprons to be worn during patient contact. To ensure compliance general unannounced inspections were performed throughout the clinic at regular intervals and feed-back given to the staff, in all categories.

Statistics

Possible predictors for SWI were compared in patients with and without SWI. Nominal data were analysed using the $X2$ test. The Kolmogorov–Smirnov goodness-of-fit test was used to analyse data distribution for the remaining risk factors. If distributions deviated significantly ($p < 0.05$) from the normal distribution the data were analysed using the Mann–Whitney U or Kruskal–Wallis tests. Those variables not deviating from the normal distributions were analysed using Student's t-test or one-way analysis of variance (ANOVA). Variables are given as mean (and SD, standard deviation), categorical variables as percentages.

Ethics, consent and permissions

The current work is the result of quality improvement work performed at Department of Cardiothoracic Surgery and Anesthesia, Uppsala University Hospital, Sweden and adheres to the Declaration of Helsinki [18] as well as national and local ethical guidelines for research http://www.codex.vr.se. Written, informed content was obtained from all participants.

Results

Patient demographics

Initial analysis aimed to exclude any gross differences in composition between the patient cohort selected for detailed studies of medical records ($n = 503$), and the whole study population during the period, i.e. the 1642 patients operated with CABG between 2006 and end of 2012. The populations had almost identical mean age and the distribution between sexes was similar (Table 1 and Fig. 1).

Identification of risk factors associated with sternal wound infection in the cohort

The characteristics of the cohort of patients that were selected for retrospective analysis of medical records are described in Table 2, where the patients that suffered SWI are compared to the patients that did not suffer SWI, over the whole study period. This revealed that the patients that suffered from SWI more often had diabetes ($p = 0.022$)

Table 1 Comparison between the population selected for detailed review with the whole study population ($n = 1642$)

	2006–2012		
	Review of patient medical records ($n = 503$)	No review of patient medical records ($n = 1139$)	p
Age (years)	67 ± 9	67 ± 9	0.907
Sex M/F	410/93	923/241	0.874

and more often received blood transfusions on postoperative day 2 ($p = 0.007$) (Table 2). There was a strong trend ($p = 0.086$) that lower preoperative hemoglobin and higher levels of preoperative IGF-1 ($p = 0.070$) were more prevalent in the SWI group. Noteworthy is that the SWI group had a tendency to be younger than the non-infected group ($p = 0.053$) (Table 2).

Patient profiles in period one compared to period two

To exclude that any potential differences in the rates of SWI following CABG in the two study periods, i.e. before and after the intervention, were an epiphenomena due to differences in the study populations, assessment of the profiles of the patient populations in the two periods was performed. We therefore compared the whole groups, i.e. both infected and non-infected patients grouped together, from the two periods. This suggested that the two study populations were largely similar with regard to patient-related factors (Table 3). But there were some differences, for instance in period one the preoperative IGF-1 was slightly, but significantly higher, on the other hand, there were significantly more patients in period two that were on corticosteroid treatment. The groups were also similar with regard to intraoperative factors (Table 3). However, in the postoperative parameters there was one major difference between the groups, and this was the amount of blood transfusions had significantly been reduced, from 18 to 9 %. Another minor difference was that the perioperative blood glucose was slightly higher in the second period (Table 3).

Effect of the hygienic intervention of the frequency of SWI

We next assessed whether the intervention program decreased the number of postoperative SWI; this was done by comparing the incidence of SWI in period one, before the intervention, with period two, after the intervention. This demonstrated that the frequency of all kinds of SWI, that is both deep and superficial, decreased from 12.2 % in period one to 2.8 % (Table 4) in period two.

In period two the patients that suffered from SWI were significantly younger than the healthy group, whereas in period one there was no age difference between the infected and non-infected (Table 4). Smoking was a risk factor for developing SWI throughout the study period (Table 4). Viewed over the whole study period, diabetes was more common in the infected patients (Table 2), whereas after the intervention there was no significant difference in the frequency of SWI between the patients with or without diabetes (Table 4), although the number of infected patients was small. In period one erythrocyte transfusion on day 2 was associated with increased risk of SWI, whereas this was not significant in period two (Table 4).

Table 2 Characteristics of the infected and non-infected groups (n = 503) seen over the whole study period

	Patients without infection (n = 455)	Patients with infections (n = 48)	p-value
Patient related riskfactors			
Age (years)	67 ± 9	65 ± 10	0.053
Sex M/F	374/81	36/12	0.222
Body mass index (kg/m^2)	28 ± 4	28 ± 4	0.954
Preoperative insulin-like growth factor 1 (mmol/mol)	45 ± 11 (n = 438)	51 ± 17 (n = 46)	0.070
Diabetes (%)	119/455 (26.5 %)	20/48 (41.7 %)	**0.022 (*)**
Preoperative hemoglobin concentrations (g/L)	141 ± 14 (451)	137 ± 11 (n = 47)	0.086
Preoperative serum creatinine concentrations (µg/L)	86 ± 28 (n = 452)	85 ± 23 (n = 47)	0.597
Corticoid steroid treatment (%)	12/455 (2.6 %)	2/48 (4.2 %)	0.540
Current smoking no/smoked the last 2 months/never smoked	54/314/87	7/36/5	0.319
Chronic Obstructive Pulmonary Disease (%)	12/455 (2.6 %)	1/48 (2.1 %)	0.818
Ejection fraction (%)	48 ± 9 (n = 348)	49 ± 10 (n = 35)	0.272
Intraoperative risk factors			
Number of saphenous vein grafts (n)	3 ± 1 (n = 424)	3 ± 1	0.693
Internal mammary artery 0/1/2	41/412/2	2/46/0	0.621
Duration of cardiopulmonary by-pass time (min)	85 ± 29 (n = 453)	85 ± 27	0.683
Duration of aortic cross clamp time (min)	47 ± 19 (n = 453)	49 ± 19	0.634
Postoperative risk factors			
Erythrocyte transfusion day 0 (%)	135/455 (29.7 %)	19/48 (39.6 %)	0.156
Erythrocyte transfusion day 1 (%)	71/455 (15.6 %)	10/48 (20.1 %)	0.349
Erythrocyte transfusion day 2 (%)	65/455 (14.3 %)	14/48 (29.2 %)	**0.007 (**)**
Mean blood glucose concentration day 0 (mmol/L)	7.8 ± 1.3 (n = 453)	7.5 ± 1.0	0.295
Mean blood glucose concentration day 1 (mmol/L)	8.2 ± 1.6 (n = 453)	8.5 ± 1.8	0.213
Mean blood glucose concentration day 2 (mmol/L)	9.0 ± 2.2 (n = 380)	9.4 ± 3.0 (n = 46)	0.788

*= p <0.05, **= p <0.01, **=p <0.001

Microbial flora over time
Lastly, we investigated whether the hygienic intervention could cause a shift or selection in the pathogenic microflora involved in the SWI. The results are more thoroughly described in (Lytsy et al. [19], in press doi:10.1016/j.jhin.2015.08.021). In summary there was no difference in the proportion of the two most common pathogens *Staphylococcus aureus* and Coagulase Negative Staphylococci in the pre- and post-intervention wound cultures.

Discussion
In this study we demonstrate our experience from implementing an intervention program on reducing the incidence of sternal wound infection following CABG. A methodological and structured root cause analysis was performed according to a standardized protocol. This meant that a cross-professional review of the medical-, care- and hygiene procedures, with a system of continuous monitoring and feed-back was introduced. The discussion and work that followed are continuous processes that ultimately aim to enforce a higher level of alertness' to all staff in the optimization of the care of the patient. The aim of the

current study was not to primarily study risk factors for developing SWI after CABG, as this has been extensively performed before, but to assess whether the intervention was meaningful, and to exclude that potential differences were instead caused by a change in patient demographics.

Risk factor profiling
Analysis of the general risk factor profile of the patients demonstrated that the burden of co-morbidities generally associated with increased risk of postoperative infection were not markedly different in period one compared to period two, except for that there were half as many blood transfusions in period two as in period one. This probably contributes to some of the improvement seen in the frequency of SWI after the hygienic intervention. Re-operation for bleeding is a known risk-factor for developing SWI [19], and the reduction in the number of blood transfusions could potentially have reflected a reduced number of re-explorations for bleeding. However, when reviewing the medical records of the 48 patients that suffered SWI, none of them were re-operated for bleeding. So, the reduction in blood transfusion does not reflect

Table 3 Risk factors for self-reported sternal wound infection after coronary artery by-pass graft surgery in patients with review of medical records (n = 503), comparison between into period one and two

	2006–2010 to week 26 (Period 1) n = 362	2010 from week 27–2012 (Period 2) n = 141	p-value
Patient related riskfactors			
Age (years)	67 ± 9	67 ± 9	0.610
Sex M/F	73/289	121/20	0.121
Body mass index (kg/m^2)	28 ± 4	28 ± 4	0.998
Preoperative insulin-like growth factor 1 (mmol/mol)	46 ± 12	44 ± 11	**0.014 (*)**
Diabetes (%)	94/268 (26 %)	45/96 (32 %)	0.180
Preoperative hemoglobin concentrations (g/L)	140 ± 14	141 ± 14	0.880
Preoperative serum creatinine concentrations (μg/L)	86 ± 28	87 ± 38	0.747
Chronic obstructive pulmonary disease (%)	12/350 (3.3 %)	1/140 (0.7 %)	0.098
Corticoid steroid treatment (%)	6/356 (1.7 %)	8/133 (5.7 %)	**0.014 (*)**
Current smoking/smoked the last 2 months/never smoked	46/246/70	15/104/22	0.444
Ejection fraction (%)	48 ± 9	49 ± 8	**0.041 (*)**
Intraoperative risk factors			
Number of saphenous vein grafts (n)	3 ± 1	3 ± 1	0.982
Internal mammary artery 0/1/2	30/330/2	13/128/0	0.646
Duration of cardiopulmonary by-pass time (min)	85 ± 28	85 ± 29	0.744
Duration of aortic cross clamp time (min)	47 ± 19	48 ± 20	0.818
Postoperative risk factors			
Erythrocyte transfusion day 0 (%)	118/244 (32.6 %)	36/105 (25.5 %)	0.123
Erythrocyte transfusion day 1 (%)	61/301 (16.9 %)	20/121 (14.2 %)	0.465
Erythrocyte transfusion day 2 (%)	66/296 (18.2 %)	13/128 (9.2 %)	**0.013 (*)**
Mean blood glucose concentration day 0 (mmol/L)	7.7 ± 1.3	8.2 ± 1.7	**0.000 (***)**
Mean blood glucose concentration day 1 (mmol/L)	8.2 ± 1.6	8.3 ± 1.8	0.408
Mean blood glucose concentration day 2 (mmol/L)	9.0 ± 2.3	8.9 ± 2.3	0.634

*= p <0.05, **= p <0.01, **=p <0.001

a reduced re-operation for bleeding in the infected group. But blood transfusion *per se* has also been linked to development of mediastinitis, often synonymous with DSWI [21]. Consequently, the decline in transfusion rates in period two may have contributed to the decrease in postoperative infections, however, the 50 % reduction in blood transfusions does not solely explain the almost 80 % reduction in SWI. This suggests that the action program had significant additional effect, on top of that which could be attributed reduced transfusion. It also suggests that introduction of the action program as a positive side-effect reduced the amount of blood transfusions, which in any case is a desirable consequence.

Furthermore we saw that diabetes and erythrocyte transfusions on day 2 after surgery were no longer associated with increased risk of SWI after the intervention, suggesting that the changes implemented perhaps were especially effective for these patients, although these numbers should be interpreted with caution as the infected group in period two is small.

We did not see any association between higher blood glucose and SWI, although the general ambition of controlling blood glucose levels is high at our department and both the infected and non-infected groups were well regulated in this regard. With this said, it is therefore still possible that poor glycemic control may be a risk for SWI [22], although contradicting evidence exists, as intense perioperative glucose monitoring has been shown to not affect the rates of wound infection following cardiac surgery, but to decrease mortality [23]. Other commonly studied factors like cross-clamp time or ECC time were in our data not significant risk factors for developing SWI.

The tendency for lower age in the infected group as compared to the healthy group is somewhat surprising, but could reflect a dimension not mirrored by the other parameters, for instance genetic factors [24]. And since they are operated with CABG at a young age, this may suggest a more aggressive disease, rather than young age being a risk factor *per se* for suffering SWI.

Table 4 Risk factors for self-reported sternal wound infection after coronary artery by-pass graft surgery in patients with review of medical records (n = 503), comparison between into period one and two divided into infected and non-infected patients

	2006–2010 to week 26 n = 362			2010 from week 27–2012 n = 141		
	Patients without infection (n = 318) 87.8 %	Patients with infections (n = 44) 12.2 %	p-value	Patients without infection (n = 137) 97.2 %	Patients with infections (n = 4) 2.8 %	p-value
Patient related riskfactors						
Age (years)	67 ± 9	65 ± 10	0.198	68 ± 9	56 ± 7	**0.032 (*)**
Sex M/F	256/62	33/11	0.394	118/19	3/1	0.529
Body mass index (kg/m^2)	28 ± 4	27.1 ± 4	0.606	28 ± 4	32 ± 4	0.051
Preoperative insulin-like growth factor 1 (mmol/mol)	46 ± 11 (n = 307)	52 ± 18 (n = 42)	0.115	44 ± 11 (n = 131)	44 ± 8	0.917
Diabetes (%)	75/318 (23.6 %)	19/4443.2 %	**0.005 (*)**	44/137 (32.1 %)	1/4 (25 %)	0.763
Preoperative hemoglobin concentrations (g/L)	141 ± 14 (n = 315)	137 ± 11 (n = 43)	0.115	141 ± 14 (n = 136)	136 ± 11	0.467
Preoperative serum creatinine concentrations (μg/L)	86 ± 22 (n = 243)	86 ± 23 (n = 43)	0.908	87 ± 39	70 ± 11	0.094
Chronic obstructive pulmonary disease (%)	11/318 (3.5 %)	1/44 (2.3 %)	0.680	1/137 (0.7 %)	0/4	0.864
Corticoid steroid treatment (%)	5/318 (1.6 %)	1/44 (2.3 %)	0.733	7/137 (5.1 %)	1/4 (25 %)	0.090
Current smoking/smoked the last 2 months/ never smoked	39/211 /68	7/35/2	**0.029 (*)**	15/103/19	0/1/3	**0.004 (**)**
Ejection fraction (%)	47 ± 10 (n = 217)	49 ± 11 (n = 31)	0.222	49 ± 8 (n = 131)	51 ± 7	0.481
Intra-operative risk factors						
Number of saphenous vein grafts (n)	3 ± 1 (n = 317)	3 ± 1	0.893	3 ± 1 (107)	4 ± 1	0.117
Internal mammary artery 0/1/2	28/288/2	2/42/0	0.675	13/124/0	0/4/0	0.518
Duration of cardiopulmonary by-pass time (min)	84 ± 2 (n = 317)	84 ± 28	0.886	85 ± 29 (n = 136)	90 ± 6	0.748
Duration of aortic cross clamp time (min)	47 ± 18 (n = 317)	48 ± 19	0.929	48 ± 20 (n = 136)	53 ± 6	0.582
Postoperative risk factors						
Erythrocyte transfusion day 0 (%)	100/318 (31.4 %)	18/44 (40.9 %)	0.209	35/137 (25.5 %)	1/4 (25 %)	0.980
Erythrocyte transfusion day 1 (%)	52/318 (16.4 %)	9/44 (20.5 %)	0.496	19/137 (13.9 %)	1/4 (25 %)	0.529
Erythrocyte transfusion day 2 (%)	53/318 (16.7 %)	13/44 (29.5 %)	**0.038 (*)**	12/137 (8.8 %)	1/4 (25 %)	0.268
Mean blood glucose concentration day 0 (mmol/L)	7.5 ± 1.1 (n = 317)	7.5 ± 1.0	0.916	8.2 ± 1.7 (n = 136)	7.6 ± 0.4	0.585
Mean blood glucose concentration day 1 (mmol/L)	8.1 ± 1.4 (n = 316)	8.5 ± 1.9	0.504	8.3 ± 1.8	8.1 ± 0.9	0.821
Mean blood glucose concentration day 2 (mmol/L)	9.0 ± 2.1 (n = 267)	9.4 ± 3.1 (n = 42)	0.902	8.9 ± 2.4 (n = 113)	9.1 ± 1.9	0.887

*= p <0.05, **= p <0.01, **=p <0.001

In summary, the selected risk factors that proved to differ significantly between the infected and healthy group were not new, although IGF-1 seems an interesting molecule to study further in these contexts, as there was a strong trend (p = 0.07) for higher levels in the infected group. There is to our knowledge no studies assessing the link between high levels of IGF-1 and SWI. IGF-1 is a good marker for nutritional status and anabolic responses [25] and IGF-1 is often considered beneficial in wound healing [26, 27], even though it has been shown detrimental in parasitic skin infections [28]. IGF-1 is also strongly linked to glucose-insulin pathways, however, the link to diabetes is not altogether easy, as both high and low levels of IGF-1 have been shown to correlate with subsequent onset of diabetes [29]. Also, alterations in the IGF-1 gene leads to lower levels of IGF-1, in turn linked to a higher risk of developing both diabetes and myocardial infarction [30]. The strong trend for elevated levels of IGF-1 in the SWI group are therefore difficult to interpret. And although we believe that, in our setting, elevated levels of IGF-1 could be seen as a marker for poor metabolic control, this may be an over-simplification, and instead reflect something more complex.

A general impression at the clinic was that the proportion of *S.aureus* decreased and the proportion of CoNS increased in the infected wounds after the intervention. However, statistical analysis of the wound cultures from the patients that were surgically revised revealed no differences, as further discussed in (Lytsy et al. 2015, in press doi:10.1016/j.jhin.2015.08.021). However, we lack wound cultures from a majority of the superficial SWI, as they were treated at other hospitals than Uppsala University Hospital, and we can therefore not say if the intervention affected the microbial population in the superficial SWI. This constitutes an interesting question for further studies, especially as it has been shown that the use of a 4 % chlorhexidine detergent solution can reduce the amount of *S.aureus* colonization [31]. Even though this was in the setting of pediatrics it could suggest that the extra preoperative shower with chlorhexidine that was added as a part of the intervention could lead to less *S.aureus* infections. Regarding chlorhexidine skin scrub, there is also evidence from orthopedic surgery that postoperative scrub of the wound with chlorhexidine may be effective in reducing wound infections [32]. So we believe the chlorhexidine skin scrub at the end of surgery was an easy and cost-effective measure to introduce, which may have contributed to the beneficial outcome.

The complexity of assessing interventions
A weakness with the study is that the findings are correlative, as no randomization or control group existed. Even though the importance of hygiene in the setting of surgery cannot be considered controversial, the degree of impact can be discussed. The present study therefore to some grade objectifies the significance of hygienic interventions. Another aspect is that we have not analyzed the cost-effectiveness of the program, merely the medical aspects. Although we deem it most likely that the undertaken actions have been a good investment, not only in decreased patient suffering, but also economically as the cost of a CABG with postoperative deep SWI is almost 3-fold to that of a CABG without SWI [5], and many of the introduced changes did not cost extra. However, this could be the topic of further research.

It is difficult to assess the influence of individual interventions when multiple changes are introduced simultaneously. We can therefore not say which of the changes in the perioperative routines had the most significant effect. It is possible that some of the changes *de facto* were negative, but that this penetrance could have been blunted by the stronger positive effect of another change. It is therefore important to constantly aim to improve, and not settle for a final solution. To ultimately study the impact of individual actions randomized clinical trials are warranted.

As often with patient-based collection of data there is a risk for selection bias; it is possible that the patients that suffered from SWI in a higher extent chose, or were not able, to respond to the post-discharge evaluation. But for the patients that were re-admitted for surgery, i.e. the most severe infections, this data exists and is reliable, no matter if the patient answered the evaluation or not. Also, the response rate was very good throughout the study period, with no clear yearly variation. We therefore find it reasonable to believe that the frequency of non-responders were the same in the two periods, and that the potential selection bias would affect both periods similarly.

It should also be noted that the study includes all kinds of SWI which means that a large spectrum of disease severity exists within the infected group. However, main the purpose of the current study was not to specifically study SWI morbidity or mortality, which has been well studied before, but rather to evaluate the effect of the intervention on the frequency of all types, i.e. both superficial and deep, postoperative SWI. Ultimately all kinds of SWI are best avoided, both for the sake of the patients and the health care system.

Conclusions
The risk factors associated with developing SWI after CABG are well studied but still not fully understood, and tend to differ between materials [8]. The aim of the current study was not to primarily study risk factors, this was done with the goal to exclude that any differences in outcome/SWI after the intervention were confounded by differences in the study populations. This was to some extent the case as the number of blood transfusions were significantly reduced after the intervention. However, this did not explain the full difference, so it is still possible to conclude that the program had effect in reducing SWI, and as a positive side-effect reduced the number of blood transfusions.

The problem of SWI is multifactorial, and it is not possible to say where in the chain of events that surround a CABG operation the infectious course starts. We therefore believe it is of essence that all levels of the clinic, from operating surgeon to nurse assistant are engaged in the process. Another important aspect, and difficulty, is to maintain the increased discipline and accuracy with time, and not settle for a final solution, after the changes have been implemented and initial success achieved. With the current study we show that a structured root cause analysis and a purposeful and stringent intervention program can reduce the problem, although the exact importance of each single change is difficult to define.

Competing interests
The authors declare that they have no competing interests.

Authors' contributions
RL wrote the manuscript and analyzed the data. BL and UR analyzed the data and participated in the design of the study. CS, NL and BL collected the data. CLS collected and analyzed the data and edited the manuscript. All authors were active in conceiving the study. All authors read and approved the final manuscript.

Acknowledgements
We express the sincere gratitude to our loyal patients who contributed to the excellent response rate of the postoperative questionnaire. This work was supported by Uppsala County Association against Heart and Lung Diseases, Erik, Karin och Gösta Selanders Foundation and Dr Åke Olssons Foundation for Education. The funders had no role in study design, data collection and analysis, decision to publish, or preparation of the manuscript.

Author details
[1]Department of Cardiothoracic Surgery and Anesthesia, Uppsala University Hospital, 751 85 Uppsala, Sweden. [2]Department of Medical Sciences, Unit for Clinical Microbiology and Infectious Medicine, Uppsala University, Uppsala, Sweden. [3]Department of Public Health and Caring Sciences, Uppsala University, Uppsala, Sweden.

References
1. Garcia S, Sandoval Y, Roukoz H, Adabag S, Canoniero M, Yannopoulos D, et al. Outcomes after Complete versus Incomplete Revascularization of Patients with Multivessel Coronary Artery Disease: A Meta-Analysis of 89,883 Patients Enrolled in Randomized Clinical Trials and Observational Studies. J Am Coll Cardiol. 2013;62(16):1421-31.
2. Fortuna D, Nicolini F, Guastaroba P, De Palma R, Di Bartolomeo S, Saia F, et al. Coronary artery bypass grafting vs percutaneous coronary intervention in a 'real-world' setting: a comparative effectiveness study based on propensity score-matched cohorts. Eur J Cardiothorac Surg. 2013;44(1):e16–24.
3. Farkouh ME, Domanski M, Sleeper LA, Siami FS, Dangas G, Mack M, et al. Strategies for multivessel revascularization in patients with diabetes. N Engl J Med. 2012;367(25):2375–84.
4. Kubota H, Miyata H, Motomura N, Ono M, Takamoto S, Harii K, et al. Deep sternal wound infection after cardiac surgery. J Cardiothorac Surg. 2013;8:132.
5. Graf K, Ott E, Vonberg RP, Kuehn C, Schilling T, Haverich A, et al. Surgical site infections–economic consequences for the health care system. Langenbecks Arch Surg. 2011;396(4):453–9.
6. Swenne CL, Lindholm C, Borowiec J, Carlsson M. Surgical-site infections within 60 days of coronary artery by-pass graft surgery. J Hosp Infect. 2004; 57(1):14–24.
7. Berg TC, Kjorstad KE, Akselsen PE, Seim BE, Lower HL, Stenvik MN, et al. National surveillance of surgical site infections after coronary artery bypass grafting in Norway: incidence and risk factors. Eur J Cardiothorac Surg. 2011;40(6):1291–7.
8. Bryan CS, Yarbrough WM. Preventing deep wound infection after coronary artery bypass grafting: a review. Tex Heart Inst J. 2013;40(2):125–39.
9. Borer A, Gilad J, Meydan N, Riesenberg K, Schlaeffer F, Alkan M, et al. Impact of active monitoring of infection control practices on deep sternal infection after open-heart surgery. Ann Thorac Surg. 2001;72(2):515–20.
10. Haycock C, Laser C, Keuth J, Montefour K, Wilson M, Austin K, et al. Implementing evidence-based practice findings to decrease postoperative sternal wound infections following open heart surgery. J Cardiovasc Nurs. 2005;20(5):299–305.
11. Batalden P, Splaine M. What will it take to lead the continual improvement and innovation of health care in the twenty-first century? Qual Manag Health Care. 2002;11(1):45–54.
12. Vincent C, Batalden P, Davidoff F. Multidisciplinary centres for safety and quality improvement: learning from climate change science. BMJ Qual Saf. 2011;20 Suppl 1:i73–78.
13. Durkin MJ, Dicks KV, Baker AW, Lewis SS, Moehring RW, Chen LF, et al. Seasonal variation of common surgical site infections: does season matter? Infect Control Hosp Epidemiol. 2015;36(9):1011 6.

14. Bagian JP, Lee C, Gosbee J, DeRosier J, Stalhandske E, Eldridge N, et al. Developing and deploying a patient safety program in a large health care delivery system: you can't fix what you don't know about. Jt Comm J Qual Improv. 2001;27(10):522–32.
15. Casha AR, Gauci M, Yang L, Saleh M, Kay PH, Cooper GJ. Fatigue testing median sternotomy closures. Eur J Cardiothorac Surg. 2001;19(3):249–53.
16. Casha AR, Yang L, Kay PH, Saleh M, Cooper GJ. A biomechanical study of median sternotomy closure techniques. Eur J Cardiothorac Surg. 1999;15(3):365–9.
17. Haynes AB, Weiser TG, Berry WR, Lipsitz SR, Breizat AH, Dellinger EP, et al. A surgical safety checklist to reduce morbidity and mortality in a global population. N Engl J Med. 2009;360(5):491–9.
18. World Medical Association Declaration of Helsinki: ethical principles for medical research involving human subjects. Jama 2013. 310(20):2191–2194
19 Lytsy B, Lindblom RP, Ransjö U, Leo-Swenne CJ .Hygienic interventions to decrease deep sternal wound infections following coronary artery bypass grafting. Hosp Infect. 2015. pii: S0195-6701(15)00343-6. doi:10.1016/j.jhin. 2015.08.021.
20. Salehi Omran A, Karimi A, Ahmadi SH, Davoodi S, Marzban M, Movahedi N, et al. Superficial and deep sternal wound infection after more than 9000 coronary artery bypass graft (CABG): incidence, risk factors and mortality. BMC Infect Dis. 2007;7:112.
21. Ang LB, Veloria EN, Evanina EY, Smaldone A. Mediastinitis and blood transfusion in cardiac surgery: a systematic review. Heart Lung. 2012;41(3):255–63.
22. Omar AS, Salama A, Allam M, Elgohary Y, Mohammed S, Tuli AK, et al. Association of time in blood glucose range with outcomes following cardiac surgery. BMC Anesthesiol. 2015;15(1):14.
23. Giakoumidakis K, Eltheni R, Patelarou E, Theologou S, Patris V, Michopanou N, et al. Effects of intensive glycemic control on outcomes of cardiac surgery. Heart Lung. 2013;42(2):146–51.
24. Braenne I, Reiz B, Medack A, Kleinecke M, Fischer M, Tuna S, et al. Whole-exome sequencing in an extended family with myocardial infarction unmasks familial hypercholesterolemia. BMC Cardiovasc Disord. 2014;14:108.
25. Clemmons DR, Underwood LE, Dickerson RN, Brown RO, Hak LJ, MacPhee RD, et al. Use of plasma somatomedin-C/insulin-like growth factor I measurements to monitor the response to nutritional repletion in malnourished patients. Am J Clin Nutr. 1985;41(2):191–8.
26. Toulon A, Breton L, Taylor KR, Tenenhaus M, Bhavsar D, Lanigan C, et al. A role for human skin-resident T cells in wound healing. J Exp Med. 2009; 206(4):743–50.
27. Balaji S, LeSaint M, Bhattacharya SS, Moles C, Dhamija Y, Kidd M, et al. Adenoviral-mediated gene transfer of insulin-like growth factor 1 enhances wound healing and induces angiogenesis. J Surg Res. 2014;190(1):367–77.
28. Goto H, Gomes CM, Corbett CE, Monteiro HP, Gidlund M. Insulin-like growth factor I is a growth-promoting factor for Leishmania promastigotes and amastigotes. Proc Natl Acad Sci U S A. 1998;95(22):13211–6.
29. Schneider HJ, Friedrich N, Klotsche J, Schipf S, Nauck M, Volzke H, et al. Prediction of incident diabetes mellitus by baseline IGF1 levels. Eur J Endocrinol. 2011;164(2):223–9.
30. Vaessen N, Heutink P, Janssen JA, Witteman JC, Testers L, Hofman A, et al. A polymorphism in the gene for IGF-I: functional properties and risk for type 2 diabetes and myocardial infarction. Diabetes. 2001;50(3):637–42.
31. Meberg A, Schoyen R. Bacterial colonization and neonatal infections. Effects of skin and umbilical disinfection in the nursery. Acta Paediatr Scand. 1985; 74(3):366–71.
32. W-Dahl A, Toksvig-Larsen S. Pin site care in external fixation sodium chloride or chlorhexidine solution as a cleansing agent. Arch Orthop Trauma Surg. 2004;124(8):555–8.

4

Transplantation of EPCs overexpressing PDGFR-β promotes vascular repair in the early phase after vascular injury

Hang Wang[1†], Yang-Guang Yin[2†], Hao Huang[3], Xiao-Hui Zhao[4], Jie Yu[4], Qiang Wang[4], Wei Li[4], Ke-Yin Cai[1] and Shi-Fang Ding[5*]

Abstract

Background: Endothelial progenitor cells (EPCs) play important roles in the regeneration of the vascular endothelial cells (ECs). Platelet-derived growth factor receptor (PDGFR)-β is known to contribute to proliferation, migration, and angiogenesis of EPCs, this study aims to investigate effects of transplantation of EPCs overexpressing PDGFR-β on vascular regeneration.

Methods: We transplanted genetically modified EPCs overexpressing PDGFR-β into a mouse model with carotid artery injury. After 3 days of EPCs transplantation, the enhanced green fluorescent protein (EGFP)-expressing cells were found at the injury site and the lining of the lumen by laser scanning confocal microscope (LSCM). At 4, 7, and 14 days of the carotid artery injury, reendothelialization was evaluated by Evans Blue staining. Neointima formation was evaluated at day 14 with hematoxylin and eosin (HE) staining by calculating the neointimal area, medial area, and neointimal/media (NI/M) ratio. Intimal cell apoptosis was evaluated using TUNEL assay. Then we tested whether PDGF-BB-induced VSMC migration and PDGF-BB's function in reducing VSMC apoptosis can be attenuated by EPCs overexpressing PDGFR-β in a transwell co-culture system.

Results: Our results showed that EPCs overexpressing PDGFR-β accelerates reendothelialization and mitigates neointimal formation at 14 days after injury. Moreover, we found that there is great possibility that EPCs overexpressing PDGFR-β enhanc VSMC apoptosis and suppress VSMC migration by competitive consumption of PDGF-BB in the early phase after carotid artery injury in mice.

Conclusions: We report the first in vivo and in vitro evidence that transplantation of genetically modified EPC can have a combined effect of both amplifying the reendothelialization capacity of EPCs and inhibiting neointima formation so as to facilitate better inhibition of adverse remodeling after vascular injury.

Keywords: EPCs, PDGFR-β, Reendothelialization, Neointima, Gene therapy

Background

The normal arterial vessel wall is mostly composed of endothelial cells (ECs), vascular smooth muscle cells (VSMCs), and macrophages. Endothelial impairment is believed to be a major contributor to atherosclerosis and restenosis after percutaneous coronary intervention (PCI) [1, 2]. Reendothelialization can effectively inhibit VSMC migration and proliferation and decrease neointimal thickening [3]. Therefore, acceleration of reendothelialization is of special interest with regard to reducing neointima formation to prevent postangioplasty restenosis and development of atherosclerosis.

Endothelial progenitor cells (EPCs) include cells in multiple stages from mother cells to mature ECs. Both early EPCs that can repair the blood vessels and the late EPCs that have strong proliferation ability are involved in angiogenesis. Indeed, the numbers of EPCs in a patient with atherosclerotic vascular disease, who needs endothelial repair, are much lower

* Correspondence: dsfmd2015@163.com
†Equal contributors
5Institute of Cardiovascular Science, Wuhan General Hospital of Guangzhou Military Command, Wuhan 430070, China
Full list of author information is available at the end of the article

than that in a normal person [4–6]. Recently, several studies showed that EPCs can be recruited to the sites of endothelial injury, be differentiated into mature ECs, and can play important roles in reendothelialization after vascular injury [7–10]. Platelet-derived growth factor (PDGF) can enhance VSMC function and injury-induced neointima formation. PDGF-BB gene knockout mice show pathological defects such as heart and blood vessel dilations, proving that PDGF-BB plays a vital role in the establishment of the circulatory system in the body [11]. Recently, it was reported that PDGF-BB was locally produced by injured arteries, and it contributed to the promotion of migration, proliferation, and neointima formation of local VSMCs for participation in vascular repair/ remodeling in human and animal vascular injury models [12]. However, inhibition of PDGF-BB signaling has been shown to reduce neointima formation and inhibit vascular repair/remodeling after angioplasty [13–15]. Our previous study also showed that overexpression of PDGF-receptor (PDGFR)-β promoted PDGF-BB-induced proliferation, migration, and angiogenesis of EPCs [16].

Based on known knowledge regarding PDGF-BB and PDGFR-β on the biological functions of VSMCs and EPCs, we propose that EPCs overexpressing PDGFR-β may have effects on reendothelialization during arterial repairment after injury. To test this, we transplanted genetically modified EPCs overexpressing PDGFR-β into a mouse model with carotid artery injury and evaluated whether locally released PDGF-BB can stimulate homing of the transplanted EPCs to the site of endothelial injury and improve their biological functions. We further investigated whether the homed EPCs overexpressing PDGFR-β can compete for the locally produced PDGF-BB produced by injured arteries with the VSMCs to inhibit the local VSMC migration, proliferation, and neointima formation. Our results showed that transplantation of genetically modified EPC may have a combined effect of both amplifying the reendothelialization capacity of EPCs for repairing injured arteries as well as inhibiting the capacity of EPCs in neointima formation so as to facilitate better inhibition of adverse remodeling after vascular injury.

Methods
Animals and protocols
All procedures were performed in compliance with the Ethic Committee of Third Military Medical University and the National Institute of Health Guide for the Care and Use of Laboratory. Animals Male C57BL/6 mice (weight: 25–30 g, age: 6–8 weeks) were obtained from the Laboratory Animal Center at the Third

Military Medical University (Chongqing, China). Mice were firstly anaesthetized by 40 mg/kg sodium pentobarbital (Sigma-Aldrich, St Lois, MO, USA) via iintraperitoneal (IP) injection. The extent of anaesthesia was assessed by mouse's reaction to the toe pinching during the splenectomy or the carotid artery injury surgery. Then they received 3 mg/kg ketorolac tromethamine (Newtime, Shandong, China) by per os(PO) to minimize the postoperative pain. At last all mice were euthanized by IP injection of 240 mg/kg sodium pentobarbital.

Splenectomy
Splenectomy was performed as described in our previous study [17]. Vessels of the mice were carefully ligated using 6–0 silk ligatures via a lateral incision of the left abdomen, followed by ablation of the spleen. The abdomen was immediately closed layer by layer with single sutures using 6–0 silk. The mice were allowed to recover for 14 days after which the carotid arterial injury was induced.

EPC culturing and characterization
Culturing and characterization of mouse spleen-derived EPCs was performed as described previously [16, 18]. To determine the endothelial phenotype of EPCs, the cells were incubated with 2.4 μg/mL acLDL-DiI (Invitrogen, CA, USA) for 4 h, fixed with 4 % paraformaldehyde (PFA), and then incubated with 10 μg/mL FITC-UEA-1 (Sigma-Aldrich, St. Louis, MO, USA) for 1 h. The cells positive for both acLDL-DiI and UEA-1 were identified as differentiating EPCs. In addition, the phenotypes of EPCs were evaluated by flow cytometry (FCM). Cells (1×106) were incubated with the following monoclonal antibodies: PE-conjugated anti-VEGFR-2 (eBiosciences, San Diego, CA, USA), FITC-conjugated anti-Sca-1 (abCAM, Cambridge, MA, USA), or their corresponding isotype controls (eBiosciences).

EPCs gene transfer
The plasmids pEGFP-N2 and pEGFP-N2-PDGFR-β were kindly provided by Dr. Shangcheng Xu at the Third Military Medical University. Transfection was performed, as described previously [16], with the Lipofectamine™ 2000 reagent (Invitrogen, Shanghai, China), according to the manufacturer's instruction. The EPCs of the pEGFP-N2 or pEGFP-N2-PDGFR-β groups were collected 24 h after transfection.

VSMC culturing and characterization
VSMCs were isolated from the thoracic aorta of mice through explantation and cultured in Dulbecco's Modified Eagle Medium: nutrient mixture F-12

(DMEM/F-12) culture medium (Gibco BRL, NY, USA) supplemented with 20 % fetal calf serum (FCS, Gibco BRL, NY, USA), 100 U/mL penicillin, and 100 U/mL streptomycin. Cells were kept at 37 °C in a 5 % CO_2 atmosphere. Cultures were confirmed by smooth muscle α-actin (SMαA, NeoMarkers, CA, USA). Cells from 3 to 6 passages were used for all experiments.

Carotid artery injury model and EPC transplantation

Injury of carotid artery was induced 14 days after splenectomy, as described in our previous study [19]. Briefly, the bifurcation of the left carotid artery was exposed through a midline incision on the ventral side of the neck. A 6–0 silk slipknot was placed around the common carotid artery and the internal carotid artery to block their blood flow. Two ligatures were placed proximally and distally around the external carotid artery, and the distal ligature was then tied off. A tailored hook made from a syringe (1 mL) was used to place the silk around the external and the internal carotid arteries. An incision was made between the two ligatures to introduce the denudation device. The tailored flexible wire (0.014-in. diameter, the tip of the wire was relatively thinner) was introduced into the common carotid artery. The endothelium was denuded by passing the wire back and forth through the vessel three times. After removal of the wire, the proximal ligature of the external carotid artery was tied off. The slipknots were removed, and the blood flow was restored. The skin incision was sutured with 6–0 silk. Then, the mice were administered 200 µL saline alone or 200 µL saline containing enhanced green fluorescent protein (EGFP)-labeled EPCs (1×10^6) or EPCs overexpressing PDGFR-β (1×10^6) via tail vein injection directly after endothelial injury of the carotid artery and again after 24 h.

EPC tracing in vivo

To observe whether the transfected EPCs were capable of homing to the site of injury, labeled pEGFP-N2-EPCs and pEGFP-N2- PDGFR-β-EPCs (1×10^6) were incubated with 2.4 µg/ml acLDL-DiI (Invitrogen, CA, USA) for 1 h. Then the cells were washed with PBS 3 times and injected into the mice' tail vein in 200 µL saline after induction of arterial injury and again after 24 h. 7 days later, EPC tracking and immunohistochemistry were performed. Images of the stained cells were obtained by a fluorescence microscope (Leica).

RNA extraction and semi-quantitative reverse transcription-polymerase chain reaction (RT-PCR)

Total RNA was extracted from the arteries by using RNA-out (Tianenze Biotech, Beijing, China), and the cDNA was

obtained through RT-PCR with the PrimeScript™ RT Reagent Kit (Takara, Biotechnology, Dalian, China) by using total RNA as a template, followed by amplification. The primers used were as follows: PDGFR-β (sense) 5′-CCGGCGCTGGCGAGTTAGTTT-3′, (antisense) 5′-ACACCTACTTTTGAGGTCTCTGCAGG-3′; product length 296 bp. PDGF-BB (sense) 5′-TGCTGAGCGAC-CACTCCATC-3′, (antisense) 5′-TGTGCTCGGGTCAT GTTCAAG-3′; product length 109 bp. Glyceraldehyde 3-phosphate dehydrogenase (GAPDH) (sense) 5′- AAC TTTGGCATTGTGGAAGGGCTC-3′, (antisense) 5′- AC CCTGTTGCTGTAGCCGTATTCA-3′; product length 473 bp. All primers were obtained from Invitrogen (Shanghai, China).

Western blotting

The protein concentration of tissue lysates was estimated by the Bradford method, and the proteins were transferred onto polyvinylidene fluoride (PVDF) membranes. The membranes were blocked with 5 % non-fat milk, probed with anti-PDGFR-β (Abcam, USA), anti-PDGF-BB (Santa Cruz Biotechnology, USA), and anti-GAPDH (Cell Signaling Biotechnology, Beverly, MA, USA), followed by staining with horseradish peroxidase-coupled secondary antibodies. The protein bands were visualized by enhanced chemiluminescence (Amersham Pharmacia Biotech, UK) and quantified by using the Quantity One software (Bio-Rad, Hercules, USA).

Immunofluorescence

Before and 7 days after the carotid artery injury, the carotid arteries were snap-frozen in liquid nitrogen in optimal cutting temperature (OCT)-embedding medium and stored at –80 °C. Six cross-sections were cut (5-µm thickness) from the approximate middle portion of the artery and used for the detection of PDGF-BB by immunofluorescence. For fluorescence staining, the sections were first incubated with an anti-PDGF-BB primary mAb (1:100) and then with a FITC-labeled secondary antibody (Beyotime, Shanghai, China). Images of the sections were obtained by a laser scanning confocal microscope (LSCM; Leica).

Measurement of reendothelialization

After 4, 7, and 14 days of the carotid artery injury, endothelial regeneration was evaluated by staining the denuded areas by injecting 200 µL of 5 % Evans Blue dye with saline via the tail vein into the heart. The left common carotid artery was then harvested 5 mm away from the carotid bifurcation. The reendothelialized area appeared white in color (unstained), whereas the non-endothelialized lesions appeared blue (stained). The unstained-areas (in white) and the total carotid artery areas were measured. The ratio of reendothelialized areas (unstained area) versus the total carotid artery area were calculated.

Assessment of neointimal and medial areas

For histological analysis, hematoxylin and eosin (HE) staining was performed, according to the standard protocols; three sections taken from the middle portion of each artery, 14 days after the carotid artery injury, were examined; and the neointimal area, medial area, and neointima/media (NI/M) ratio were calculated.

Apoptosis assay in the intima

Seven days after the carotid artery injury, the carotid arteries were snap-frozen in liquid nitrogen in OCT-embedding medium and stored at –80 °C. Six cross-sections (5-μm thick), cut from the approximate middle portion of the artery, were used for the detection of intimal apoptotic cells by immunofluorescence for terminal deoxynucleotidyl transferase dUTP nick-end labeling (TUNEL) by using the in situ Cell Death Detection Kit (Roche), according to the manufacturer's instructions, and then SmαA staining of VSMCs, DAPI staining of the nuclei of cells was performed. After the fluorescence staining, the numbers of TUNEL-positive and-negative nuclei were counted in five different high-power fields (HPFs) in each section under the LSCM. Apoptosis activity was expressed in terms of TUNEL-labeling index, calculated by dividing the positively labeled cells by the total cell number.

VSMCs and EPCs co-culture

For the settlement of the VSMC/EPC system, VSMCs were seeded on Transwell filters (4 μm pores or 8 μm pores, Corning Costar, USA). A total of 2.5 × 10^5 EPCs were cultured and were transfected in a separate well, on the lower chamber of the system. After both types of cells reached confluency, the inserts with VSMCs were added to the wells where EPCs were cultured (resulting). Three groups of cells were VSMCs and EPCs co-cultured (Fig. 1): (1) control group: no cells were cultured on the lower chamber of the system; (2) pEGFP-N2 group : EPCs with the plasmid pEGFP-N2 transfection were cultured on the lower chamber of the system; (3) pEGFP-N2-PDGFR-β group : EPCs with the plasmid pEGFP-N2-PDGFR-β transfection were cultured on the lower chamber of the system.

VSMC migration assay

The co-culture migration assay was examined using the VSMC/EPC system containing 8 μm polycarbonate filter inserts in 24-well plates. Three groups of cells were filled in various concentrations (0, 20, 40,

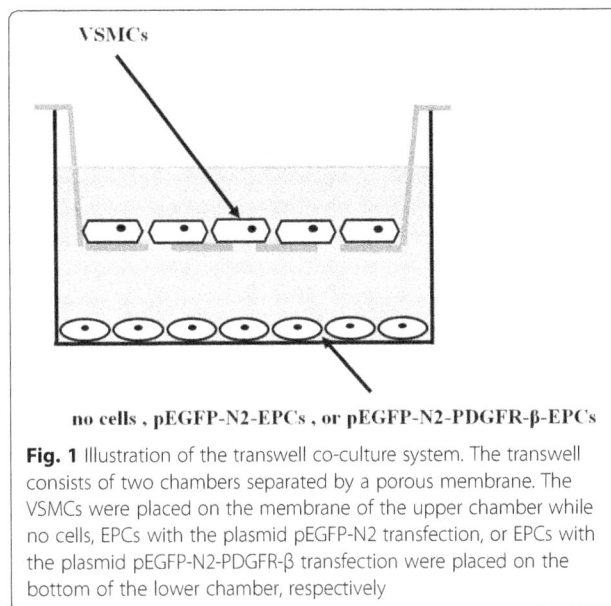

Fig. 1 Illustration of the transwell co-culture system. The transwell consists of two chambers separated by a porous membrane. The VSMCs were placed on the membrane of the upper chamber while no cells, EPCs with the plasmid pEGFP-N2 transfection, or EPCs with the plasmid pEGFP-N2-PDGFR-β transfection were placed on the bottom of the lower chamber, respectively

60, or 80 ng/mL) PDGF-BB respectively. After 12 h in culture, VSMCs on the bottom of the Transwell membrane were fixed with 4 % PFA at 37 °C for 20 min and stained with 1 % crystal violet at 37 °C for 5 min. The number of migrating cells on the bottom of the Transwell in 5 randomly HPFs (×200) was counted manually. Results were representative of three independent experiments.

VSMC apoptosis assay

The co-culture apoptosis assay was identified by immunofluorescence for TUNEL by using the in situ Cell Death Detection Kit (Roche, USA), according to the manufacturer's instructions. Briefly, the VSMC/EPC system containing 4 μm polycarbonate filter inserts in 24-well plates were used. Three groups of cells were treated with various concentrations (0, 20, 40, 60, or 80 ng/mL) PDGF-BB in DMEM/F-12 with 1 % FCS (apoptotic condition) for 72 h. VSMCs were fixed in 4 % PFA for 20 min and then treated with permeabilization solution (0.2 % Triton X-100 solution in PBS) for 5 min at room temperature. Labeling reactions were performed with 100 μL of reaction buffer for 60 min at 37 °C in a in the dark. DAPI staining of the nuclei of VSMCs was performed. After the fluorescence staining, the numbers of TUNEL-positive and-negative nuclei were counted in five HPFs (×200). Results were representative of three independent experiments. The TUNEL-labeling index was counted manually.

Statistical analysis

Data from independent experiments were expressed as mean ± standard deviation (SD). Statistical analyses were performed with the SPSS 13.0 software (SPSS Inc, Chicago, USA). Comparisons between the groups were performed by two-tailed Student's *t*-test or analysis of variance (ANOVA). Comparisons between multiple groups were tested by Multi-Way ANOVA. $P < 0.05$ was considered statistically significant.

Results

Overexpression of PDGFR-β in transfected EPCs

EPCs were transfected with either pEGFP-N2 or pEGFP-N2-PDGFR-β. After 10 days of transfection, the mRNA level of PDGFR-β in the pEGFP-N2-PDGFR-β group (0.38 ± 0.02) was significantly increased as compared to that in the non-transfected group $(0.24 \pm 0.03, p < 0.05)$ or the pEGFP-N2 group $(0.23 \pm 0.04, p < 0.05)$, as determined by semi-quantitative RT-PCR (Fig. 2a). Similarly, significantly increased protein level of PDGFR-β was also found in the pEGFP-N2-PDGFR-β group (1.30 ± 0.41) compared to that in the non-transfected group $(0.60 \pm 0.16, p < 0.05)$ and the pEGFP-N2 group $(0.63 \pm 0.26, p < 0.05)$, as determined by western blotting (Fig. 2b). Our results showed that this overexpression was maintained for at least 10 days.

Expression of PDGF-BB after wire-mediated carotid artery injury in mice

Localization of the PDGF-BB in injured vessels was investigated by immunofluorescence. PDGF-BB was rarely observed in uninjured carotids (Fig. 3a), but observed in the intima of local injured carotids at day 7 (Fig. 3b).

We analyzed the PDGF-BB expression during vascular injury following wire-mediated carotid artery injury in mice. As shown in Fig. 3c, the PDGF-BB mRNA expression was detected at low levels in uninjured control arteries (0 h), and started reducing rapidly at 6 h (3.51-fold). However, the PDGF-BB mRNA level was significantly enhanced at day 7 (3.80-fold) after the vascular injury, followed by a gradual decline at day 14 (1.67-fold).

The PDGF-BB protein expression was assessed by western blotting. The protein level started reducing rapidly at 6 h (7.80-fold) and 12 h (2.82-fold). However, the level began increasing gradually at day 2 (2.67-fold), with significant enhancement at day 7 (4.26-fold; Fig. 3d).

Labeled EPCs were observed in injured artery

After 7 days of EPC transplantation, acLDL-DiI-labeled EPCs were identified as red fluorescence cells (Fig. 4a, b). Labeled cells were seen lining the lumen that co-stained for endothelial markers FITC-UEA-1. No acLDL-DiI-labeled cells were identified in uninjured control arteries (data not shown).

Transplantation of EPCs overexpressing PDGFR-β promoted reendothelialization

To investigate whether PDGFR-β overexpression could accelerate reendothelialization, Evans Blue staining was performed (Fig. 5a). At day 4, the reendothelialized area in the pEGFP-N2-PDGFR-β-EPCs transplanted arteries $(17.76 \pm 3.35 \%)$ was significantly larger than in the saline control group $(8.83 \pm 3.16 \%, p < 0.01)$ but

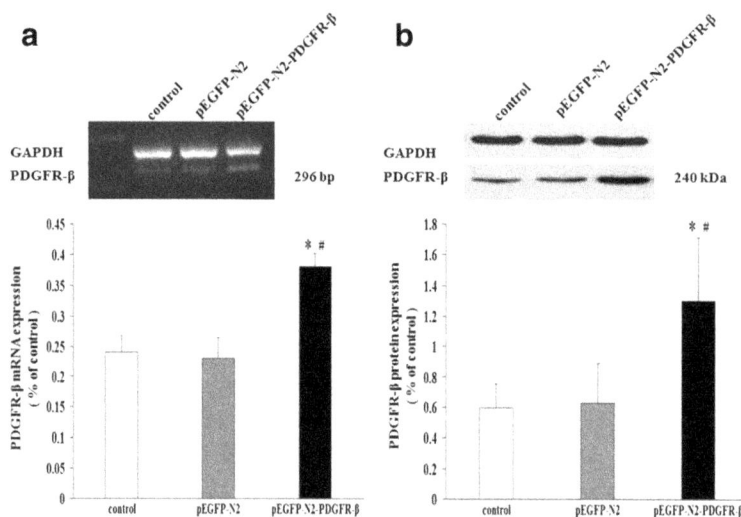

Fig. 2 Overexpression of PDGFR-β in transfected EPCs. At 10 days after transfection, PDGFR-β mRNA level (**a**) and protein levels (**b**) in the pEGFP-N2-PDGFR-β group were significantly higher than those in the control group and pEGFP-N2 group.*$P < 0.05$ vs. control or #$P < 0.05$ vs. pEGFP-N2 ($n = 3$)

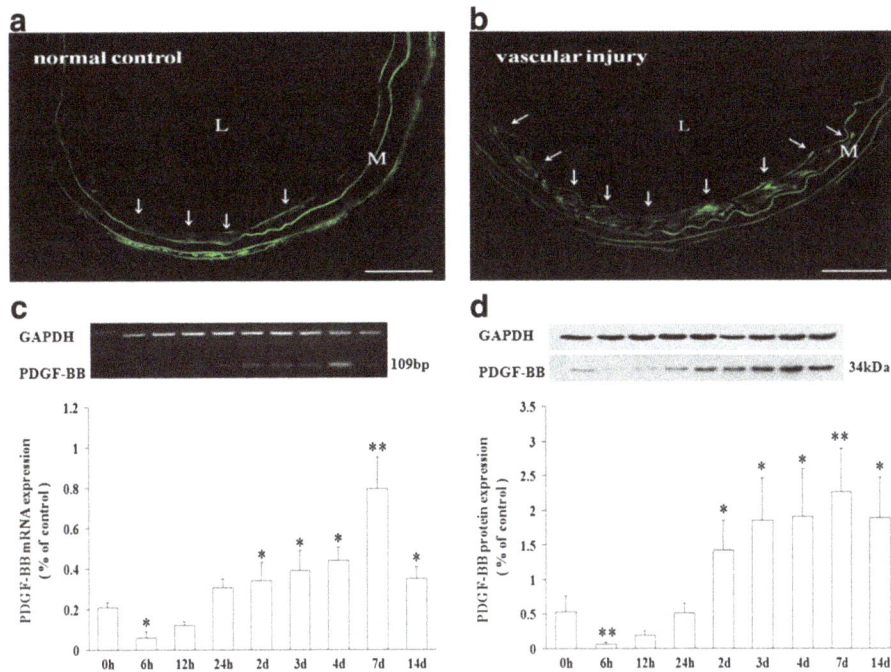

Fig. 3 Comparison of expression of PDGF-BB in normal and vascular injured mice. Arrows indicate immunofluorescence staining for PDGF-BB (green) in normal (**a**) and wire-mediated carotid artery injury mice (**b**). **c** Semi-quantitative RT-PCR revealed that PDGF-BB was significantly enhanced at day 7. **d** Top: Representative images from western blotting. Bottom: Protein level of PDGF-BB, as assessed by densitometric analysis. $*P < 0.05$ vs. 0 h; $**P < 0.01$ vs. 0 h ($n = 3$). L, lumen; M, media. Scale bar = 50 μm

was not significantly larger ($P > 0.05$) than that in the pEGFP-N2-EPCs transplanted arteries (16.56 ± 4.46 %; Fig. 5b). At day 7, the reendothelialized area in the pEGFP-N2-PDGFR-β-EPCs transplanted arteries (58.55 ± 7.17 %) was significantly larger than that in the pEGFP-N2-EPCs transplanted arteries (48.62 ± 4.55 %; $p < 0.05$; Fig. 5b) and that in the saline control group (29.15 ± 7.07 %, $p < 0.01$). At day 14, the reendothelialized area in the pEGFP-N2-PDGFR-β-EPCs transplanted arteries

(76.41 ± 10.16 %) was significantly larger than that in the pEGFP-N2-EPCs transplanted arteries (53.00 ± 7.98 %, $p < 0.01$) and that in the saline control group (34.6 ± 6.06 %, $p < 0.01$). These results demonstrate that reendothelialization of injured carotid arteries is promoted by EPC transplantation and further enhanced by transplantation with EPCs overexpressing PDGFR-β at days 7 and 14 after wire-mediated carotid artery injury.

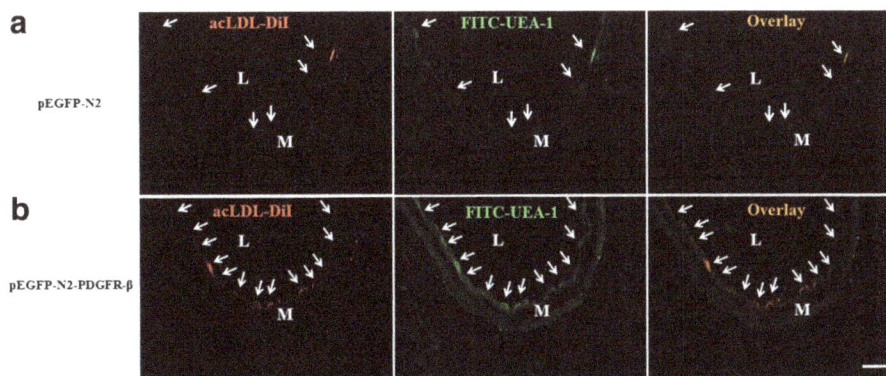

Fig. 4 EPCs tracing in vivo. **a** Labeled pEGFP-N2-EPCs and **b** pEGFP-N2- PDGFR-β-EPCs were injected into the mice after vascular injury and attached to the vascular injury site on day 7. Arrows indicate EPCs ($n = 5$). L, lumen; M, media. Scale bar = 50 μm

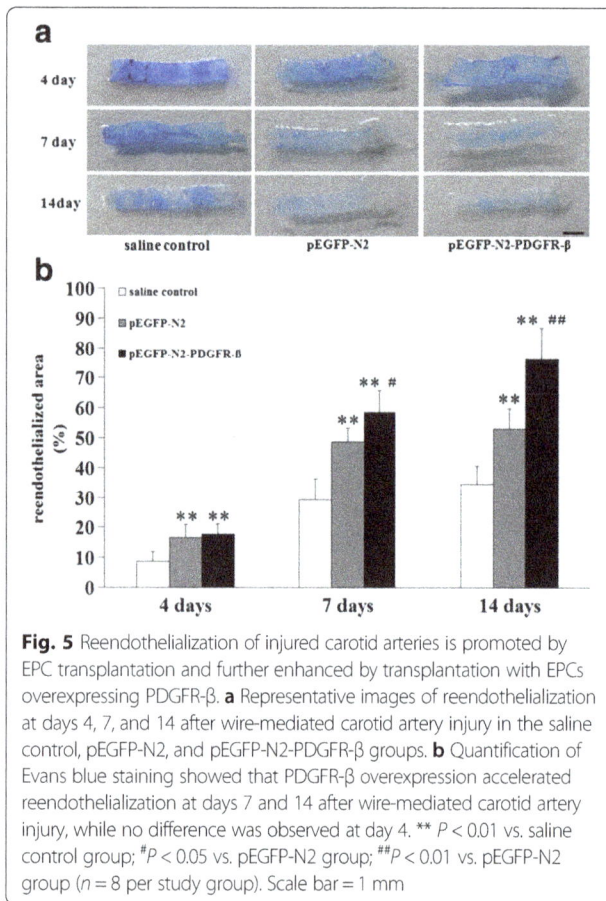

Fig. 5 Reendothelialization of injured carotid arteries is promoted by EPC transplantation and further enhanced by transplantation with EPCs overexpressing PDGFR-β. **a** Representative images of reendothelialization at days 4, 7, and 14 after wire-mediated carotid artery injury in the saline control, pEGFP-N2, and pEGFP-N2-PDGFR-β groups. **b** Quantification of Evans blue staining showed that PDGFR-β overexpression accelerated reendothelialization at days 7 and 14 after wire-mediated carotid artery injury, while no difference was observed at day 4. ** $P < 0.01$ vs. saline control group; # $P < 0.05$ vs. pEGFP-N2 group; ## $P < 0.01$ vs. pEGFP-N2 group ($n = 8$ per study group). Scale bar = 1 mm

Transplantation of EPCs overexpressing PDGFR-β attenuated neointima formation

The effect of transplantation of EPCs overexpressing PDGFR-β on neointima formation was evaluated by HE staining at 14 days after the carotid injury. At day 14, a significant decrease ($P < 0.05$) in NI/M ratio was noted in the pEGFP-N2-PDGFR-β-EPCs group (0.29 ± 0.07) as compared with that in the pEGFP-N2-EPCs group (0.43 ± 0.08; Fig. 6a, b) and in the saline control group (0.73 ± 0.13, $p < 0.01$). Our results indicate that the transplantation of EPCs overexpressing PDGFR-β can inhibit neointima formation in the early phase after carotid artery injury.

Transplantation of EPCs overexpressing PDGFR-β increased intima cells apoptosis

We next examined the effects of transplantation of EPCs overexpressing PDGFR-β on intima cells apoptosis/necrosis by TUNEL staining (Fig. 7a, b and c). After 7 days of the carotid injury, the TUNEL-labeling index was significantly greater in the pEGFP-N2-PDGFR-β-EPCs group (36.45 ± 5.83) than in the pEGFP-N2-EPCs group (24.45 ± 6.08, $p < 0.01$, Fig. 7d), indicating increased

intima cell apoptosis was associated with PDGFR-β overexpression.

Effects of EPCs overexpressing PDGFR-β on PDGF-BB-induced VSMC migration

To examine the effects of PDGF-BB-induced VSMCs, co-culture Transwell system was used. The main effect of concentration (F = 271.088, $P < 0.01$) and group (F = 335.35, $P < 0.01$), as well as their interaction (F = 34.699, $P < 0.01$), were all significant. The maximum migration induced by recombinant PDGF-BB occurred at 20 ng/mL in the control group and pEGFP-N2-PDGFR-β groups and at 60 ng/mL in the pEGFP-N2 group (Fig. 8b). Interestingly, in the pEGFP-N2-PDGFR-β group, VSMCs migration decreased significantly with increase in PDGF-BB concentration ($P < 0.01$) (Fig. 8a, b), indicating that PDGF-BB-induced VSMCs migration is attenuated by EPCs overexpressing PDGFR-β.

Effects of EPCs overexpressing PDGFR-β on PDGF-BB treatments reduced VSMCs apoptosis

VSMCs apoptosis plays an important role in vascular remodeling. We then used the in situ Cell Death Detection Kit to examine the effects of PDGF-BB treatments reduced VSMCs apoptosis. The main effects of concentration (F = 17.798, $P < 0.01$) and group (F = 74.428, $P < 0.01$), as well as their interaction (F = 10.376, $P < 0.01$), were all significant. The minimum TUNEL-labeling index was at 20 ng/mL PDGF-BB in the control group and at 80 ng/mL PDGF-BB in the pEGFP-N2 group respectively (Fig. 9a). In contrast, in the pEGFP-N2-PDGFR-β group, TUNEL-labeling index remained unchanged under different concentrations of PDGF-BB ($P > 0.05$) (Fig. 9b), indicating that PDGF-BB treatments reduced VSMCs apoptosis is attenuated by EPCs overexpressing PDGFR-β.

Discussion

In this study, we found that transplantation of EPCs overexpressing PDGFR-β significantly promoted reendothelialization in the early phase after carotid artery injury in mice. Additionally, EPCs overexpressing PDGFR-β inhibited neointima formation via increasing apoptosis and suppressing proliferation of VSMCs. The cause of limited neointima formation might be that homed EPCs overexpressing PDGFR-β can compete for the locally produced PDGF-BB which is a result of injured arteries with the VSMCs, therefore inhibiting the local VSMC migration, proliferation, antiapoptotic function, and reduced neointima formation. This assumption then confirmed by our experimental results in vitro. This study first reported that transplantation of genetically modified

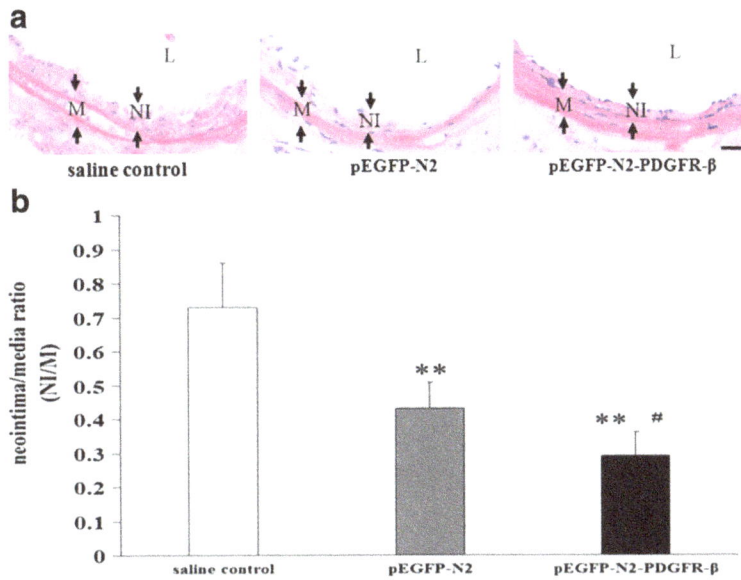

Fig. 6 Transplantation of EPCs overexpressing PDGFR-β inhibited neointima formation at day 14 after carotid artery injury. **a** Representative photos of carotid artery were stained with HE. **b** Neointima/media ratios in the injured vessels of the saline-treated, pEGFP-N2-EPCs-transplanted, and pEGFP-N2-PDGFR-β-EPCs-transplanted groups. **P < 0.01 vs. saline control group; #P < 0.05 vs.pEGFP-N2-EPCs group (n = 12 per study group). L, lumen; M, media; NI, neointima. Scale bar = 50 μm

EPC can have a combined effect of both amplifying the reendothelialization capacity of EPCs and inhibiting neointima formation so as to facilitate better inhibition of adverse remodeling after vascular injury.

EPCs can differentiate into mature ECs in vivo and therefore play an important role in vascular endothelial repair and angiogenesis in the ischemic tissues [17, 20–23].

The number and biological function of the body's circulating EPCs largely reflect the ability of vascular repair and microvascular reconstruction of the ischemic tissues [6, 8, 24, 25]. In certain diseases such as diabetes, coronary heart disease, and chronic renal failure, the number and/or biological function of the circulating EPCs decreases significantly, causing and/or facilitating

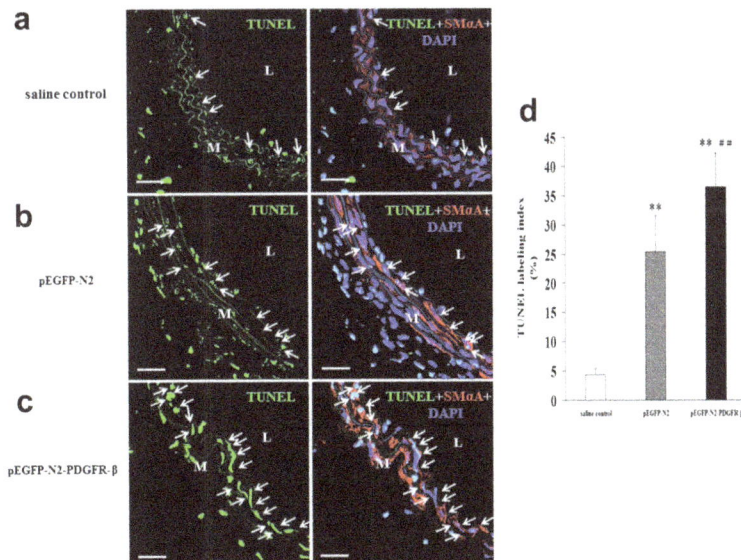

Fig. 7 Transplantation of EPCs overexpressing PDGFR-β induces apoptosis of medial cells (VSMCs). Fluorescent TUNEL staining in injured arteries of the **a** saline control group, **b** pEGFP-N2-EPCs group, and **c** pEGFP-N2-PDGFR-β-EPCs group. Arrows indicate TUNEL-positive cells (green). Red: VSMCs stained with SmαA; Blue: nuclei stained with DAPI. **d** TUNEL-labeling index. **P < 0.01 vs. saline control group; ##P < 0.01 vs. pEGFP-N2-EPCs group (n = 5). L, lumen; M, media. Scale bar = 50 μm

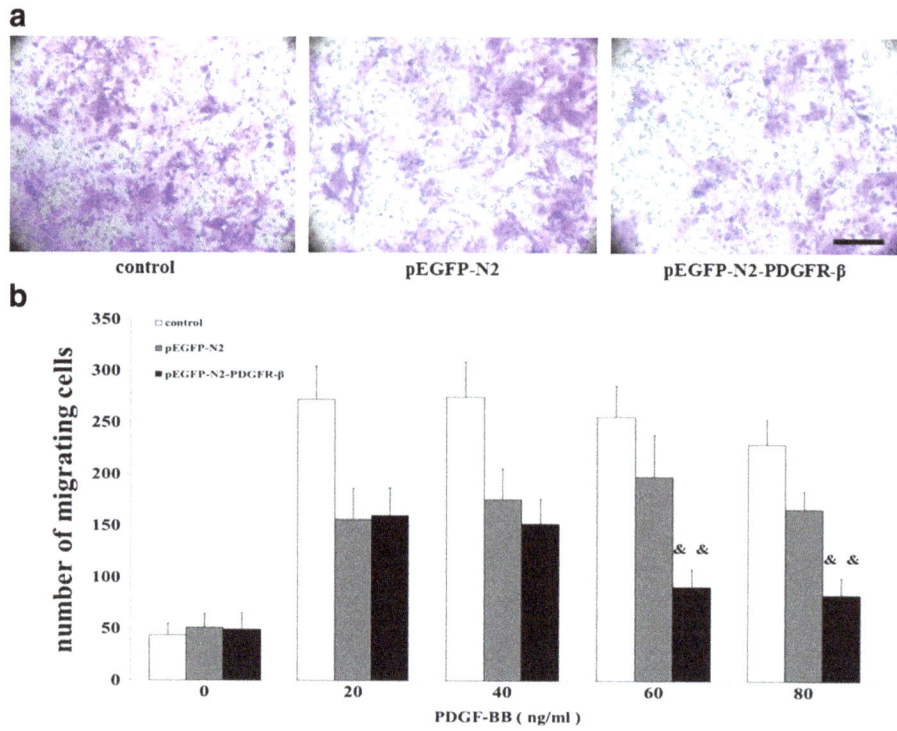

Fig. 8 Effects of PDGF-BB induced VSMC migration. **a** Representative images from VSMCs migration by recombinant PDGF-BB occurred at 60 ng/mL. **b** VSMC migration was examined by the co-culture migration assay.&& $P < 0.01$ vs. pEGFP-N2-PDGFR-β cells under 0 ng/mL PDGF-BB stimulation. Scale bar = 100 μm

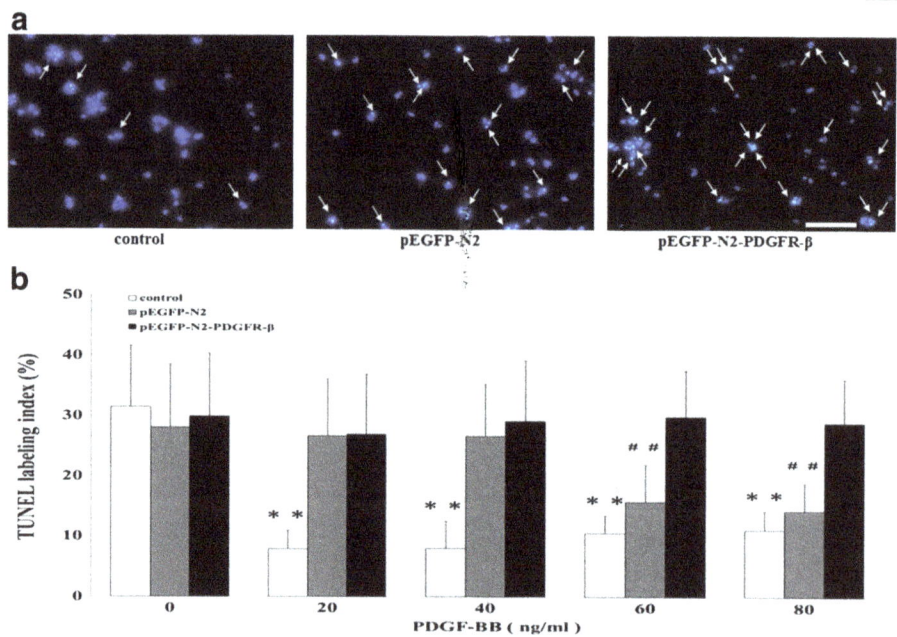

Fig. 9 Effects of PDGF-BB treatments reduced VSMC apoptosis. **a** Representative images from VSMCs apoptosis when recombinant PDGF-BB occurred at 80 ng/mL. Arrows indicate TUNEL-positive cells (green). **b** VSMC apoptosis was examined by using the in situ Cell Death Detection Kit. ** $P < 0.01$ vs. Control cells under 0 ng/mL PDGF-BB stimulation. ##$P < 0.01$ vs. pEGFP-N2 cells under 0 ng/mL PDGF-BB stimulation. Scale bar = 100 μm

the occurrence and development of these diseases [6, 8, 24–26]. Even under the normal physiological condition, in case of acute vascular injury or acute tissue ischemia (e.g., vascular endothelial damage due to a surgery), short-time blocking of the blood flow to organs, and shock leading to systemic perfusion, the number of circulating EPCs in the body are insufficient for the repair of the damaged vascular endothelium, for remodeling of the microvascular network, and for angiogenesis [17, 21, 27–29].

Previous studies have confirmed that EPC mobilization or transplantation to increase the number of circulating EPCs can promote the repair of damaged vascular endothelium [17, 21, 22, 30–36]. Transplantation of EPCs, whose biological functions have been improved by genetic modification or cytokine induction, could further enhance the repair of damaged blood vessels, as observed in some previous studies [37, 38]. In addition, a few studies reported that applying the receptor–ligand interaction mechanism to promote directional chemotaxis of EPCs could increase the number of EPCs homing to the damaged blood vessels [16, 38–40]. Both these approaches, acting on a single link, can achieve a certain effect, but not the desired effect. Presently, the homing, proliferation, and differentiation of circulating EPCs as well as the interaction of these cells with the surrounding tissue cells remain to be investigated.

Recent data have shown that remote ischaemic preconditioning reduced the incidence of periprocedural myocardial infarction following PCI [41]. Vascular interventional therapy as well as several other factors such as blood flow stress can lead to vascular intima damage, which can result in adhesion and aggregation of a large number of platelets in the intimal lesion. The adhesion of platelets releases a large amount of PDGF. Meanwhile, vascular intimal injury induces transformation of local VSMCs from contractile cells to secretory cells, leading to synthesis and secretion of a large amount of PDGF [42, 43]. PDGF exerts biological activity through the paracrine and/or autocrine glands. The PDGF family, especially PDGF-BB, is closely involved with the restenosis of the target vessels after PCI, atherosclerosis, and other vascular intimal proliferative diseases. Under normal physiological conditions, the normal artery walls have very low PDGF-BB expression level, but the PDGF-BB expression level in the target vascular tissue after PCI or in atherosclerotic vascular lesions is increased [44–46].

The local production and release of PDGF-BB exert its function in an autocrine and/or paracrine manner on the local VSMCs after vascular injury. It promotes proliferation, migration, and phenotype transformation of VSMCs [47]. In addition, it promotes postoperative restenosis after PCI and the formation of atherosclerosis plate [14, 48]. A recent study has also shown that PDGF-BB can induce proliferation, migration, and angiogenesis of EPCs over-expressing PDGFR- β receptor [16].

PDGF-BB functions mainly by acting on its specific receptor. PDGFR is a transmembrane glycoprotein possessing protein tyrosine kinase activity composed of two subunits, alpha and beta. The beta subunit PDGFR-β plays an important role in the occurrence and development of vascular intimal proliferative diseases induced by PDGF-BB [14, 48]. PDGFR-β-specific receptor blockers can effectively inhibit neointimal hyperplasia induced by PDGF-BB and reduce the degree of stenosis after vascular injury [49, 50].

Our result is consistent with previous report that the local expression and release of PDGF-BB increased during the acute period after carotid artery injury in mice and that this increase was sustained for a long time (approximately 2 weeks) [51, 52]. After transplantation of EPCs overexpressing PDGFR-β or EPCs with blank plasmid, we found that the number of EPCs homing to the injured arteries was significantly higher in the PDGFR-β overexpression group than in the PDGFR-β non-overexpression group (blank plasmid-transfected EPCs group). Evans Blue staining revealed that the reendothelialization area of injured carotid arteries was significantly higher in the PDGFR-β overexpression group than in the PDGFR-β non-overexpression group at both day 7 and day 14 and improved reendothelialization was more dramatic at day 14 compared to day 7.

Reendothelialization at sites of spontaneous or iatrogenic disruption has classically been thought to be a result from the migration and proliferation of ECs from viable endothelium adjacent to the sites of injury. Circulating EPCs as optimal candidates in cell-based therapies for vascular diseases has been well documented in contributing to the maintenance of endothelial integrity, function, and regeneration of injured endothelium [7–10]. The number, migratory capacity, and proliferative capacity of circulating EPCs are the main factors determine their ability to home to and incorporate into sites of reendothelialization. Our previous study has shown that a stably high expression of PDGFR-β of EPCs can be achieved by transfecting EPCs with pEGFP-N2-PDGFR-β. The stimulus of exogenous PDGF-BB can significantly enhance the capability of proliferation, migration, and angiogenesis in EPCs overexpressing PDGFR-β in vitro [16]. These could explain why both the number of EPCs homing to the injured arteries and the reendothelialization area of injured carotid arteries were significantly higher in the PDGFR-β overexpression group than in the PDGFR-β non-overexpression group.

We further asked whether increased reendothelialization has an impact on neointima formation. We performed HE staining and found the inhibition of neointima formation at day 14 after arterial injury in the

PDGFR-β overexpression group. This result suggests that PDGFR-β mediated reendothelialization is reversely correlated with neointima formation during vascular regeneration at the injury site. To seek the cause of decreased neointima formation, we further performed TUNEL staining to evaluate cell apoptosis to analyze inhibition of neointimal hyperplasia by transplanted EPCs overexpressing PDGFR-β after arterial injury. We found that transplanted EPCs with PDGFR-β overexpression can promote local VSMCs apoptosis in the injured carotid artery in mice at day 7 after cell transplantation. Then, we established the VSMC/EPC co-culture system in vitro. Our data shown that PDGF-BB-induced VSMC migration and PDGF-BB treatments VSMC antiapoptotic function is attenuated by EPCs overexpressing PDGFR-β competitively consume the PDGF-BB.

There are some limitations in our paper: First, our observations are based on a relatively simple animal model (young and healthy mice), and thus, the study conclusions may be limited to non-atherosclerotic arteries. Second, we did not observe the enhancing effects of the endogenous PDGF-BB, released locally by the injured carotid arteries in mice, on the recruitment of EPCs over-expressing PDGFR-β. The above-mentioned limitations would be addressed in our future studies.

Conclusions

Our present study suggests that the interaction between the transplanted EPCs overexpressing PDGFR-β and the PDGF-BB expressed and released locally by the injured carotid arteries of mice can promote homing of EPCs overexpressing PDGFR-β to the injured arteries, accelerate reendothelialization of the injured artery, and inhibit neointimal proliferation of the injured arteries after vascular injury. In addition, overexpression of PDGFR-β in the recruited EPCs can competitively consume the PDGF-BB generated locally by the injured arteries, promoting proliferation, migration, and anti-apoptosis of vascular VSMCs, which in turn can strengthen the inhibition of neointimal hyperplasia induced after vascular injury. Thus, our results suggest that the transplantation of EPCs overexpressing PDGFR-β can be used as a novel therapeutic approach for the treatment of vascular injury diseases.

Abbreviations

ANOVA: Analysis of variance; DMEM/F-12: Dulbecco's modified eagle medium: nutrient mixture F-12; ECs: Endothelial cells; EGFP: Enhanced green fluorescent protein; EPCs: Endothelial progenitor cells; FCS: Fetal calf serum; HE: Hematoxylin and eosin; HPFs: High-power fields; IP: Iintraperitoneal; NI/M: Neointimal /media; OCT: Optimal cutting temperature; PDGFR: Platelet-derived growth factor receptor; PO: Per os; PVDF: Polyvinylidene fluoride; RT-PCR: Reverse transcription-polymerase chain reaction; SMaA: Smooth muscle α-actin; TUNEL: Transferase dUTP nick-end labeling; VSMCs: Vascular smooth muscle cells

Acknowledgements
We thank Meng-yang Deng and Hua-li Kang for excellent technical help.

Funding
This work was supported by grants from the National Natural Science Foundation of China (No. 30900620, No. 81100112 and No. 81300153) and grants from the Natural Science Fund Project of Hubei Province (2014 CFA066).

Authors' contributions
HW performed the experiments and draft the manuscript, YY performed the animal experiments and draft the manuscript. XZ carried out the cell culture, participated in the immunofluorescence assay, JY participated in the cell culture, QW carried out the animal model and EPC transplantation. WL participated in the design of the study and performed the statistical analysis. KC participated in the statistical analysis. HH conceived of the study, participated in its design and helped th draft the manuscript. SD conceived of the study, and participated in its design and coordination and helped to draft the manuscript. All authors read and approved the final manuscript.

Competing interests
The authors declare that they have no competing interests.

Author details
[1]Cadre Ward Two, Wuhan General Hospital of Guangzhou Military Command, Wuhan 430070, China. [2]Intensive Care Unit, The sixth people's hospital of Chongqing, Nan'an District, Chongqing 400060, China. [3]Clinic center, Shenzhen Hornetcorn Biotechnology Company, Ltd, Shenzhen 518400, China. [4]Institute of Cardiovascular Science, Xinqiao Hospital, Third Military Medical University, Chongqing 400037, China. [5]Institute of Cardiovascular Science, Wuhan General Hospital of Guangzhou Military Command, Wuhan 430070, China.

References
1. Kipshidze N, Dangas G, Tsapenko M, Moses J, Leon MB, Kutryk M, Serruys P. Role of the endothelium in modulating neointimal formation: vasculoprotective approaches to attenuate restenosis after percutaneous coronary interventions. J Am Coll Cardiol. 2004;44(4):733–9.
2. Ong AT, McFadden EP, Regar E, de Jaegere PP, van Domburg RT, Serruys PW. Late angiographic stent thrombosis (LAST) events with drug-eluting stents. J Am Coll Cardiol. 2005;45(12):2088–92.
3. Hutter R, Carrick FE, Valdiviezo C, Wolinsky C, Rudge JS, Wiegand SJ, Fuster V, Badimon JJ, Sauter BV. Vascular endothelial growth factor regulates reendothelialization and neointima formation in a mouse model of arterial injury. Circulation. 2004;110(16):2430–5.
4. Gulati R, Jevremovic D, Peterson TE, Witt TA, Kleppe LS, Mueske CS, Lerman A, Vile RG, Simari RD. Autologous culture-modified mononuclear cells confer vascular protection after arterial injury. Circulation. 2003;108(12):1520–6.
5. Griese DP, Ehsan A, Melo LG, Kong D, Zhang L, Mann MJ, Pratt RE, Mulligan RC, Dzau VJ. Isolation and transplantation of autologous circulating endothelial cells into denuded vessels and prosthetic grafts: implications for cell-based vascular therapy. Circulation. 2003;108(21):2710–5.
6. Werner N, Kosiol S, Schiegl T, Ahlers P, Walenta K, Link A, Bohm M, Nickenig G. Circulating endothelial progenitor cells and cardiovascular outcomes. N Engl J Med. 2005;353(10):999–1007.
7. Caporali A, Pani E, Horrevoets AJ, Kraenkel N, Oikawa A, Sala-Newby GB, Meloni M, Cristofaro B, Graiani G, Leroyer AS, et al. Neurotrophin p75 receptor (p75NTR) promotes endothelial cell apoptosis and inhibits angiogenesis: implications for diabetes-induced impaired neovascularization in ischemic limb muscles. Circ Res. 2008;103(2):e15–26.
8. Giannotti G, Doerries C, Mocharla PS, Mueller MF, Bahlmann FH, Horvath T, Jiang H, Sorrentino SA, Steenken N, Manes C, et al. Impaired endothelial repair capacity of early endothelial progenitor cells in prehypertension: relation to endothelial dysfunction. Hypertension. 2010;55(6):1389–97.
9. Kawabe-Yako R, Ii M, Masuo O, Asahara T, Itakura T. Cilostazol activates function of bone marrow-derived endothelial progenitor cell for re-endothelialization in a carotid balloon injury model. PLoS One. 2011;6(9):e24646.
10. Piatkowski A, Grieb G, Simons D, Bernhagen J, van der Hulst RR. Endothelial progenitor cells–potential new avenues to improve neoangiogenesis and

reendothelialization. Int Rev Cell Mol Biol. 2013;306:43–81.

11. Leveen P, Pekny M, Gebre-Medhin S, Swolin B, Larsson E, Betsholtz C. Mice deficient for PDGF B show renal, cardiovascular, and hematological abnormalities. Genes Dev. 1994;8(16):1875–87.

12. Siow RC, Churchman AT. Adventitial growth factor signalling and vascular remodelling: potential of perivascular gene transfer from the outside-in. Cardiovasc Res. 2007;75(4):659–68.

13. Ferns GA, Raines EW, Sprugel KH, Motani AS, Reidy MA, Ross R. Inhibition of neointimal smooth muscle accumulation after angioplasty by an antibody to PDGF. Science. 1991;253(5024):1129–32.

14. Deguchi J, Namba T, Hamada H, Nakaoka T, Abe J, Sato O, Miyata T, Makuuchi M, Kurokawa K, Takuwa Y. Targeting endogenous platelet-derived growth factor B-chain by adenovirus-mediated gene transfer potently inhibits in vivo smooth muscle proliferation after arterial injury. Gene Ther. 1999;6(6):956–65.

15. Levitzki A. PDGF receptor kinase inhibitors for the treatment of restenosis. Cardiovasc Res. 2005;65(3):581–6.

16. Wang H, Yin Y, Li W, Zhao X, Yu Y, Zhu J, Qin Z, Wang Q, Wang K, Lu W, et al. Over-expression of PDGFR-beta promotes PDGF-induced proliferation, migration, and angiogenesis of EPCs through PI3K/Akt signaling pathway. PLoS One. 2012;7(2):e30503.

17. Zhao X, Huang L, Yin Y, Fang Y, Zhou Y. Autologous endothelial progenitor cells transplantation promoting endothelial recovery in mice. Trans int. 2007;20(8):712–21.

18. Wang H, Cai KY, Li W, Huang H. Sphingosine-1-Phosphate Induces the Migration and Angiogenesis of Epcs Through the Akt Signaling Pathway via Sphingosine-1-Phosphate Receptor 3/Platelet-Derived Growth Factor Receptor-beta. Cell molecular bio letters. 2015;20(4):597–611.

19. Yin Y, Zhao X, Fang Y, Huang L. Carotid artery wire injury mouse model with a nonmicrosurgical procedure. Vascular. 2010;18(4):221–6.

20. Asahara T, Murohara T, Sullivan A, Silver M, VanderZee R, Li T, Witzenbichler B, Schatteman G, Isner JM. Isolation of putative progenitor endothelial cells for angiogenesis. Science. 1997;275(5302):964–7.

21. Werner N, Junk S, Laufs U, Link A, Walenta K, Bohm M, Nickenig G. Intravenous transfusion of endothelial progenitor cells reduces neointima formation after vascular injury. Circ Res. 2003;93(2):e17–24.

22. Chen L, Wu F, Xia WH, Zhang YY, Xu SY, Cheng F, Liu X, Zhang XY, Wang SM, Tao J. CXCR4 gene transfer contributes to in vivo reendothelialization capacity of endothelial progenitor cells. Cardiovasc Res. 2010;88(3):462–70.

23. Lee SH, Lee JH, Yoo SY, Hur J, Kim HS, Kwon SM. Hypoxia inhibits cellular senescence to restore the therapeutic potential of old human endothelial progenitor cells via the hypoxia-inducible factor-1alpha-TWIST-p21 axis. Arterioscler Thromb Vasc Biol. 2013;33(10):2407–14.

24. Sung SH, Wu TC, Chen JS, Chen YH, Huang PH, Lin SJ, Shih CC, Chen JW. Reduced number and impaired function of circulating endothelial progenitor cells in patients with abdominal aortic aneurysm. Int J Cardiol. 2013;168(2):1070–7.

25. Yamagishi S, Maeda S, Ueda S, Ishibashi Y, Matsui T. Serum pigment epithelium-derived factor levels are independently associated with decreased number of circulating endothelial progenitor cells in healthy non-smokers. Int J Cardiol. 2012;158(2):310–2.

26. Pelliccia F, Pasceri V, Cianfrocca C, Vitale C, Speciale G, Gaudio C, Rosano GM, Mercuro G. Angiotensin II receptor antagonism with telmisartan increases number of endothelial progenitor cells in normotensive patients with coronary artery disease: a randomized, double-blind, placebo-controlled study. Atherosclerosis. 2010;210(2):510–5.

27. Werner N, Wassmann S, Ahlers P, Schiegl T, Kosiol S, Link A, Walenta K, Nickenig G. Endothelial progenitor cells correlate with endothelial function in patients with coronary artery disease. Basic Res Cardiol. 2007;102(6):565–71.

28. Spadaccio C, Pollari F, Casacalenda A, Alfano G, Genovese J, Covino E, Chello M. Atorvastatin increases the number of endothelial progenitor cells after cardiac surgery: a randomized control study. J Cardiovasc Pharmacol. 2010;55(1):30–8.

29. Zhang XY, Su C, Cao Z, Xu SY, Xia WH, Xie WL, Chen L, Yu BB, Zhang B, Wang Y, et al. CXCR7 upregulation is required for early endothelial progenitor cell-mediated endothelial repair in patients with hypertension. Hypertension. 2014;63(2):383–9.

30. Yu J, Wang Q, Wang H, Lu W, Li W, Qin Z, Huang L. Activation of liver X receptor enhances the proliferation and migration of endothelial progenitor cells and promotes vascular repair through PI3K/Akt/eNOS signaling pathway activation. Vasc Pharmacol. 2014;62(3):150–61.

31. Wang CH, Lee MF, Yang NI, Mei HF, Lin SY, Cherng WC. Bone marrow rejuvenation accelerates re-endothelialization and attenuates intimal hyperplasia after vascular injury in aging mice. Circ j: official j Japanese Circ Soc. 2013;77(12):3045–53.

32. Yu Y, Gao Y, Qin J, Kuang CY, Song MB, Yu SY, Cui B, Chen JF, Huang L. CCN1 promotes the differentiation of endothelial progenitor cells and reendothelialization in the early phase after vascular injury. Basic Res Cardiol. 2010;105(6):713–24.

33. Ikesue M, Matsui Y, Ohta D, Danzaki K, Ito K, Kanayama M, Kurotaki D, Morimoto J, Kojima T, Tsutsui H, et al. Syndecan-4 deficiency limits neointimal formation after vascular injury by regulating vascular smooth muscle cell proliferation and vascular progenitor cell mobilization. Arterioscler Thromb Vasc Biol. 2011;31(5):1066–74.

34. Wang Z, Moran E, Ding L, Cheng R, Xu X, Ma JX. PPARalpha regulates mobilization and homing of endothelial progenitor cells through the HIF-1alpha/SDF-1 pathway. Invest Ophthalmol Vis Sci. 2014;55(6):3820–32.

35. Kong D, Melo LG, Gnecchi M, Zhang L, Mostoslavsky G, Liew CC, Pratt RE, Dzau VJ. Cytokine-induced mobilization of circulating endothelial progenitor cells enhances repair of injured arteries. Circulation. 2004;110(14):2039–46.

36. Iwakura A, Luedemann C, Shastry S, Hanley A, Kearney M, Aikawa R, Isner JM, Asahara T, Losordo DW. Estrogen-mediated, endothelial nitric oxide synthase-dependent mobilization of bone marrow-derived endothelial progenitor cells contributes to reendothelialization after arterial injury. Circulation. 2003;108(25):3115–21.

37. Yamauchi A, Kawabe J, Kabara M, Matsuki M, Asanome A, Aonuma T, Ohta H, Takehara N, Kitagawa T, Hasebe N. Apurinic/apyrimidinic endonucelase 1 maintains adhesion of endothelial progenitor cells and reduces neointima formation. Am J Physiol Heart Circ Physiol. 2013;305(8):H1158–67.

38. Li D, Yan D, Liu W, Li M, Yu J, Li Y, Qu Z, Ruan Q. Foxc2 overexpression enhances benefit of endothelial progenitor cells for inhibiting neointimal formation by promoting CXCR4-dependent homing. J Vasc Surg. 2011;53(6):1668–78.

39. Hristov M, Zernecke A, Bidzhekov K, Liehn EA, Shagdarsuren E, Ludwig A, Weber C. Importance of CXC chemokine receptor 2 in the homing of human peripheral blood endothelial progenitor cells to sites of arterial injury. Circ Res. 2007;100(4):590–7.

40. Hristov M, Erl W, Weber PC. Endothelial progenitor cells: mobilization, differentiation, and homing. Arterioscler Thromb Vasc Biol. 2003;23(7):1185–9.

41. D'Ascenzo F, Moretti C, Omede P, Cerrato E, Cavallero E, Er F, Presutti DG, Colombo F, Crimi G, Conrotto F, et al. Cardiac remote ischaemic preconditioning reduces periprocedural myocardial infarction for patients undergoing percutaneous coronary interventions: a meta-analysis of randomised clinical trials. EuroIntervention : j EuroPCR collab Working Group Interventional Cardiol Eur Soc Cardiol. 2014;9(12):1463–71.

42. Rubin P, Williams JP, Riggs PN, Bartos S, Sarac T, Pomerantz R, Castano J, Schell M, Green RM. Cellular and molecular mechanisms of radiation inhibition of restenosis. Part I: role of the macrophage and platelet-derived growth factor. Int J Radiat Oncol Biol Phys. 1998;40(4):929–41.

43. Osherov AB, Gotha L, Cheema AN, Qiang B, Strauss BH. Proteins mediating collagen biosynthesis and accumulation in arterial repair: novel targets for anti-restenosis therapy. Cardiovasc Res. 2011;91(1):16–26.

44. Barrett TB, Benditt EP. sis (platelet-derived growth factor B chain) gene transcript levels are elevated in human atherosclerotic lesions compared to normal artery. Proc Natl Acad Sci U S A. 1987;84(4):1099–103.

45. Tanizawa S, Ueda M, van der Loos CM, van der Wal AC, Becker AE. Expression of platelet derived growth factor B chain and beta receptor in human coronary arteries after percutaneous transluminal coronary angioplasty: an immunohistochemical study. Heart. 1996;75(6):549–56.

46. Suzuki J, Baba S, Ohno I, Endoh M, Nawata J, Miura S, Yamamoto Y, Sekiguchi Y, Takita T, Ogata M, et al. Immunohistochemical analysis of platelet-derived growth factor-B expression in myocardial tissues in hypertrophic cardiomyopathy. Cardiovascular pathol: offic j S Cardiovascular

Pathol. 1999;8(4):223–31.

47. Raines EW. PDGF and cardiovascular disease. Cytokine Growth Factor Rev. 2004;15(4):237–54.

48. Sirois MG, Simons M, Edelman ER. Antisense oligonucleotide inhibition of PDGFR-beta receptor subunit expression directs suppression of intimal thickening. Circulation. 1997;95(3):669–76.

49. Nabel EG, Yang Z, Liptay S, San H, Gordon D, Haudenschild CC, Nabel GJ. Recombinant platelet-derived growth factor B gene expression in porcine arteries induce intimal hyperplasia in vivo. J Clin Invest. 1993;91(4):1822–9.

50. Noiseux N, Boucher CH, Cartier R, Sirois MG. Bolus endovascular PDGFR-beta antisense treatment suppressed intimal hyperplasia in a rat carotid injury model. Circulation. 2000;102(11):1330–6.

51. Uchida K, Sasahara M, Morigami N, Hazama F, Kinoshita M. Expression of platelet-derived growth factor B-chain in neointimal smooth muscle cells of balloon injured rabbit femoral arteries. Atherosclerosis. 1996;124(1):9–23.

52. Lindner V, Giachelli CM, Schwartz SM, Reidy MA. A subpopulation of smooth muscle cells in injured rat arteries expresses platelet-derived growth factor-B chain mRNA. Circ Res. 1995;76(6):951–7.

5

Metabolomic profiling in patients undergoing Off-Pump or On-Pump coronary artery bypass surgery

H. Kirov[1], M. Schwarzer[1], S. Neugebauer[3,4], G. Faerber[1], M. Diab[1,2] and T. Doenst[1*]

Abstract

Background: Coronary artery bypass surgery can be performed without (Off-Pump) or with cardiopulmonary bypass (On-Pump). Extracorporeal circulation and cardioplegic arrest may cause alterations in the plasma metabolome. We assessed metabolomic changes in patients undergoing On-Pump or Off-Pump coronary artery bypass surgery.

Methods: We assessed five analyte classes (41 acylcarnitines, 14 amino acids, 92 glycerophospholipids, 15 sphingolipids, sugars, lactate) using a mass-spectrometry-based kit (Biocrates Absolute*IDQ*® p150) in paired arterial and coronary sinus blood obtained from 10 consecutive On-Pump and 10 Off-Pump patients. Cardioplegia for On-Pump was warm blood Calafiore. On-Pump outcomes were corrected for hemodilution through crystalloid priming.

Results: Demographic data were equal in both groups with normal ejection fraction, renal and liver function. Patients received 2.25 ± 0.64 bypass grafts. All postoperative courses were uneventful. Of 164 measured metabolites, only 13 (7.9%) were altered by cardiopulmonary bypass. We found more long-chain acylcarnitines Off-Pump and more short-chain acylcarnitines On-Pump. Glycerophospholipids showed lower concentrations On-Pump and arginine (as the only different amino acid) Off-Pump. Interestingly, plasma arginine (nitric oxide precursor) concentration at the end of surgery correlated inversely with postoperative vasopressor need ($r = -0.7$; $p < 0.001$). Assessing arterial/venous differences revealed phosphatidylcholine-production and acylcarnitine-consumption. These findings were unaffected by cardiopulmonary bypass, cardioplegia or temporary vessel occlusion during Off-Pump surgery.

Conclusions: Cardiopulmonary bypass and warm blood cardioplegia cause only minor changes to the metabolomic profile of patients undergoing coronary artery bypass surgery. The observed changes affected mainly acylcarnitines. In addition, there appears to be a relationship between arginine and vasopressor need after bypass surgery.

Keywords: Metabolomics, Cardiac surgery, Vasopressor

Background

Novel molecular technologies have been applied to assess the impact of metabolic intermediates on outcome in cardiac surgery. Recent studies have shown that specific metabolic profiles may independently predict adverse events after coronary artery bypass grafting (CABG) [1] or in heart failure patients and after left ventricular assist device (LVAD) implantation [2]. While these investigations addressed the metabolic signatures either before and/or after the surgical procedure, the direct impact of cardiopulmonary bypass surgery has thus far not been addressed. However, cardiopulmonary bypass has been implicated with a plethora of alterations and changes in many systems of the human organism (e.g. inflammatory cascades, coagulation system, individual organ function) [3]. It is therefore well conceivable that the use of cardiopulmonary bypass also results in significant alterations in the metabolomic plasma profile.

CABG without cardiopulmonary bypass (Off-Pump) has been one area, where surgeons have tried to avoid the potentially detrimental effects of cardiopulmonary bypass (On-Pump) [4]. However, the controversial

---
* Correspondence: doenst@med.uni-jena.de
[1]Department of Cardiothoracic Surgery, Friedrich Schiller University Jena, University Hospital, Am Klinikum 1, 07747 Jena, Germany
Full list of author information is available at the end of the article

benefits and risks of Off-Pump compared to On-Pump CABG are still a subject of an ongoing discussion [5, 6].

We thus hypothesized that patients undergoing CABG On-Pump and those operated Off-Pump would show substantial differences in their plasma metabolomic profile. We tested our hypothesis in a proof-of-principle type study using targeted metabolomic analysis.

Methods
Patient population
A total of 20 consecutive patients undergoing CABG were included in the study. The first 10 patients were operated Off-Pump and the next 10 with cardioplegic arrest. The institutional ethic review committee approved the study protocol (reference number: 3194-07/11) and all patients provided written informed consent. Inclusion criteria were age between 30 and 80 years, Body Mass Index < 30, left ventricular ejection fraction between 50 and 80% and planned elective, isolated, coronary bypass surgery. End stage liver and renal insufficiency, ongoing infection, immunosuppressive therapy and tumours were exclusion criteria.

Study protocol and sample collection
All patients included in this study received standardized preoperative anaesthetic preparation. The technical approach was similar and in all cases, distal anastomoses were performed before the proximal ones. The patients received insulin infusions as required to attain euglycemia.

In the On-Pump group, immediately after cardiopulmonary bypass was established, a retrograde cardioplegia catheter was inserted in the coronary sinus (CS) and used to gather blood samples. Its correct position was verified manually. Antegrade warm blood cardioplegia was used every 20 min. No retrograde cardioplegia was given, as the retrograde catheter was used only for drawing blood. In both groups, paired arterial and CS blood samples were collected simultaneously at baseline (immediately after CS catheter placement and before aortic cross clamping in the On-Pump group) and immediately after each distal anastomosis was completed. Samples were taken slowly to avoid haemolysis and the first 1 ml was discarded to avoid possible contamination with right atrial blood. They were drawn into EDTA- treated tubes (S-Monovette® EDTA K$_2$ Gel, Saarstedt, Nuembrecht, Germany). All samples were immediately centrifuged at 4 °C and 5000 rpm for 10 min and plasma aliquots were stored in liquid nitrogen.

Analytical rationale
We used the obtained samples to perform the following analyses. First, a comparison of arterial blood samples from on- and off pump surgery in order to obtain information on the influence of cardiopulmonary bypass on

the plasma metabolome. Second, we compared arterial and coronary sinus blood samples in oder to obtain information on the transcoronary changes in the metabolome with and without cardiopulmonary bypass. Finally, we attempted to assess the influence of regional (off pump) and global ischemia (on pump with cardioplegia) with respect to changes in the plasma metabolome.

Plasma metabolite analyses
Determination of laboratory parameters glucose and lactate was performed using routine diagnostic procedures at an Abbott Architect analyzer (Abbott GmbH, Ludwigshafen, Germany). Glucose was determined with a hexokinase method according to the manufacturer's recommendations. A colorimetric assay was used for measurement of lactate concentrations.

Metabolite concentrations of five analytic classes (Additional file 1: Table S1) - 41 acylcarnitines, 14 amino acids, 92 glycerophospholipids, 15 sphingolipids and 1 sugar - were measured after preparation of serum according to the manufacturer's protocol using the Absolute*IDQ*® p150 kit (Biocrates Life Science AG, Innsbruck, Austria) on an API4000™ LC/MS/MS System (AB SCIEX, USA) equipped with an electrospray ionization source, an Agilent G1367B autosampler, and the Analyst 1.51 software (AB SCIEX, USA). In brief, 10 μl of serum was added onto the center kit plate and was dried using a nitrogen evaporator for 30 min. Subsequently, 20 μl of a 5% solution of phenylisothiocyanate (Merck) was added. After incubation of 20 min at room temperature, the plate was dried again using an evaporator for 45 min. The metabolites were extracted using 300 μl of a 5 mM ammonium acetate solution in methanol (Merck, Roth). The extracts were obtained after incubation for 30 min on a shaker (450 rpm) by centrifugation at 100 g for 2 min followed by a dilution step with 600 μl of kit MS running solvent. The plate was measured by flow injection analysis and detection of fragments was performed in multiple reaction monitoring mode. Two subsequent 20 μl injections (one for positive and one for negative mode analysis) were injected directly to the MS at a flow of 30 μl/min with MS running solvent. Concentrations for metabolites were determined using the MetIQ™ software package, which is an integral part of the Absolute*IDQ*® kit. These data were exported for following statistical analysis. For analysis only metabolites which appear in at least 50% of the patients were included. Outcomes in the On-Pump group were corrected for hemodilution through crystalloid priming (assessed by the drop in haematocrit). Heatmaps were created with MetaboAnalyst 3.0 software [7, 8]. Data were normalized for each metabolite (autoscaling method, mean-centered and divided by the standard deviation of each variable). A hierarchical clustering in form of a dendrogram for the metabolites using the Pearson distance and the average algorithm was performed.

Statistical analysis

Statistical analysis was performed via SPSS Statistics 22 (IBM, USA). Normal distribution of the metabolite concentrations was tested. Depending on the outcome either the student-t-test (normal distribution) or the Mann-Whitney-u-test (no normal distribution) was chosen for determination of statistical significance. Pearson correlation was used to investigate the correlation between two variables. Statistical significance was considered for p-values < 0.05.

Results

Table 1 shows the demographic and laboratory data of the patients. There were no differences between the groups. The majority of patients were around 60 years of age and male. There was mild obesity among the patients and approximately one third were diabetic. Ejection fraction was normal in both groups. Preoperative laboratory values showed no evidence of renal or liver dysfunction as well as the absence of major lipid disorders.

Table 2 shows laboratory values and preoperative blood-gas analyses. There were no relevant differences in acid-base homeostasis, glucose, lactate or electrolyte concentrations.

Table 3 shows the operative characteristics of the study population. The majority of patients received two or three bypass grafts. All had uneventful operations and were successfully discharged. There was no cardiopulmonary bypass time in the Off-Pump group. The duration of the operative procedure was 50 min longer On-Pump.

Figure 1 shows the metabolomic comparison of On-Pump and Off-Pump arterial blood samples, drawn at the beginning of the operation. Of the 164 measured metabolites, only 7.9% ($n = 13$) were altered by the establishment

of cardiopulmonary bypass (CPB). These differences are presented in the figure in form of a heatmap (Fig. 1a) – and by quantitative comparison of acylcarnitines (Panel B), arginine (Panel C) and glycerophospholipids (Panel D). The heatmap shows significant differences in the colour patterns. More long-chain acylcarnitines (C18:1) were present in the Off-Pump group and more short chain acylcarnitines (C5-DC (C6-OH) and C5-OH (C3-DC-M)) were present in the On-Pump group (Fig. 1b). C14:2 –OH was the only long-chain acylcarnitine that was elevated On-Pump, but here the concentration differences were minor. From the 14 measured amino acids, only arginine was significantly different. Its concentration was higher On-Pump and lower Off-Pump (Fig. 1c). Glycerophospholipid concentrations were higher Off-Pump and lower On-Pump (Fig. 1d).

Figure 2 shows the arterio-venous (coronary sinus) difference measured at the beginning of the operation. Panel A (quantitative comparison) and Panel B (heatmap) display this differences in the On-Pump group (with established CPB). Panel C (quantitative comparison) and Panel D (heatmap) represent the arterial to coronary sinus difference in the Off-Pump group. On-Pump, during CPB, the heart produced mainly phosphatidylcholines (PCaaC42:6), lysophosphatidylcholines (lysoPCaC26:1) and acylcarnitines (C5:1, C12, C12-DC, C16-2-OH) and consumed only acylcarnitines (C5-1-DC, C5-OH). In general, the changes were similar in the Off-Pump patients with production of mainly phosphatidylcholines (PCaaC26:0, PCaaC24:0, PCaaC42:6), lysophosphatidylcholines (lysoPCaC24:0, lysoPCaC28:0, lysoPCaC26:1) acylcarnitines (C12) and consumption of acylcarnitines (C5:1-DC, C7-DC, C9, C16:1-OH, C5-OH) and only one lysophosphatidylcholine- lysoPcaC6:0.

Table 1 Demographic and laboratory characteristics of the study population

	On-Pump ($n = 10$)	Off-Pump ($n = 10$)	p value
Age (years)	67.1 ± 7.53	62.8 ± 3.96	0.133
Male sex (%)	80	90	0.531
BMI (kg/m^2)	27.84 ± 1.95	27.75 ± 2.2	0.920
Diabetes mellitus (%)	40	30	0.660
Left ventricular ejection fraction (%)	59.3 ± 8.43	63.3 ± 8.6	0.309
Creatinine (μmol/l)	75.3 ± 9.47	78.8 ± 7.05	0.361
CRP (mg/l)	4.51 ± 6.19	2.22 ± 4.53	0.358
ASAT (μmol/l*s)	0.53 ± 0.1	0.57 ± 0.34	0.699
ALAT (μmol/l*s)	0.73 ± 0.23	0.734 ± 0.4	0.979
γ-GT (μmol/l*s)	0.94 ± 0.56	0.67 ± 0.37	0.222
Cholesterol (mmol/l)	4.54 ± 1.07	5.06 ± 1.21	0.332
Triglycerides (mmol/l)	3.02 ± 2.37	2.17 ± 1.45	0.350

Values are mean ± standard deviation or percent of patients
BMI body mass index, *CRP* C-reactive protein, *ASAT* aspartate aminotransferase, *ALAT* alanine transaminase, *γ-GT* γ-Glutamyltransferase

Table 2 Preoperative laboratory values and arterial blood gas analyses

	On-Pump (n = 10)	Off-Pump (n = 10)	p value
Standard bicarbonate (mmol/l)	25.04 ± 1.06	24.93 ± 1.91	0.891
Base excess (mmol/l)	0.55 ± 1.85	0.43 ± 2.18	0.896
pH	7.42 ± 0.28	7.41 ± 0.53	0.821
pCO$_2$ (kPa)	5.06 ± 0.18	5.13 ± 0.64	0.733
pO$_2$ (kPa)	15.77 ± 12.56	10.38 ± 2.3	0.213
O$_2$ Saturation,	97.24 ± 1.73	95.7 ± 1.96	0.084
Hb (mmol/l)	8.55 ± 1.13	8.16 ± 1.78	0.461
Na $^+$ (mmol/l)	137.88 ± 3.25	136.4 ± 3.65	0.364
K $^+$ (mmol/l)	4.01 ± 0.32	4.03 ± 0.5	0.924
Ca $^{2+}$ (mmol/l)	1.20 ± 0.2	1.18 ± 0.24	0.131
Glucose (mmol/l)	6.35 ± 1.17	6.65 ± 2.31	0.719
Lactate (mmol/l)	1.29 ± 0.46	1.29 ± 0.45	1.00

Values are mean ± standard deviation
pCO$_2$ carbon dioxide partial pressure, pO$_2$ arterial oxygen partial pressure, O$_2$Saturation arterial oxygen saturation, Hb arterial haemoglobin

Figure 3 illustrates the arterio-coronary sinus differences, similar to Fig. 2, but from samples taken from the end of the second anastomosis- i.e. after an expected ischemic event. Again, panels A and B represent the On-Pump group and panels C and D the Off-Pump group. The already observed trends in the arterial to coronary sinus difference remained similar and were not affected by blood cardioplegia or by temporary vessel occlusion during Off-Pump surgery.

Figure 4 shows a comparison between the arterial plasma arginine concentrations in the Off-Pump and On-Pump groups at all measured time points (panel A) as well as the correlation between arterial arginine concentration and vasopressor need (Panel B). The Off-Pump patients had lower arginine concentrations. This difference increased with time and was greatest at the last measured time point (A). This difference in concentration was related to postoperative vasopressor requirements (B). There was a strong correlation between the noradrenaline concentration administered at the end of the operation and the last measured intraoperative arginine value. Thus, the On-Pump patients had high arginine concentrations and low postoperative

noradrenaline doses and, vice versa, Off-Pump patients had low arginine concentrations but higher postoperative noradrenaline requirements.

Discussion

We demonstrate in this manuscript that cardiopulmonary bypass and warm blood cardioplegia cause only minor changes to the metabolomic profile of patients undergoing bypass surgery and that acylcarnitines are elevated in both Off-Pump and On-Pump, but chain lengths differ. Furthermore, we demonstrate that there appears to be a correlation between arterial arginine concentration and vasopressor need after bypass surgery.

One would expect that establishing cardiopulmonary bypass leads to major changes in the metabolomic composition of the blood. However, the overall changes we observed were rather minor. Less than 10% of metabolites were altered (Fig. 1). This is striking because investigations addressing the activation of signalling cascades through cardiopulmonary bypass show substantial derangements [9, 10]. For instance, inflammatory processes have been suggested to be activated by the exposure of blood to external surfaces [10, 11]. Since inflammatory

Table 3 Operative characteristics of the study population

	On-Pump (n = 10)	Off-Pump (n = 10)	p value
Single bypass (n)	1	1	
Double bypass (n)	5	6	
Triple bypass (n)	4	3	
Bypass, mean (n)	2.3 ± 0.68	2.2 ± 0.63	0.736
Cardiopulmonary bypass time (min)	92.7 ± 13.81	0	
Aortic cross clamping time (min.)	57.8 ± 14.05	0	
Operating time (min.)	205.6 ± 13.09	154.2 ± 35.7	0.001

Values are presented as mean ± standard deviation or number of patients

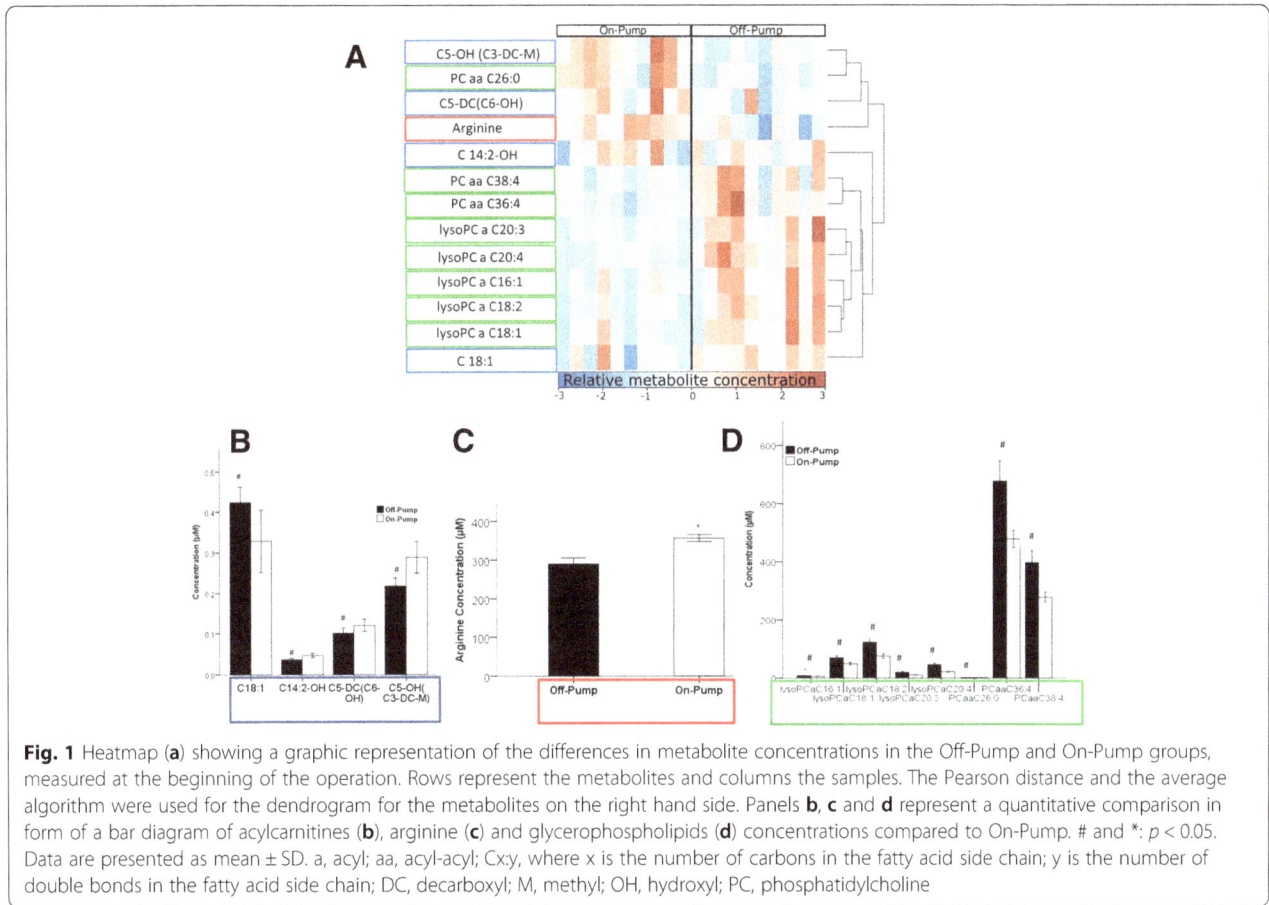

Fig. 1 Heatmap (**a**) showing a graphic representation of the differences in metabolite concentrations in the Off-Pump and On-Pump groups, measured at the beginning of the operation. Rows represent the metabolites and columns the samples. The Pearson distance and the average algorithm were used for the dendrogram for the metabolites on the right hand side. Panels **b**, **c** and **d** represent a quantitative comparison in form of a bar diagram of acylcarnitines (**b**), arginine (**c**) and glycerophospholipids (**d**) concentrations compared to On-Pump. # and *: $p < 0.05$. Data are presented as mean ± SD. a, acyl; aa, acyl-acyl; Cx:y, where x is the number of carbons in the fatty acid side chain; y is the number of double bonds in the fatty acid side chain; DC, decarboxyl; M, methyl; OH, hydroxyl; PC, phosphatidylcholine

cascades directly influence the expression of genes and the function of the cell [12], it would be no surprise to see measureable changes in metabolites associated with such activations. Some of those genes for example are relevant for the facilitation of glucose transport in tissues with a high glucose demand (Solute carrier family 2, member 3) or gluconeogenesis (Phosphoenolpyruvate carboxykinase 2) [13]. That would mean that we could expect changes in the levels of glucose or the metabolites connected with glycolysis and gluconeogenesis. However, the levels of glucose and lactate were not different between On-Pump and Off-pump in our analysis. Thus, it may be one conclusion that the use of cardiopulmonary bypass is less relevant than the type of surgery (i.e. bypass surgery) or the surgical approach. Irrespective of the magnitude of the overall changes, we still identified several changes in individual metabolite classes that may be relevant for long or short-term outcome and therefore require further discussion.

We demonstrate that patients on cardiopulmonary bypass have significantly elevated levels of short-chain acylcarnitines and lower levels of long-chain acylcarnitines such as C18:1 compared to Off-Pump patients (Fig. 1b). Plasma acylcarnitines are products of incomplete β-

oxidation and might be elevated due to inborn or other errors of mitochondrial fatty acid oxidation. Short- and medium-chain acylcarnitines are significantly increased in acute myocardial infarction and chest pain patients whereas the levels of long-chain acylcarnitines such as C18:1 and C18:2 are insignificantly decreased in these patients [14]. Short-chain acylcarnitines are also known to be predictive of myocardial infarction, repeat revascularisation or death at any time following CABG [1]. Applying these data to our results may suggest that On-Pump patients are possibly at higher risk of myocardial infarction, repeat revascularization or death, compared to Off-Pump patients. However, in heart failure patients, long-chain acylcarnitines have been associated with poor long term outcomes [2]. Thus, it appears that chain length may not be the most important part of this association. In addition, these studies assessed the role of acylcarnitines before surgery and/or during follow-up and did not address the changes during surgery as we did. Since current evidence does not support any major differences in long term outcome between On- and Off-Pump CABG, it is unlikely that the observed metabolomic alterations during surgery may have substantial impact.

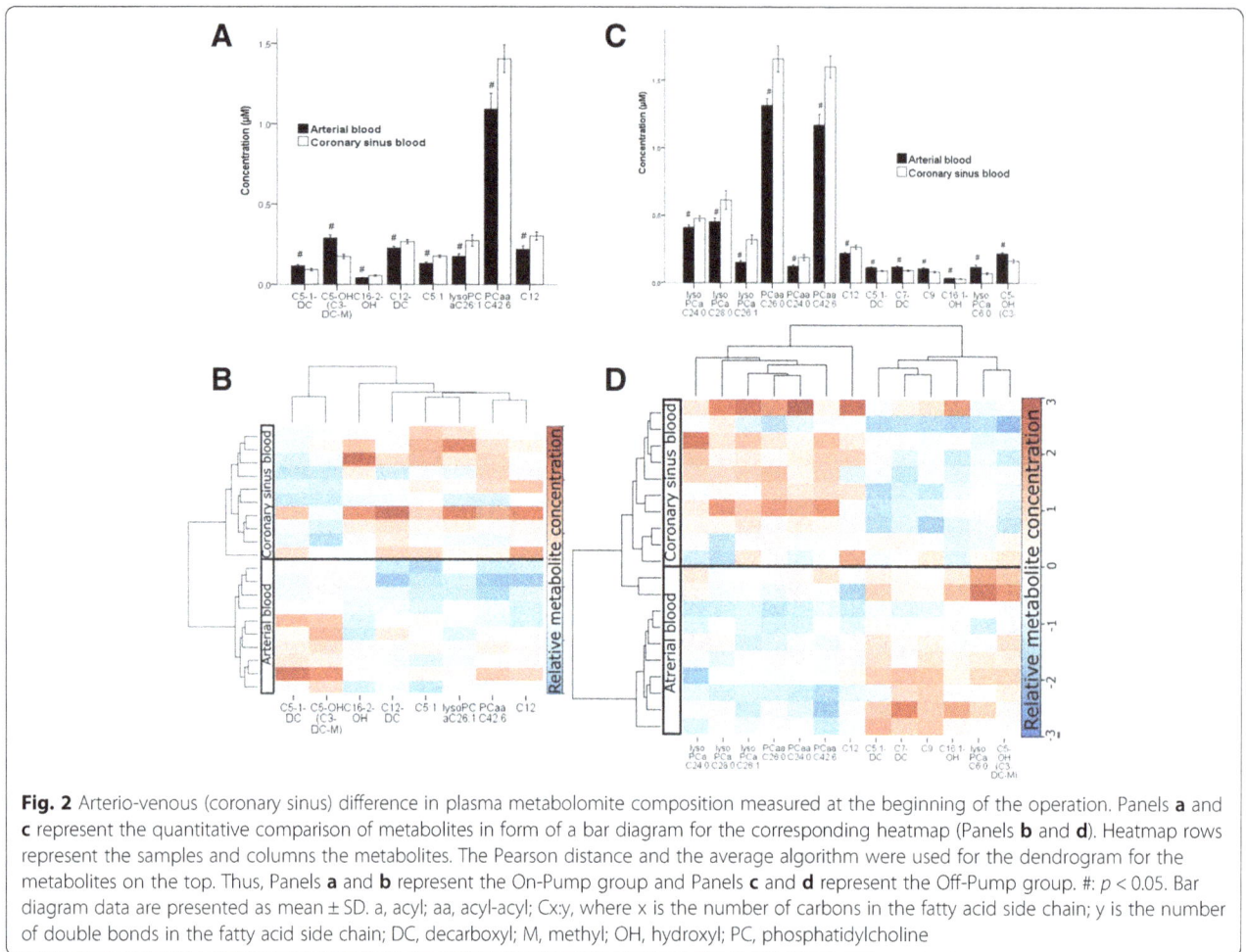

Fig. 2 Arterio-venous (coronary sinus) difference in plasma metabolomite composition measured at the beginning of the operation. Panels **a** and **c** represent the quantitative comparison of metabolites in form of a bar diagram for the corresponding heatmap (Panels **b** and **d**). Heatmap rows represent the samples and columns the metabolites. The Pearson distance and the average algorithm were used for the dendrogram for the metabolites on the top. Thus, Panels **a** and **b** represent the On-Pump group and Panels **c** and **d** represent the Off-Pump group. #: $p < 0.05$. Bar diagram data are presented as mean ± SD. a, acyl; aa, acyl-acyl; Cx:y, where x is the number of carbons in the fatty acid side chain; y is the number of double bonds in the fatty acid side chain; DC, decarboxyl; M, methyl; OH, hydroxyl; PC, phosphatidylcholine

We also demonstrate a significant correlation between arterial arginine concentration at the end of surgery and postoperative vasopressor needs in the immediately following time period in the intensive care unit (Fig. 4). Off-Pump patients had lower arginine concentrations and required more vasopressor therapy. In contrast, On-Pump patients had higher arginine concentrations but lower vasopressor needs. Arginine is the primary substrate for the synthesis of nitric oxide in the human body. Nitric oxide is produced from arginine through the enzyme nitric oxide synthase, which has three isoforms: endothelial (eNOS), neuronal (nNOS), and inducible (iNOS). Arginine deficiency is suggested to be the result of decreased arginine uptake or an impaired arginine de novo synthesis from citrulline [15]. The latter may appear in combination with an enhanced arginine catabolism by the upregulation of arginase and the inflammatory nitric oxide synthase (iNOS; NOS2) in the immune response [15]. It is also known that activated through the immune response, macrophages actively import arginine to synthesize NO by NOS2 [16, 17]. However, the NOS2 in the macrophages can also be inhibited through interleukins, such as IL-10

[18, 19]. We did not measure IL-10 in this study but this has been done before by others in the past [20–22]. Several authors have shown higher IL-10 levels On-Pump than Off-Pump at the end of surgery and early postoperatively [20–22]. Assuming that same is true in our patients, it is conceivable that IL-10 at the end of the operation inhibits iNOS in On-Pump CABG, resulting in less NO production and decreased arginine catabolism through iNOS. The consequence is higher arginine in plasma and less vascular dilatation requiring less vasopression from noradrenaline. Irrespective of the above described potential mechanism, it is not clear whether arginine is truly involved in the mechanism leading to vasopressor requirements. However, the significant correlation shown in Fig. 4 is striking and requires further investigation because it may reveal new understanding for the postoperative vasopressor management of patients undergoing cardiac surgery On- or Off-Pump.

Conclusions

In conclusion, we demonstrate in this study that cardiopulmonary bypass and warm blood cardioplegia cause

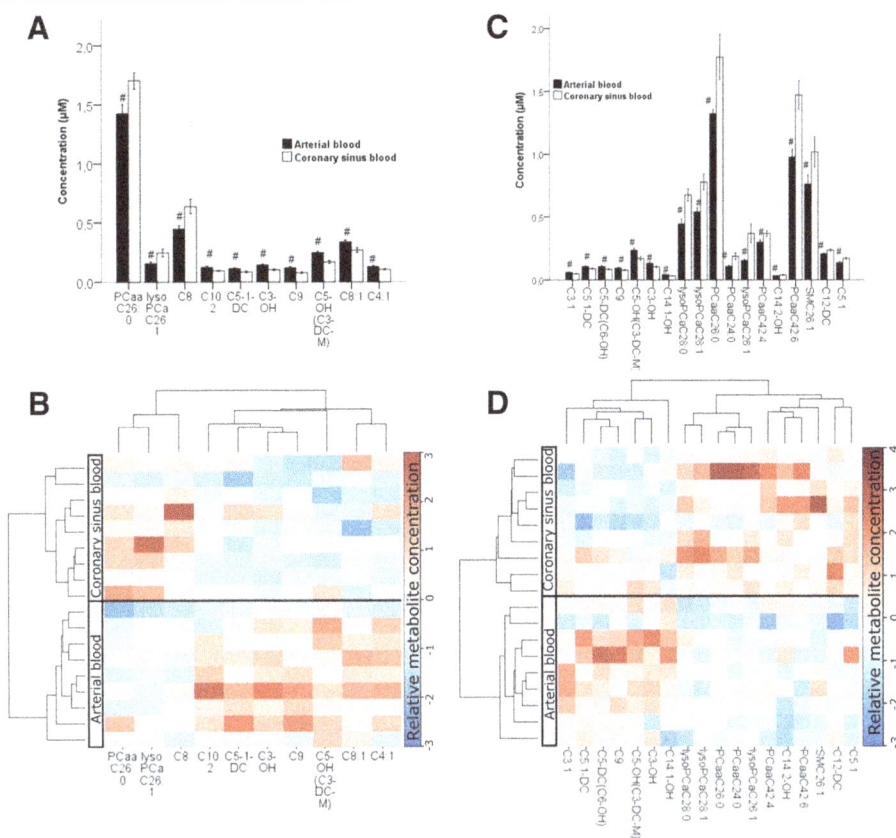

Fig. 3 Arterio-venous (coronary sinus) difference in plasma metabolomite composition measured at the end of the second distal anastomosis. Panels **a** and **c** represent the quantitative comparison of metabolites in form of a bar diagram for the corresponding heatmap (Panels **b** and **d**). Heatmap rows represent the samples and columns the metabolites. The Pearson distance and the average algorithm were used for the dendrogram for the metabolites on the top. Thus, Panels **a** and **c** represent the On-Pump group and Panels **b** and **d** represent the Off-Pump group. #: $p < 0.05$. Bar diagram data are presented as mean ± SD. a, acyl; aa, acyl-acyl; Cx:y, where x is the number of carbons in the fatty acid side chain; y is the number of double bonds in the fatty acid side chain; DC, decarboxyl; M, methyl; OH, hydroxyl; PC, phosphatidylcholine; SM, sphingomyelin

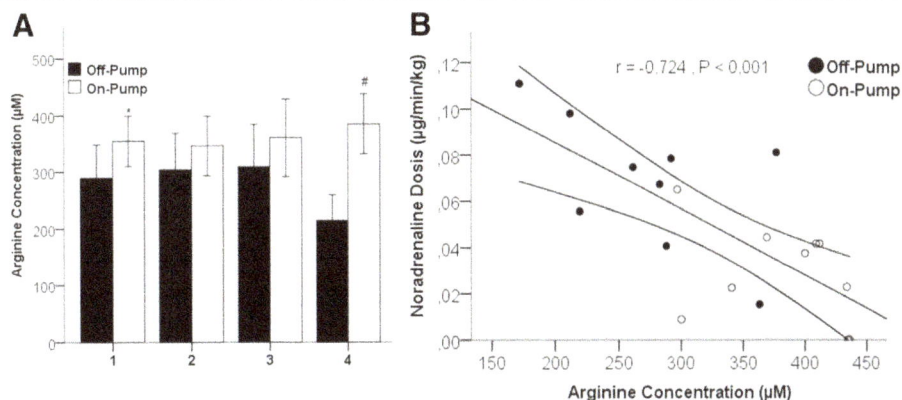

Fig. 4 a Comparison of mean arterial arginine concentration measured at the beginning of the operation (1), after the first (2), second (3) and third (4) distal anastomosis in the On-Pump (*white*) and Off-Pump (*black*) group.* $p < 0.001$ and # $p < 0.05$. Data are presented as mean ± SEM. **b** Pearson correlation between postoperative noradrenaline doses and arterial arginine concentration measured at the time of the last distal anastomosis in the On-Pump (o) and Off-Pump (•) group including regression line and 95% confidence interval

only minor changes to the metabolomic profile of patients undergoing bypass surgery and that acylcarnitines are elevated in both Off-Pump and On-Pump cases, but chain lengths differ. Furthermore, we demonstrate that there appears to be a correlation between arterial arginine concentration and vasopressor need after bypass surgery.

Acknowledgements

The authors wish to thank Benjamin Gloy for editorial assistance.

Funding

The study was supported by grants from the DFG to TD (Do602/9-1) and from the German Center for Sepsis Control and Care (CSCC) and the Federal Ministry of Education and Research (BMBF) (grant number: 01 E0 1002).

Authors' contributions

HK created with TD the study design, application for approval from the ethic committee, organized the work processes and logistics, enrolled all the patients included in the study; provided written informed consent to all patients, controlled all steps in the study process; analyzed the results and wrote the manuscript with the help of TD. MS helped in analyzing the study results. SN performed the laboratory measurements of the metabolites, did the statistic work, proofreading and correction of the manuscript. GF and MD performed the operative procedures. TD gave the idea, provided financial support, took part in creating the study design, analyzed the study results, took part in writing and correcting the manuscript and provided active support through all parts of the study process. All authors read and approved the final manuscript.

Competing interest

The authors declare that they have no competing interests.

Author details

[1]Department of Cardiothoracic Surgery, Friedrich Schiller University Jena, University Hospital, Am Klinikum 1, 07747 Jena, Germany. [2]Department of Cardiothoracic Surgery, Cairo University, Cairo, Egypt. [3]Department of Clinical Chemistry and Laboratory Medicine, Friedrich-Schiller-University Jena, University Hospital, Jena, Germany. [4]Integrated Research and Treatment Center, Center for Sepsis Control and Care (CSCC), Jena, Germany.

References

1. Shah AA, Craig DM, Sebek JK, Haynes C, Stevens RC, Muehlbauer MJ, Granger CB, Hauser ER, Newby LK, Newgard CB, et al. Metabolic profiles predict adverse events after coronary artery bypass grafting. J Thorac Cardiovasc Surg. 2012;143(4):873–8.
2. Ahmad T, Kelly JP, McGarrah RW, Hellkamp AS, Fiuzat M, Testani JM, Wang TS, Verma A, Samsky MD, Donahue MP, et al. Prognostic implications of long-chain acylcarnitines in heart failure and reversibility with mechanical circulatory support. J Am Coll Cardiol. 2016;67(3):291–9.
3. Murphy GJ, Angelini GD. Side effects of cardiopulmonary bypass: what is the reality? J Card Surg. 2004;19(6):481–8.
4. Polomsky M, Puskas JD. Off-pump coronary artery bypass grafting–the current state. Circ J. 2012;76(4):784–90.
5. Lazar HL. Should off-pump coronary artery bypass grafting be abandoned? Circulation. 2013;128(4):406–13.
6. Doenst T, Struning C, Moschovas A, Gonzalez-Lopez D, Essa Y, Kirov H, Diab M, Faerber G. Cardiac surgery 2015 reviewed. Clin Res Cardiol. 2016;105:801–14.
7. Xia JG, Sinelnikov IV, Han B, Wishart DS. MetaboAnalyst 3.0-making metabolomics more meaningful. Nucleic Acids Res. 2015;43(W1):W251–7.
8. Xia JG, Psychogios N, Young N, Wishart DS. MetaboAnalyst: a web server for metabolomic data analysis and interpretation. Nucleic Acids Res. 2009;37: W652–60.
9. Levy JH, Tanaka KA. Inflammatory response to cardiopulmonary bypass. Ann Thorac Surg. 2003;75(2):S715–20.
10. Kraft F, Schmidt C, Van Aken H, Zarbock A. Inflammatory response and extracorporeal circulation. Best Pract Res Clin Anaesthesiol. 2015;29(2):113–23.
11. Day JR, Taylor KM. The systemic inflammatory response syndrome and cardiopulmonary bypass. Int J Surg. 2005;3(2):129–40.
12. Natoli G, Ghisletti S, Barozzi I. The genomic landscapes of inflammation. Genes Dev. 2011;25(2):101–6.
13. Ruel M, Bianchi C, Khan TA, Xu S, Liddicoat JR, Voisine P, Araujo E, Lyon H, Kohane IS, Libermann TA, et al. Gene expression profile after cardiopulmonary bypass and cardioplegic arrest. J Thorac Cardiovasc Surg. 2003;126(5):1521–30.
14. Khan HA, Alhomida AS, Al Madani H, Sobki SH. Carnitine and acylcarnitine profiles in dried blood spots of patients with acute myocardial infarction. Metabolomics. 2013;9(4):828–38.
15. Wijnands KAP, Castermans TMR, Hommen MPJ, Meesters DM, Poeze M. Arginine and citrulline and the immune response in sepsis. Nutrients. 2015; 7(3):1426–63.
16. Yeramian A, Martin L, Arpa L, Bertran J, Soler C, McLeod C, Modolell M, Palacin M, Lloberas J, Celada A. Macrophages require distinct arginine catabolism and transport systems for proliferation and for activation. Eur J Immunol. 2006;36(6):1516–26.
17. MacMicking J, Xie QW, Nathan C. Nitric oxide and macrophage function. Annu Rev Immunol. 1997;15:323–50.
18. Cunha FQ, Moncada S, Liew FY. Interleukin-10 (IL-10) inhibits the induction of nitric oxide synthase by interferon-gamma in murine macrophages. Biochem Biophys Res Commun. 1992;182(3):1155–9.
19. Huang CJ, Stevens BR, Nielsen RB, Slovin PN, Fang X, Nelson DR, Skimming JW. Interleukin-10 inhibition of nitric oxide biosynthesis involves suppression of CAT-2 transcription. Nitric oxide. 2002;6(1):79–84.
20. Tomic V, Russwurm S, Moller E, Claus RA, Blaess M, Brunkhorst F, Bruegel M, Bode K, Bloos F, Wippermann J, et al. Transcriptomic and proteomic patterns of systemic inflammation in on-pump and off-pump coronary artery bypass grafting. Circulation. 2005;112(19):2912–20.
21. Dybdahl B, Wahba A, Haaverstad R, Kirkeby-Garstad I, Kierulf P, Espevik T, Sundan A. On-pump versus off-pump coronary artery bypass grafting: more heat-shock protein 70 is released after on-pump surgery. Eur J Cardiothorac Surg. 2004;25(6):985–92.
22. Czerny M, Baumer H, Kilo J, Lassnigg A, Hamwi A, Vikovich T, Wolner E, Grimm M. Inflammatory response and myocardial injury following coronary artery bypass grafting with or without cardiopulmonary bypass. Eur J Cardiothorac Surg. 2000;17(6):737–42.

6

Seven years of use of implantable cardioverter-defibrillator therapies: a nationwide population-based assessment of their effectiveness in real clinical settings

Arn Migowski[1*], Antonio Luiz Ribeiro[2], Marilia Sá Carvalho[3], Vitor Manuel Pereira Azevedo[1], Rogério Brant Martins Chaves[1], Lucas de Aquino Hashimoto[4], Carolina de Aquino Xavier[4] and Regina Maria de Aquino Xavier[1]

Abstract

Background: The efficacy of implantable cardioverter-defibrillator (ICD) and cardiac resynchronization therapy-defibrillator (CRT-D) therapy has already been established in clinical trials but their effectiveness in several clinical settings remains undetermined. This study aimed to assess the effectiveness of ICD and CRT-D therapies within the Brazilian National Health System (SUS).

Methods: All patients who underwent ICD or CRT-D implantation within the SUS from 2001 to 2007 were included in the study. We compared estimated Kaplan-Meier survival curves using the Peto's test. Prognostic factors were selected using Cox's models.

Results: There were included 3,295 patients in the ICD group and 681 patients in the CRT-D group. Cardiac causes accounted for 79% of all deaths in both groups and Chagas' heart disease accounted for 31% of these deaths. In the CRT-D group, survival significantly decreased around the fourth year of follow-up, with a decrease from 59.5% to 38.3% in 5.5 months. Transvenous implantation technique was used in 62% of CRT-D patients. In-hospital case-fatality rates were higher in those undergoing surgical implantation (5.3%) than those undergoing transvenous implantation (1.6%) (p = 0.02).

Conclusions: The results show that short-term, medium-term and long-term effectiveness of ICD therapy appears to be similar to that evidenced in clinical trials. In the CRT-D group, in-hospital case-fatality and 30-day case-fatality were higher than those reported in other studies. Surgical epicardial implantation technique was performed in this group at a higher frequency than that reported in the literature and was associated with poorer short-term prognosis.

Keywords: Implantable defibrillators, Cardiac resynchronization therapy devices, Chagas cardiomyopathy, Survival analysis, Medical record linkage, Brazil, Database, Technology assessment, Hospital mortality, High-cost technology

---

* Correspondence: arnmigowski@yahoo.com.br
[1]Instituto Nacional de Cardiologia - INC (National Institute of Cardiology, Ministry of Health), Coordenação de Ensino e Pesquisa, Divisão de Saúde Coletiva, rua das Laranjeiras 374, Laranjeiras, Rio de Janeiro, RJ, Brazil
Full list of author information is available at the end of the article

Background

The efficacy of implantable cardioverter-defibrillator (ICD) therapy for primary and secondary prevention of sudden cardiac death has been established in several clinical scenarios in patients with both ischemic and nonischemic heart disease [1]. The efficacy of cardiac resynchronization therapy combined with ICD (cardiac resynchronization therapy-defibrillator, CRT-D) in reducing overall mortality has also been shown in some clinical settings compared with optimal pharmacological therapy [2], ICD alone [3] or even with the CRT-alone [4].

However, clinical trials do not assess the effectiveness of these therapies under real life conditions of use where patient follow-up is a common problem [5]. Other common issues include inappropriate indications, suboptimal adherence to guidelines and off-label uses [6], more heterogeneous patient populations, and potential provider- or device-related technical shortcomings. Furthermore, evidence showing long-term effectiveness of these therapies is scarce [7] and some controversial issues have not been properly addressed in clinical trials, including indications of dual-chamber ICD [8], use of ICD and CRT-D in children and adolescents [9] and in patients with Chagas' heart disease [10].

In the light of these issues and scarcity of population-based data on ICD implantation [11] particularly lack of national registries—administrative databases have increasingly gained importance as a source of information complementary to data obtained from clinical trials and specific records [12].

Therefore, probabilistic record linkage techniques have been used in cardiology research to analyze population data from routine hospital administrative databases and nationwide death records [13]. These national databases are essential sources of information in countries with great population heterogeneity and a wide range of patterns of therapy utilization.

The present study aimed to assess short-term, medium-term and long-term survival of ICD and CRT-D therapies within the Brazilian National Health System (SUS) using record linkage between two national databases.

Methods

Study population and data sources

Two national databases were used as data sources for the study: the Brazilian Mortality Database (known by its Portuguese acronym SIM) and the Brazilian Hospital Information Database (known by its Portuguese acronym SIH). SIM was created in 1975 and covers the entire population nationwide. Mortality data is considered reliable from the qualitative point of view, as accurate as that of other countries with a long tradition in these statistics [14]. SIH was created in 1981 and covers the entire Brazilian National Health System (SUS), which provides universal health coverage for over 200 million people, with 75% of them covered exclusively by it. The accuracy of the SIH variables related to the diagnosis, medical procedures, sex, age-group and in-hospital outcomes are considered satisfactory [15].

Our study cohort consisted of all patients admitted to SUS hospitals (either public or SUS-affiliated private) undergoing transvenous ICD or CRT-D implantation from 2001 to 2007. The main clinical indications (Class I) for ICD implantation within SUS during the study period following the Brazilian Ministry of Health guidelines included: cardiac arrest due to ventricular tachycardia or ventricular fibrillation from irreversible causes in patients with EF ≤35%; spontaneous sustained ventricular tachycardia from irreversible causes in patients with EF ≤35%; non-sustained ventricular tachycardia with previous acute myocardial infarction, left ventricular dysfunction (EF ≤40%) and sustained ventricular tachycardia or ventricular fibrillation inducible at programmed ventricular stimulation. CRT-D therapy was primarily indicated for patients meeting one of the above criteria for ICD implantation and QRS duration equal to or greater than 130 ms, functional class III or IV (The New York Heart Association [NYHA] Functional Classification) and left ventricle end-diastolic diameter equal to or greater than 55 mm and EF ≤0.30.

A probabilistic record linkage technique was used to find death records for each patient in the national SIM database during the study period. We chose to apply the probabilistic record linkage as there is no unique identifier between SIM and SIH databases. The linkage method applied showed 90.6% sensitivity and 100% specificity [16].

Data analysis

We performed an overall survival and cardiac survival analysis considering only deaths from any underlying cardiac cause (including Chagas' heart disease and congenital heart disease), procedure-related complications or other causes potentially related to sudden cardiac death according to the following codes: T821; I00-I528; B570-B572; Q200-Q249; R570; R960, and R98 (International Statistical Classification of Diseases and Related Health Problems, 10th Revision).

Patients who did not die by the end of the study period (12/31/2007) were censored. No patient was lost to follow-up during the study period assuming universal coverage of SIM nationwide and no deaths occurring abroad. As for cardiac survival rates, patients whose underlying cause of death was not defined as of cardiac origin were also censored and were included in the analysis on the date of death or on the last date of observation. The start time of observation for each individual (T_0) was the date of hospitalization for the implantation procedure. If a patient underwent more than one ICD or CRT-D implantation, only the first procedure was analyzed. Generator replacement and/or lead revision procedures or any other procedures not related to device implantation were disregarded.

Due to differences in clinical eligibility criteria, patients were divided into two therapy groups for the analysis: ICD alone and CRT-D. Survival curves were estimated using the Kaplan-Meier method and compared using Peto's test at a significance level of $p < 0.05$. The variables selected in the univariate Cox proportional hazards regression models—adjusted for age in years—were included in the multivariate models to estimate the independent effect of the variables. The following variables were studied in the models in both groups: age; gender; hospital category; year of device implantation; and hospital location (state). We analyzed type of device (dual- or single-chamber) in the ICD-alone group and implantation technique (transvenous or mini-thoracotomy) in the CRT-D group. Separate models were constructed for overall and cardiac survival analysis stratified by therapy group (ICD alone or CRT-D). We estimated hazard ratios (HR) and their related 95% confidence intervals. Schoenfeld residuals were used to test the proportional hazards assumption of Cox models.

In Brazil, hospital admissions authorization (AIH) forms include a field for the principal diagnosis of current admission and a second one for secondary diagnosis. In the ICD-alone group, 91.83% of admission forms included the arrhythmia code as principal diagnosis but did not provide any information on the underlying disease. In the CRT-D group, a greater proportion of patient forms (33.3%) included information on the underlying disease at admission. Since there was no information on the underlying disease for many patients, we thus chose not to include this variable in the Cox models. We therefore included a new variable for underlying cardiac disease using all the disease codes from the two AIH fields and the five SIM fields, including the "contributing cause", which may also display several codes for diseases not directly associated with the death. As a result, we were able to determine underlying disease for another 581 patients.

In-hospital case fatality was estimated based on deaths occurring during the admission when the first ICD or CRT-D implantation was performed. We calculated mean length of stay of these admissions.

For the comparison of means, we performed Student's t-test for variables with normal distribution or otherwise the Mann-Whitney U-test. For the comparison of proportions, we used the chi-squared test. The statistical significance was set at $p < 0.05$. Data analyses were performed using the R Statistical Package, version 2.6.2.

This study was approved by the research ethics committee (name: Comitê de Ética em Pesquisa COEP-UFMG, protocol number 0084.0.203.000-09) and followed the principles of the Declaration of Helsinki. The ethics committee waived the requirement for written informed consent due to the study's design.

Results

The ICD group comprised 3,295 patients from 85 hospitals with a mean observation time of about 2.5 years, maximum follow-up time of approximately 7 years and 799 deaths were observed. CRT-D therapy became available to SUS patients in 2002, and 681 patients from 50 hospitals had received the device by 2007. The mean follow-up time in the CRT-D group was 16 months, maximum follow-up time was slightly over 5 years and 197 deaths were observed.

Single-chamber ICDs were more often implanted (64%) than dual-chamber devices. Dual-chamber devices became available to SUS patients in 2004 and accounted for 65% of all devices implanted in the ICD-alone group during 2005–2007. In general, the variables studied were similar in patients receiving single-chamber ICDs, dual-chamber ICDs and CRT-D (Table 1). The mean age was lower in the ICD-alone than CRT-D group (58 vs. 61 years, $p < 0.001$). The CRT-D group had a higher proportion of elderly (70 years or older) ($p < 0.01$) and lower proportion of patients aged 10 to 49 years ($p < 0.001$) when compared to the ICD-alone group. A comparison of device implant between Brazilian states showed that most procedures—especially CRT-D—were performed in care facilities in São Paulo, which is the richest and most industrialized state in Brazil. We found a lower proportion of supraventricular tachycardia among patients receiving dual-chamber compared to single-chamber ICDs ($p < 0.001$).

Among patients with information about underlying disease, in the ICD-alone group (n = 760), 36% were diagnosed with Chagas' heart disease and 25.1% with ischemic heart disease (Table 2). In the CRT-D group (n = 310), 12.3% were diagnosed with Chagas' heart disease (Table 2). The underlying cardiac diseases by age groups were described in Table 3. Cardiac causes accounted for 79% of deaths in both groups (Table 4), and Chagas' heart disease accounted for 33% and 23% of cardiac deaths in the ICD-alone and CRT-D groups, respectively ($p < 0.05$). Of all deaths, there were only six unattended deaths in the ICD-alone group and one in the CRT-D group.

The mean length of hospital stay for device implantation was shorter in ICD-alone compared to CRT-D patients (5.8 vs. 7.7 days, $p < 0.001$). The in-hospital case fatality was 0.3% in the ICD group and 2.9% in the CRT-D group ($p < 0.001$). The in-hospital case fatality of CRT-D patients over 70 was 8.5%. Overall short-term, medium-term and long-term survival and short-, medium- and long-term cardiac survival (30 days, 1 year and 5 years, respectively) are presented in Figures 1 and 2, stratified by type of therapy. The differences found in survival times of

Table 1 Baseline patient characteristics stratified by type of ICD

Characteristics		Type of ICD					
		Single-chamber ICD (n = 2,109)		Dual-chamber ICD (n = 1,186)		CRT-D (n = 681)	
Age (years), mean (SD)		56	(±14)	57	(±14)	60	(±12)
Age group, n (%)							
	<10 years	6	(0.3)	3	(0.3)	2	(0.3)
	10 to 49 years	580	(27.5)	321	(27.1)	127	(18.7)
	50 to 59 years	580	(27.5)	310	(26.1)	189	(27.8)
	60 to 69 years	587	(27.8)	362	(30.5)	219	(32.2)
	70 years or more	356	(16.9)	190	(16.0)	143	(21.0)
Sex, n (%)							
	Female	626	(29.7)	365	(30.8)	176	(25.8)
	Male	1482	(70.3)	821	(69.2)	505	(74.2)
Arrhythmia, n (%)							
	Ventricular Flutter or Fibrillation	407	(19.3)	356	(30.0)	13	(1.9)
	Ventricular Tachycardia	914	(43.3)	618	(52.1)	242	(35.5)
	Supraventricular Tachycardia	514	(24.4)	101	(8.5)	2	(0.3)
Hospital location (state), n (%)							
	São Paulo	1069	(50.7)	703	(59.3)	486	(71.4)
	Other	1040	(49.3)	483	(40.7)	195	(28.6)
Category of hospital, n (%)							
	Charity Hospital	814	(38.6)	587	(49.5)	377	(55.4)
	Private Hospital (non-philanthropic)	245	(11.6)	175	(14.8)	38	(5.6)
	Public Hospital	1050	(49.8)	424	(35.8)	266	(39.1)
Implant technique – mini-thoracotomy, n (%)		0		0		227	(38.0)

the ICD and CRT-D groups were statistically significant for all periods studied, for both overall and cardiac survival (Figures 1 and 2). Patients in the CRT-D group showed poorer prognosis (Figure 1). A marked drop in survival was evident in the CRT-D group around the fourth year of observation (Figure 1), with a decrease in survival rates from 59.5% (95% CI 54.3–65.3) to 38.3% (95% CI 27.7–52.9) in only 5.5 months.

The analysis of overall survival of ICD patients showed that age was associated with the outcome (HR 1.03, 95%

Table 2 Underlying cardiac disease by type of ICD

Underlying cardiac disease, n (%)	Type of ICD			
	ICD		CRT-D	
Cardiomyopathy	172	(22.6)	202	(65.2)
Chagas' heart disease	274	(36.1)	38	(12.3)
Congenital heart disease	45	(5.9)	0	(0.0)
Ischemic heart disease	191	(25.1)	61	(19.7)
Other causes (myocarditis, valvular heart disease, hypertensive heart disease)	78	(10.26)	9	(2.9)
Total	760	(100)	310	(100)

CI 1.03–1.04), with 3% increase in the risk of death per year. This association remained in the multivariate models for both overall and cardiac survival. There were no deaths in children in our study. In the ICD group, the 1-year survival was 93.8% (95% CI 92.2–95.5) in patients aged 10 to 49 years and 81.6% (95% CI 78.3–85.1) in those 70 years or more. No other variables studied were significantly associated with the outcome in either group.

Figure 3 shows survival curves with underlying disease information drawn from the AIH for the ICD-alone group. This Figure does not include the information on underlying disease drawn from the mortality database, because – as we used specific data on patients who died – survival would be artificially low. Kaplan-Meier survival estimates were not significantly different (Peto's test, p = 0.84) between the two groups (with and without underlying disease at SIH), suggesting random loss of these information. The cardiac survival curves were very similar to these overall survival curves, showing the same pattern.

In the CRT-D group, it was used a transvenous endocardial technique in 62% patients, epicardial in 28% and

Table 3 Underlying cardiac disease by age group

Underlying cardiac disease, n (%)	Age group, n (%)															
	<10 years		10 to 19		20 to 29		30 to 39		40 to 49		50 to 59		60 to 69		70 years or more	
Cardiomyopathy	1	(100)	6	(42.9)	12	(44.4)	22	(44.0)	50	(42.0)	93	(32.4)	111	(33.0)	78	(33.2)
Chagas' heart disease	0	(0.0)	0	(0.0)	4	(14.8)	18	(36.0)	44	(37.0)	96	(33.4)	100	(29.8)	50	(21.3)
Congenital heart disease	0	(0.0)	4	(28.6)	4	(14.8)	0	(0.0)	8	(6.7)	6	(2.1)	13	(3.9)	10	(4.3)
Ischemic heart disease	0	(0.0)	2	(14.3)	4	(14.8)	6	(12.0)	10	(8.4)	65	(22.6)	89	(26.5)	76	(32.3)
Other causes (myocarditis, valvular heart disease, hypertensive heart disease)	0	(0.0)	2	(14.3)	3	(11.1)	4	(8.0)	7	(5.9)	27	(9.4)	23	(6.8)	21	(8.9)
Total	1	(100)	14	(100)	27	(100)	50	(100)	119	(100)	287	(100)	336	(100)	235	(100)

endocardial requiring thoracotomy due to implant failure in 10%. The in-hospital case fatality was 5.3% among those undergoing epicardial lead placement, which is higher than 1.6% found among those undergoing transvenous implantation (p <0.05) considering that both groups had a similar median length of hospital stay (4 days). Those requiring thoracotomy due to implant failure accounted for 25.1% of all patients undergoing epicardial technique and 16.7% of deaths in this group. There were no significant differences in the medium-term and long-term prognosis according to implantation technique (Figure 4).

Discussion

To the best of our knowledge, this is the first study to analyze survival in all patients undergoing ICD and CRT-D implantation within a National Health System. This design allowed to avoiding selection bias and increasing the generalizability of effectiveness results.

Overall 1-year, 2-year and 3-year survival rates in the ICD-alone group were similar to those reported in the AVID study (89.3%, 81.6% and 75.4%, respectively) [17]. In addition, the rate of cardiac deaths was similar to that reported in the same study [18]. One-year, 2-year, 3-year, 4-year, and 5-year survival rates in the CRT-D and ICD

Table 4 Causes of death by type of ICD

Underlying cause of death	Type of ICD		
	Single-chamber ICD	Dual-chamber ICD	CRT-D
	(n = 2,109)	(n = 1,186)	(n = 681)
Chagas' heart disease	167 (26.0%)	42 (26.8%)	36 (18.3%)
Cardiac diseases (other)	340 (53.0%)	82 (52.2%)	119 (60.4%)
Noncardiac vascular diseases	17 (2.6%)	5 (3.2%)	8 (4.1%)
Cancer	16 (2.5%)	2 (1.3%)	4 (2.0%)
Infection	12 (1.9%)	2 (1.3%)	0 (0.0%)
Other	90 (14.0%)	24 (15.3%)	30 (15.2%)
Total	642 (100%)	157 (100%)	197 (100%)

groups were similar to those described in a large case series in the US [7]. The overall 5-year survival in our study was similar to that reported in the RAFT Trial (65.4%) among ICD patients, but considerably lower than that reported in CRT-D patients [19]. This difference in long-term prognosis may be explained by the inclusion of patients with NYHA functional class II or III in this study. The one-year survival in the CRT-D group was lower than the 88% described in the COMPANION trial, even when the group undergoing transvenous implant was considered individually [2].

The 5-year survival found among ICD patients in our study was very similar to that observed in a study of patients with Chagas' heart disease [10]. Although Chagas disease was the underlying cause in one-third of all patients who eventually died, we cannot infer that these patients had a poorer prognosis. Our survival curves by underlying disease suggests that etiology of heart disease (Chagas vs. ischemic heart disease) was not a prognostic factor. The ICD-LABOR study that also included patients with Chagas' heart disease found similar results [20]. Barbosa et al. suggested that Chagas' heart disease patients are more likely to have ventricular arrhythmias than patients with other cardiopathies, but on the other hand, they have higher rates of appropriate ICD therapy [21].

The in-hospital case fatality of 0.33% observed in the ICD group in our study was only slightly higher than the 0.2% reported in a systematic review of nonthoracotomy ICD trials [22] but considerably lower than that reported in other clinical data analyses [12,23,24]. Nevertheless, the 1.1% 30-day case fatality observed was identical to that reported in the AVID trial, but higher than the 0.6% found in a systematic review of nonthoracotomy ICD trials by Rees et al. [22]. The mean length of hospital stay among ICD patients was shorter than that reported in a large study of administrative databases in the US [12].

The in-hospital case fatality of 2.9% seen in the CRT-D group was higher than the 0.5% case fatality reported in a systematic review [25], 0.9% reported by Swindle et al. [23] and 1.1% reported in Medicare patients [24]. The COMPANION and MADIT-CRT trials also found much

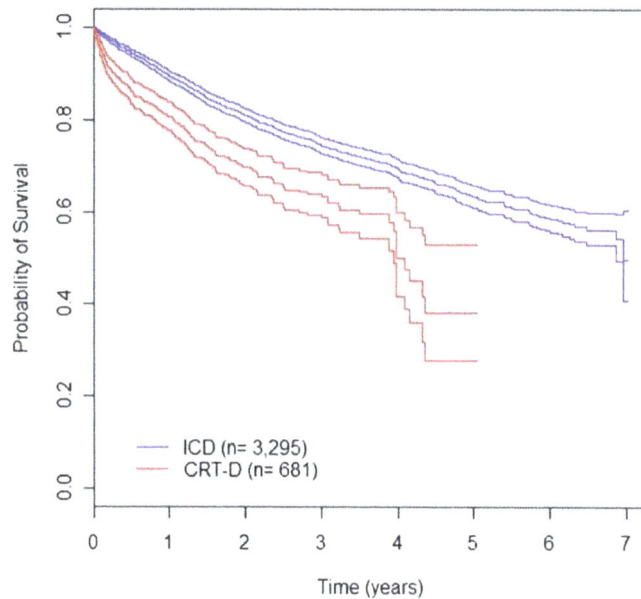

Figure 1 Overall survival by therapy (ICD-alone or CRT-D). Kaplan-Meier survival estimates were significantly different between the two groups (95% CI).

		30 days	1 year	2 years	3 years	4 years	5 years	6 years	7 years
ICD	Survival (%)	98.9	89.5	81.1	74.5	69.6	63.4	58.6	49.7
	95% CI	98.6–99.3	88.4–90.6	79.6–82.6	72.8–76.3	67.6–71.6	61.0–65.9	55.7–61.6	40.9–60.4
CRT-D	Survival (%)	95.4	80.9	69.7	63.3	50.0	38.3	–	–
	95% CI	93.9–97.0	77.8–84.0	65.8–73.9	58.8–68.2	41.8–59.8	27.7–52.9		

lower in-hospital case fatality (0.6% and 0.1%, respectively) than that found in the present study; however, both studies excluded patients with implantation with thoracotomy and the MADIT-CRT trial included only patients with NYHA Class I and II [22]. Even the in-hospital case fatality in the CRT-D sub-group undergoing transvenous implantation (1.6%) was higher than those reported in these studies. The 8.5% in-hospital case fatality in CRT-D patients older than 70 was much higher than that reported by Swindle et al. in elderly patients [23]. The 30-day mortality in those undergoing transvenous CRT-D implantation in our study (4.1%) was higher than the 1.8% observed in the COMPANION trial [2]. Even among younger patients, the mean length of stay in the CRT-D group was higher within SUS than that reported in Zhan et al. study [12]. The median length of hospital stay in our study was the same regardless of the implant technique.

Our study did not find any deaths in children undergoing ICD implantation. Other study corroborate the good prognosis in this age group [9]. Differences in survival times between ICD-alone or CRT-D patients were expected because the indication criteria for CRT-D implant included poor functional status (NYHA Class III or IV) and ventricular dyssynchrony.

The decrease in survival among CRT-D patients around the fourth year of follow-up may suggest the impact of the disease natural history or device-related problems. A study by Cleland and colleagues with patients with heart failure and dyssynchrony found among those treated with medical therapy alone a pattern of decline in survival mainly due to sudden death that is similar to that observed in our study [26]. However, this pattern of survival was not observed in Saxon and colleagues study that also assessed long-term outcomes [7]. One explanation for this pattern would be the effect of a factor affecting the long-term effectiveness of CRT-D therapy and its impact in the disease natural history. Horlbeck and colleagues showed that mean lifetime of CRT-D devices was 4 years [27]. Likewise, Biffi and colleagues demonstrated that median lifetime of CRT-D devices was approximately 4 years [28]. Thijssen and colleagues reported that mean battery lifetime of CRT-D devices was 4.7 years [29]. In an earlier study by Hauser and colleagues (1998–2005) only 4% of CRT-D pulse generators were operating normally within

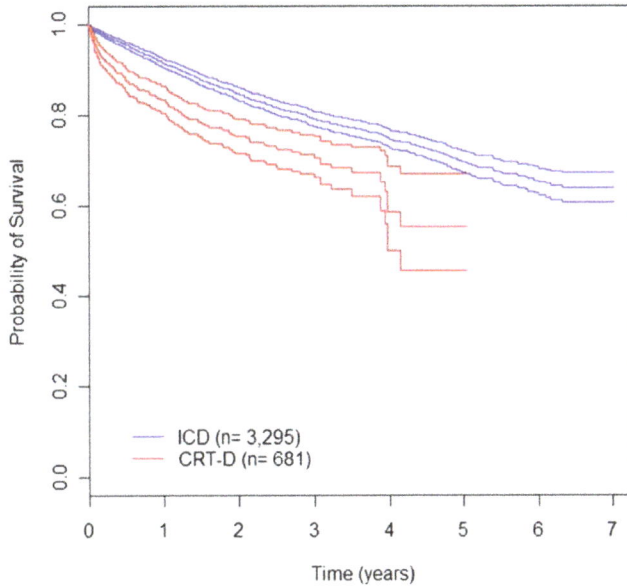

		30 days	1 year	2 years	3 years	4 years	5 years	6 years	7 years
ICD	Survival (%)	99.1	91.5	84.7	79.2	75.0	69.7	65.3	63.9
	95% CI	98.7–99.4	90.5–92.5	83.4–86.1	77.5–80.9	73.1–77.0	67.4–72.1	62.4–68.3	60.6–67.3
CRT-D	Survival (%)	95.7	83.4	75.4	70.7	58.5	55.4	–	–
	95% CI	94.2–97.3	80.5–86.4	71.7–79.3	66.3–75.3	49.9–68.6	45.8–67.1		

Figure 2 Cardiac survival by therapy (ICD-alone or CRT-D). Kaplan-Meier survival estimates were significantly different between the two groups (95% CI).

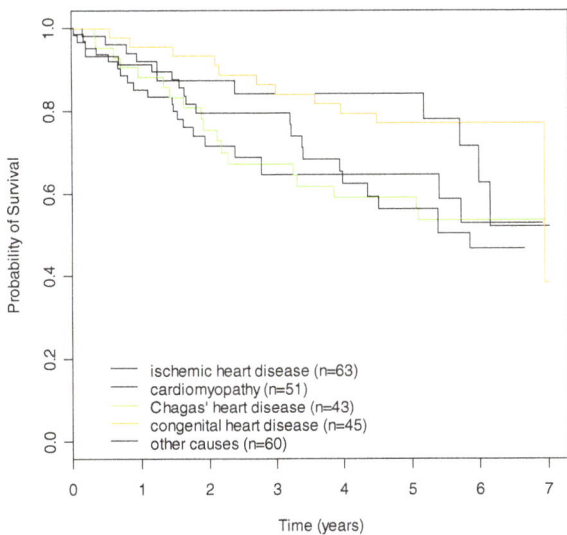

Figure 3 Overall survival by underlying cardiac disease (ICD-alone group). Kaplan-Meier survival estimates were not significantly different between groups (Peto's test p = 0.05). These survival curves with underlying disease information drawn only from the hospital admission (AIH) forms.

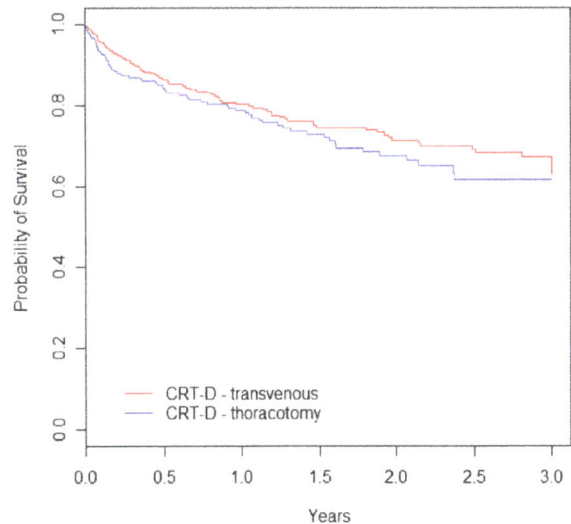

Figure 4 Overall survival by implant technique. Kaplan-Meier survival estimates were not significantly different between the two groups (Peto's test p = 0.263). The group we denominated 'thoracotomy' comprises two subgroups with survival curves overlaid: patients with surgically-implanted left ventricle leads as the first approach and patients with transvenous implantation failure, who were subsequently converted to thoracotomy.

four years of the implant [30]. A recent study by Landolina and colleagues reported that at three years slightly more than 10% of patients underwent surgical revision for battery depletion and at four years this rate rose to about 50% [31]. This same study showed that patients undergoing replacement had double the risk of infection, which could also explain the mortality observed in our study. Only ongoing monitoring can establish whether this finding was exclusive to the initial cohort of patients undergoing CRT-D implantation (long follow-up) and to what extent it was impacted by the small number of patients at-risk in the fourth year of follow-up.

Dual-chamber devices accounted for 65% of all ICD implants In the last three years studied, a percentage that is similar to that reported in the US National ICD Registry (62% from 2006 to 2007) [8]. In this study only 40.4% of patients implanted with dual-chamber ICD devices met the indications for pacemaker therapy and the use of dual-chamber ICD devices was associated with increased in-hospital complications and in-hospital case fatality rates [8]. In our study we found no differences in in-hospital case fatality and short-term, medium-term and long-term survival rates among those implanted with single- and dual-chamber devices. Those undergoing dual-chamber ICD implantation were less likely to have supraventricular tachycardia, which contrasts with that reported by Dewland and colleagues [8], suggesting that this is not a common indication for atrial lead placement in Brazilian patients.

The present study showed that the proportion of CRT-D with surgically implanted left ventricle leads as first approach (28%) seems slightly greater than that reported in other studies (24.1% to 24.9%) [32,33]. The percentage of transvenous implantation failure in our study (13.7%) was also higher than that reported in other studies with CRT-D (5.9% to 11%) [32-34]. In patients undergoing CRT-D implantation, epicardial lead placement was found associated with increased in-hospital case fatality, as suggested in other studies with CRT [35] and CRT-D [32]. Despite increased in-hospital case fatality and 30-day case-fatality, we found similar medium-term and long-term survival rates for both implantation techniques suggesting similar effectiveness of these techniques in patients surviving the initial post-implantation period, which corroborates that reported by Miller and colleagues [35] with CRT. However, conflicting results have been reported. One study showed poorer short-term and long-term prognosis with the epicardial technique [32] while other studies found no significant differences in short-term or long-term results [33,36]. The results found in our study regarding the epicardial technique may be explained by the "learning curve" of surgical teams, quality of postoperative care and potentially suboptimal drug therapy prescribed to patients with advanced heart failure referred to surgery [37].

Our study has some limitations common to studies relying on administrative databases. The lack of information on patient variables such as NYHA functional class, left ventricle ejection fraction, and history of sudden cardiac death does not allow proper adjustment for the patients' baseline risk. The proportion of underlying diseases may not reflect their actual distribution in the study population due to missing information on this variable in SIH database. Information on the underlying condition is often missing in hospital admission authorization forms because providers are required to fill out two different diagnosis fields including diagnostic codes to support the patient's eligibility for device implantation (e.g., type of arrhythmia and heart failure). The sensitivity of the probabilistic record linkage method used to find deaths registries (90.6%) may have potentially missed some death records in the database. However, there was 100% specificity in identifying deaths records and probably random loss [16].

Conclusion

Our study showed that the medium-term and long-term effectiveness of ICD therapy in Brazil appears to be similar to the efficacy found in clinical trials. However, there is an apparent slight excess of deaths within the first 30 days of implantation. Younger age at the time of implantation was a predictor of better prognosis in the ICD-alone group. In the CRT-D group, in-hospital case fatality and 30-day case fatality were higher than those reported in other studies. There was a marked drop in survival around the fourth year after implantation, and further investigation is necessary to determine its causes. In addition, the epicardial implantation technique was more frequently used in the CRT-D group than that reported in the literature and was found to be associated with poorer short-term prognosis. The study results suggest there is still room for reducing the proportion of surgical procedures within SUS, and more importantly, actions should be taken to reduce mortality associated with surgical CRT-D implantation and transvenous implantation of both ICDs and CRT-Ds.

Abbreviations
ICD: Implantable cardioverter-defibrillator; CI: Confidence interval; CRT-D: Cardiac resynchronization therapy-defibrillator; EF: Ejection fraction; HR: Hazard ratio; NYHA: New York Heart Association; SIH: Brazilian Hospital Database; SIM: Brazilian National Mortality Database; SUS: Brazilian National Health System; AIH: Hospital admission authorization forms.

Competing interests
The authors declare that they have no competing interests.

Authors' contributions
AM undertook the literature review. AM; ALR, RBMC and RMAX contributed to the study conception and design. LAH, CAX, AM and RBMC performed data cleaning and record linkage of the different databases used in the analysis. AM and MSC performed statistical analysis. AM, ALR, MSC, VMPA and RMAX drafted the manuscript. All authors read and approved the final manuscript.

Acknowledgments

This study received funding from Brazilian National Council for Scientific and Technological Development (Conselho Nacional de Desenvolvimento Científico e Tecnológico – CNPq) and from Ministry of Health (research call: MCT/CNPq/MS-SCTIE-DECIT n° 033/2007).

Author details

[1]Instituto Nacional de Cardiologia - INC (National Institute of Cardiology, Ministry of Health), Coordenação de Ensino e Pesquisa, Divisão de Saúde Coletiva, rua das Laranjeiras 374, Laranjeiras, Rio de Janeiro, RJ, Brazil. [2]University Hospital and School of Medicine, Federal University of Minas Gerais (UFMG), Minas Gerais, Brazil. [3]Oswaldo Cruz Foundation (FIOCRUZ), Rio de Janeiro, Brazil. [4]School of Medicine, Federal University of Rio de Janeiro (UFRJ), Rio de Janeiro, Brazil.

References

1. Theuns DA, Smith T, Hunink MG, Bardy GH, Jordaens L. Effectiveness of prophylactic implantation of cardioverter-defibrillators without cardiac resynchronization therapy in patients with ischaemic or non-ischaemic heart disease: a systematic review and meta-analysis. Europace. 2010;12(11):1564–70.
2. Bristow MR, Saxon LA, Boehmer J, Krueger S, Kass DA, De Marco T, et al. Cardiac-resynchronization therapy with or without an implantable defibrillator in advanced chronic heart failure. N Engl J Med. 2004;350:2140–50.
3. Bertoldi EG, Polanczyk CA, Cunha V, Ziegelmann PK, Beck-da-Silva L, Rohde LE. Mortality reduction of cardiac resynchronization and implantable cardioverter-defibrillator therapy in heart failure: an updated meta-analysis. Does recent evidence change the standard of care? J Card Fail. 2011;17(10):860–6.
4. Jiang M, He B, Zhang Q. Comparison of CRT and CRT-D in heart failure: systematic review of controlled trials. Int J Cardiol. 2012;158(1):39–45.
5. Al-Khatib SM, Mi X, Wilkoff BL, Qualls LG, Frazier-Mills C, Setoguchi S, et al. Follow-up of patients with new cardiovascular implantable electronic devices: are experts' recommendations implemented in routine clinical practice? Circ Arrhythm Electrophysiol. 2013;6(1):108–16.
6. Fein AS, Wang Y, Curtis JP, Masoudi FA, Varosy PD, Reynolds MR, et al. Prevalence and predictors of off-label use of cardiac resynchronization therapy in patients enrolled in the National Cardiovascular Data Registry Implantable Cardiac-Defibrillator Registry. J Am Coll Cardiol. 2010;56(10):766–73.
7. Saxon RA, Hayes DL, Gilliam FR, Heidenreich PA, Day J, Seth M, et al. Long-term outcome after ICD and CRT implantation and influence of remote device follow-up: the ALTITUDE survival study. Circulation. 2010;122(23):2359–67.
8. Dewland TA, Pellegrini CN, Wang Y, Marcus GM, Keung E, Varosy PD. Dual-chamber implantable cardioverter-defibrillator selection is associated with increased complication rates and mortality among patients enrolled in the NCDR implantable cardioverter-defibrillator registry. J Am Coll Cardiol. 2011;58(10):1007–13.
9. Burns KM, Evans F, Kaltman JR. Pediatric ICD utilization in the United States from 1997 to 2006. Heart Rhythm. 2011;8(1):23–8.
10. Martinelli M, de Siqueira SF, Sternick EB, Rassi Jr A, Costa R, Ramires JA, et al. Long-term follow-up of implantable cardioverter-defibrillator for secondary prevention in chagas' heart disease. Am J Cardiol. 2012;110(7):1040–5.
11. Lee DS, Birnie D, Cameron D, Crystal E, Dorian P, Gula LJ, et al. Population-Based Registry of Implantable Cardioverter Defibrillators. Design and implementation of a population-based registry of implantable cardioverter defibrillators (ICDs) in Ontario. Heart Rhythm. 2008;5(9):1250–6.
12. Zhan C, Baine WB, Sedrakyan A, Steiner C. Cardiac Device Implantation in the United States from 1997 through 2004: a Population-based Analysis. J Gen Intern Med. 2008;23 Suppl 1:13–9.
13. Smolina K, Wright FL, Rayner M, Goldacre MJ. Determinants of the decline in mortality from acute myocardial infarction in England between 2002 and 2010: linked national database study. BMJ. 2012;344:d8059.
14. Laurenti R, Mello Jorge MHP, Gotlieb SLD. Underlying cause-of-death mortality statistics: considering the reliability of data. Rev Panam Salud

Publica. 2008;23(5):349–56.
15. Escosteguy CC, Portela MC, Medronho RA, Vasconcellos MTL. The Brazilian Hospital Information System and the acute myocardial infarction hospital care. Rev Saude Publica. 2002;36(4):491–9.
16. Migowski A, Chaves RBM, Coeli CM, Ribeiro AL, Tura BR, Kuschnir MC, et al. Accuracy of probabilistic record linkage in the assessment of high-complexity cardiology procedures. Rev Saude Publica. 2011;45(2):269–75.
17. AVID Investigators. A comparison of antiarrhythmic-drug therapy with implantable defibrillators in patients resuscitated from near-fatal ventricular arrhythmias. N Engl J Med. 1997;337:1576–83.
18. AVID Investigators. Causes of death in the antiarrhythmic versus implantable defibrillators (AVID) trial. J Am Coll Cardiol. 1999;34:1552–9.
19. Tang ASL, Wells GA, Talajic M, Arnold MO, Sheldon R, Connolly S, et al. Cardiac-resynchronization therapy for mild-to-moderate heart failure. N Engl J Med. 2010;363:2385–95.
20. Dubner S, Valero E, Pesce R, Zuelgaray JG, Mateos JC, Filho SG, et al. A Latin American registry of implantable cardioverter defibrillators: the ICD-LABOR study. Ann Noninvasive Electrocardiol. 2005;10(4):420–8.
21. Barbosa MP, da Costa Rocha MO, de Oliveira AB, Lombardi F, Ribeiro AL. Efficacy and safety of implantable cardioverter-defibrillators in patients with Chagas disease. Europace. 2013;15(7):957–62.
22. van Rees JB, de Bie MK, Thijssen J, Borleffs CJ, Schalij MJ, van Erven L. Implantation-related complications of implantable cardioverter-defibrillators and cardiac resynchronization therapy devices: a systematic review of randomized clinical trials. J Am Coll Cardiol. 2011;58(10):995–1000.
23. Swindle JP, Rich MW, McCann P, Burroughs TE, Hauptman PJ. Implantable cardiac device procedures in older patients: use and in-hospital outcomes. Arch Intern Med. 2010;170(7):631–7.
24. Reynolds MR, Cohen DJ, Kugelmass AD, Brown PP, Becker ER, Culler SD, et al. The frequency and incremental cost of major complications among medicare beneficiaries receiving implantable cardioverter-defibrillators. J Am Coll Cardiol. 2006;47(12):2493–7.
25. McAlister FA, Ezekowitz J, Hooton N, Vandermeer B, Spooner C, Dryden DM, et al. Cardiac resynchronization therapy for patients with left ventricular systolic dysfunction: a systematic review. JAMA. 2007;297:2502.
26. Cleland JG, Daubert JC, Erdmann E, Freemantle N, Gras D, Kappenberger L, et al. Longer-term effects of cardiac resynchronization therapy on mortality in heart failure [the CArdiac REsynchronization-Heart Failure (CARE-HF) trial extension phase]. Eur Heart J. 2006;27(16):1928–32.
27. Horlbeck FW, Mellert F, Kreuz J, Nickenig G, Schwab JO. Real-world data on the lifespan of implantable cardioverter-defibrillators depending on manufacturers and the amount of ventricular pacing. J Cardiovasc Electrophysiol. 2012;23:1336–42.
28. Biffi M, Ziacchi M, Bertini M, Sangiorgi D, Corsini D, Martignani C, et al. Longevity of implantable cardioverter-defibrillators: implications for clinical practice and health care systems. Europace. 2008;10(11):1288–95.
29. Thijssen J, Borleffs CJ, van Rees JB, Man S, de Bie MK, Venlet J, et al. Implantable cardioverter-defibrillator longevity under clinical circumstances: an analysis according to device type, generation, and manufacturer. Heart Rhythm. 2012;9(4):513–9.
30. Hauser RG, Hayes DL, Epstein AE, Cannom DS, Vlay SC, Song SL, et al. Multicenter experience with failed and recalled implantable cardioverter-defibrillator pulse generators. Heart Rhythm. 2006;3(6):640–4.
31. Landolina M, Gasparini M, Lunati M, Iacopino S, Boriani G, Bonanno C, et al. Long-term complications related to biventricular defibrillator implantation: rate of surgical revisions and impact on survival: insights from the Italian Clinical Service Database. Circulation. 2011;123:2526–35.
32. Daoud EG, Kalbfleisch SJ, Hummel JD, Weiss R, Augustini RS, Duff SB, et al. Implantation techniques and chronic lead parameters of biventricular pacing dual-chamber defibrillators. J Cardiovasc Electrophysiol. 2002;13(10):964–70.
33. Pfau G, Schilling T, Kozian A, Lux A, Götte A, Huth C, et al. Outcome after implantation of cardiac resynchronization/defibrillation systems in patients with congestive heart failure and left bundle-branch block. J Cardiothorac Vasc Anesth. 2010;24(1):30–6.
34. Bisch L, Da Costa A, Dauphinot V, Romeyer-Bouchard C, Khris L, M'baye A, et al. Predictive factors of difficult implantation procedure in cardiac resynchronization therapy. Europace. 2010;12(8):1141–8.

35. Miller AL, Kramer DB, Lewis EF, Koplan B, Epstein LM, Tedrow U. Event-free survival following CRT with surgically implanted LV leads versus standard transvenous approach. Pacing Clin Electrophysiol. 2011;34(4):490–500.

36. Puglisi A, Lunati M, Marullo AG, Bianchi S, Feccia M, Sgreccia F, et al. Limited thoracotomy as a second choice alternative to transvenous implant for cardiac resynchronisation therapy delivery. Eur Heart J. 2004;25(12):1063–9.

37. Mair H, Sachweh J, Meuris B, Nollert G, Schmoeckel M, Schuetz A, et al. Surgical epicardial left ventricular lead versus coronary sinus lead placement in biventricular pacing. Eur J Cardiothorac Surg. 2005;27(2):235–42.

7

Feasibility and safety of early discharge after transfemoral transcatheter aortic valve implantation – rationale and design of the FAST-TAVI registry

Marco Barbanti[1*†], Jan Baan[2†], Mark S. Spence[3†], Fortunato Iacovelli[4,5], Gian Luca Martinelli[6], Francesco Saia[7], Alessandro Santo Bortone[8], Frank van der Kley[9], Douglas F. Muir[10], Cameron G. Densem[11], Marije Vis[2], Martijn S. van Mourik[2], Lenka Seilerova[12], Claudia M. Lüske[13], Peter Bramlage[13]ⓘ and Corrado Tamburino[1]

Abstract

Background: There is an increasing trend towards shorter hospital stays after transcatheter aortic valve implantation (TAVI), in particular for patients undergoing the procedure via transfemoral (TF) access. Preliminary data suggest that there exists a population of patients that can be discharged safely very early after TF-TAVI. However, current evidence is limited to few retrospective studies, encompassing relatively small sample sizes.

Methods: The Feasibility And Safety of early discharge after Transfemoral TAVI (FAST-TAVI) registry is a prospective observational registry that will be conducted at 10 sites across Italy, the Netherlands and the UK. Patients will be included if they have been scheduled to undergo TF-TAVI with the balloon-expandable SAPIEN 3 transcatheter heart valve (THV; Edwards Lifesciences, Irvine, CA). The primary endpoint is a composite of all-cause mortality, vascular-access-related complications, permanent pacemaker implantation, stroke, re-hospitalisation due to cardiac reasons, kidney failure and major bleeding, occurring during the first 30 days after hospital discharge. Patients will be stratified according to whether they were high or low risk for early discharge (≤3 days) (following pre-specified criteria), and according to whether or not they were discharged early. Secondary endpoints will include time-to-event (Kaplan–Meier) analysis for the primary outcome and its individual components, analysis of the relative costs of early and late discharge, and changes in short- and long-term quality of life. Multivariate logistic regression will be used to identify factors that indicate that a patient may be suitable for early discharge.

Discussion: The data gathered in the FAST-TAVI registry should help to clarify the safety of early discharge after TF-TAVI and to identify patient and procedural characteristics that make early discharge from hospital a safe and cost-effective strategy.

Keywords: Aortic stenosis, Hospitalisation, Length of stay, Cost-effectiveness, Transfemoral, SAPIEN

* Correspondence: mbarbanti83@gmail.com
†Equal contributors
[1]Catania Division of Cardiology, Ferrarotto Hospital, University of Catania, Via Salvatore Citelli 6, Catania, Italy
Full list of author information is available at the end of the article

Background

Transcatheter aortic valve implantation (TAVI) is a feasible alternative to surgical aortic valve replacement (SAVR) for patients who are at prohibitively high risk for open surgery. More recently, there has been a trend towards performing TAVI in lower-risk patients, with similar rates of all-cause mortality reported in a randomised trial comparing TAVI with SAVR in intermediate risk patients [1]. The cost-effectiveness of TAVI compared to SAVR has been shown to be acceptable in high-risk patients, especially when transfemoral (TF) access is utilised [2]. However, in a real-world setting, the high cost of TAVI, mainly due to the price of the transcatheter heart valve (THV), limits extension of the procedure to lower risk patients [3].

Hospitalisation is the main contributor to the costs of SAVR, and the second largest contributor to the costs of TAVI [4]. While there is limited scope for reducing the length of hospital stay after open surgery, increasing use of a minimalist approach to TAVI has the potential to significantly reduce the time to discharge. When TF access is used, the procedure can often be performed in a catheterisation laboratory, with use of local anaesthesia and conscious sedation rather than general anaesthesia. This approach reduces the costs of the procedure itself and allows for a shorter stay in the intensive care unit (ICU) and the potential for early discharge from hospital [5–7]. Indeed, there has been a significant decreasing trend in length of hospital stay after TAVI [8, 9], with a recent study reporting an average of 4 days after TF-TAVI at a centre that actively pursued early discharge [10].

A number of studies have evaluated the safety of early discharge after TAVI [8, 11, 12]. Lauck et al. retrospectively evaluated data from 393 TAVI patients, 38% of whom had been discharged within 48 h after their procedure. They found no differences in terms of 30-day mortality, rehospitalisation or disabling stroke between the early and standard discharge groups [11]. Similarly, Durand et al. reported discharge within 72 h for 36% of their 337 TF-TAVI patients, with no difference in 30-day mortality or rehospitalisation [8].

In a small prospective study ($N = 130$), early discharge was specifically targeted after elective TF-TAVI [10]. A total of 59% of patients were successfully discharged within 72 h, with one death and 3 cases of rehospitalisation occurring during the subsequent 30 days. While no death occurred in the patients that were discharged after 72 h, 7 required rehospitalisation. In a cohort of 120 patients that underwent TAVI at a single centre, 21.7% of patients were discharged on either the same day as the procedure or the following day, with a further 32.5% discharged at 2 or 3 days [6]. There were no deaths within 30 days for any of these patients, while mortality was 5.5% for those that were discharged after 4 days. Rehospitalisation rates did not differ significantly between groups.

These studies have provided preliminary data in support of the feasibility and safety of early discharge after TF-TAVI. However, if this approach is to be more widely adopted, there is a clear need for larger, prospective multicentre studies. A substantial cohort of TAVI patients would also allow for evaluation of baseline and procedural characteristics that may indicate suitability for early discharge, further decreasing the associated risks. Furthermore, the rapid advancements being made in THV and implantation technologies make up-to-date information essential.

The Feasibility And Safety of early discharge after Transfemoral-TAVI (FAST-TAVI) registry has been designed in order to provide contemporary data regarding early discharge after TAVI. This prospective, multicentre study will evaluate patients undergoing TF-TAVI with the latest generation of the balloon-expandable SAPIEN THV (SAPIEN 3; Edwards Lifesciences). In addition to assessing adverse outcomes after discharge, the dataset will enable the identification of criteria that will allow safe early discharge of patients after TF TAVI.

Methods/design

FAST-TAVI is an observational, prospective, multicentre registry that will be performed at 5 sites in Italy (Catania, Bari, Novara, Bologna and Mercogliano), 2 sites in the Netherlands (Amsterdam & Leiden), and 3 sites in the UK (Belfast, Cambridge, Middlesbrough). Approximately 50 patients undergoing TF-TAVI with the SAPIEN 3 THV will be enrolled at each site.

Patients

Patients undergoing TF-TAVI with the SAPIEN 3 THV (Edwards Lifesciences) will be enrolled on a consecutive basis. The decision to perform this procedure will be made by the Heart Team at each institution according to standard practice; it will not be influenced in any way by the investigators. Beyond the applicable criteria of the device Instructions for Use, no other inclusion or exclusion criteria will be applied.

Data collection

Data will be collected prospectively according to the timetable set out in Table 1, and will be entered in a standardised case report form (CRF). At baseline, demographic and clinical characteristics will be documented. Laboratory data from blood and urine analysis will be collected and an echocardiogram and an ECG will be performed. Patients will also undergo a full physical examination. A mini-mental state examination (MMSE) will be carried out and patients will be asked to complete the SF-12 QoL (Quality of life) questionnaire (version 2.0). Procedural characteristics, including any complications, will be collected. Post-procedure, patients will be monitored

Table 1 Data collection timetable

	Baseline	Procedure (up to 2 h post-TAVI)	Day 1	Day 2[c]	Day 3[c]	Discharge	30 ± 12 days	12 months
Informed consent	X							
Demographics	X							
Clinical characteristics	X							
Physical examination[a]	X		X	X	X	X	X	X
Laboratory analysis[b]	X		X	X	X	X		
Current medication	X					X	X	X
ECG	X	X	X	X	X	X	X	X
Echocardiogram	X	X	X			X	X	X
MMSE	X							
SF-12	X						X	X
Clinical event assessment		X				X	X	X

Legend: ECG, electrocardiogram; MMSE, mini-mental state examination; SF-12, short-form-12 quality of life questionnaire. [a]Includes symptoms, mobility, self-care; [b]includes blood and urine analysis (complete blood count, electrolytes, renal function etc.); [c]if still in hospital

according to standard practice. An echocardiogram and an ECG will be acquired within 2 h of the procedure, and at least once prior to discharge. A physical examination and blood and urine analysis will be performed at daily intervals until discharge.

Patients will be discharged when it is deemed appropriate by the treating physician. This will be unaffected by their participation in the registry. The length of hospital stay will be documented. Follow-up visits will be conducted in accordance with hospital protocol. Data regarding events during the first 30 ± 12 days after discharge will be collected at next visit after this time point. These will include the components set out in the Valve Academic Research Consortium (VARC)-2 consensus document [13]. An echocardiogram and an ECG will be obtained and a full physical examination will be carried out. Furthermore, patients will be asked to again complete the SF-12 QoL questionnaire.

Further follow-up information will be collected at 12 months post-TAVI. This will include the results of a physical examination, blood and urine analysis, echocardiography and an ECG. Any adverse events or rehospitalisation during the 12 months since TAVI will be recorded.

Patient stratification

Patients will be stratified when data collection for all patients is complete. A patient will be classified as being at low risk for early discharge if they fulfil all of the criteria at the point of leaving hospital, as displayed in Table 2. The patients will be further stratified according to whether they were discharged early (≤3 days post-TAVI) or late (<3 days). This will give 4 groups for comparison purposes. Further time points (e.g. stratification at hospital admission) as well as cut-offs (1, 2 or 4 days etc.) will be explored once data are available.

Primary endpoint

The primary endpoint is a composite of all-cause mortality, vascular-access-related complications, permanent pacemaker implantation, stroke, re-hospitalisation due to cardiac reasons, kidney failure and major bleeding, occurring during the first 30 days after hospital discharge.

Cumulative and time-dependent (Kaplan–Meier) incidence of the primary endpoint will be compared between the 4 groups stratified according to suitability for early discharge (according to protocol) and actual discharge.

Secondary endpoints

The incidence of the individual components of the primary outcome (between discharge and 30 days) will be evaluated for the 4 groups. Time-dependent (Kaplan–

Table 2 Patient stratification

A patient will be classified as being at low risk for early discharge if they fulfil all of the following criteria at the point of leaving hospital:

New York Heart Association (NYHA) class ≤ II

No chest pain attributable to cardiac ischaemia

No untreated major arrhythmias

Complications on day 0 to 1, but free of signs or symptoms on day 3

No fever during the last 24 h (infection-related)

Independent mobilisation and capability of self-care

Preserved diuresis (>40 ml/h during the last 24 h)

No unresolved acute kidney injury type 3 (according to VARC-2 criteria)

No red blood cell transfusion during the last 72 h

Stable haemoglobin in 2 consecutive samples (defined as a decrease of no more than 2 mg/dl)

No stroke or transient ischaemic attack (TIA)

No sign of systemic inflammation or infection (clinic or laboratory)

No haemodynamic instability

Meier) incidence of the primary outcome and its individual components will also be assessed between discharge and 12 months after TAVI.

Multivariate analysis will be performed in order to identify procedural outcomes associated with incidence of the primary endpoint in the patients that were discharged early. A further analysis will be performed to identify factors predictive of early discharge.

Other endpoints will include the length of ICU and overall hospital stay; the QoL scores at baseline, 30 days and 12 months. Other exploratory endpoints may be investigated.

Statistics

As there are few reliable data on early discharge after TAVI, no formal sample size calculation was performed. Based on rates of TAVI procedures being performed, it was estimated that approximately 50 patients could be recruited in one year at each site.

Intent-to-treat analysis, defined as all patients enrolled in the registry, will be employed. Subjects will be considered registry participants when they enter the catheterisation laboratory/hybrid suite/operating room. Descriptive data summaries will be used to present and summarise the collected data. For categorical variables, frequency distributions will be given. For numeric variables, means and standard deviations or medians and interquartile ranges will be calculated, depending on data distribution. Kaplan–Meier analysis will be performed for time-to-event outcomes. Multivariate logistic regression will be performed to identify predictors of the primary endpoint in the patients discharged early, and predictors of early discharge. Variables entered into the analysis will include baseline characteristics and periprocedural complications.

Discussion

The FAST-TAVI registry has been designed to provide a registry of prospectively collected data that can be used to elucidate the benefits and risks of early discharge after TF-TAVI. Analysis of the results should enable identification of certain patient and procedural characteristics that indicate whether a patient requires further in-hospital monitoring or whether they could safely be discharged within just a few days after the TAVI procedure.

Preliminary data from previous studies suggest that there exists a population of patients that can be safely discharged soon after undergoing uncomplicated TAVI via the TF route [6, 8, 10, 11]. However, the human and financial costs associated with inappropriate early discharge could be immense. Complications after TAVI include bleeding, stroke and kidney injury, each associated with a mortality risk. Furthermore, all patients that undergo TAVI are at high risk for death during open cardiac surgery. They are generally elderly and display multiple comorbidities and frailty, providing an even greater risk of mortality. In addition, unplanned rehospitalisation after TAVI is expensive and so may counteract the cost savings made by discharging a patient early [14]. Studies evaluating readmission after TAVI have consistently found that heart failure is the most common cause, although the relative contributions of other factors varied [14, 15]. Furthermore, high proportions of patients were hospitalised for non-cardiovascular reasons, highlighting the complex nature of this elderly and comorbid population.

In an attempt to identify factors that indicate that an individual patient is suitable for early discharge after TAVI, Durand et al. reviewed the records of all patients that underwent TF-TAVI using the SAPIEN XT THV during a 4-year period [8]. Of the baseline and procedural characteristics that were entered into their multivariate analysis, a requirement for blood transfusion(s) and previous balloon aortic valvuloplasty were predictive of late discharge, while a pre-existing pacemaker was associated with early discharge. There was also a wide variety of univariate predictors that may have proved more influential in a larger population. The FAST-TAVI registry will build on these initial data while investigating the most recent of the SAPIEN THVs, the SAPIEN 3.

Often overlooked aspects of recovery after TAVI are patient comfort and the mental and emotional aspects that affect their QoL during the first few days and weeks. In a recent study looking into self-reported health and QoL changes during the first month after TAVI, Olsen et al. reported a significant improvement in the physical component summary of the SF-12 questionnaire, but not in the mental component summary [16]. The main contributing factors to the insignificant increase in the mental component were social and emotional, which is in agreement with a previous study by Krane et al. [17]. Reynolds et al. reported a significant improvement in both physical and mental scores at 6 months and one-year post-TAVI compared to baseline; however, the mental component only increased slightly during the first 30-days of follow-up [18]. It is possible that early discharge from hospital may help to improve patients' emotional wellbeing in the first month after TAVI. In order to evaluate this hypothesis, the SF-12 questionnaire will be completed at baseline, 30 days and 12 months in the FAST-TAVI registry.

Potential limitations

While the multinational nature of this registry increases the applicability of the findings to other countries, the differences in healthcare systems may also introduce some difficulties. This is of particular significance when evaluating the financial implications of early discharge. Furthermore, standard procedural and aftercare protocols are likely to vary between countries, and possibly between institutions within a country. However, one significant advantage of the present registry is that all patients will receive the same THV (SAPIEN 3) via the same access route (TF), reducing the variability common to the majority of prior TAVI studies.

Potential clinical impact

The knowledge acquired from the FAST-TAVI registry should help to elucidate the relative risks and benefits of discharging a patient early after TF-TAVI. This not only includes the clinical implications for the patient, but also takes into account their QoL. Furthermore, with hospitalisation contributing significantly to the overall cost of a TAVI procedure, the potential for extending its cost-effectiveness to lower-risk patients can be explored.

Abbreviations

CRF: Case report form; FAST-TAVI : The Feasibility and Safety of early discharge after Transfemoral TAVI; ICU: Intensive care unit; MMSE: Mini-mental state examination; QoL: Quality of life; SAVR: Surgical aortic valve replacement; SF-12: Short-form-12 quality of life questionnaire; TAVI: Transcatheter aortic valve implantation; TF: Transfemoral; THV: Transcatheter heart valve; VARC-2: Valve Academic Research Consortium-2

Acknowledgements

Data were captured using the s4trials Software provided by Software for Trials Europe GmbH, Berlin, Germany. Katherine H. Smith (Institute for Pharmacology and Preventive Medicine, Terrassa, Spain) provided editorial support. Fortunato Iacovelli is currently attending the Cardiopath PhD program.

Funding

Unrestricted educational research grant provided by Edwards Lifesciences (Nyon, Switzerland) to the Institute for Pharmacology and Preventive Medicine (Cloppenburg, Germany).

Authors' contributions

MB, JB, MS, MV, PB, LS, and CT were involved in the conception and design of the registry. FI, GLM, FS, ASB, FvdK, DM, CD, MvM gave feedback on the final protocol and are including patients. MB, CL and PB drafted the manuscript and all other authors have been revising the article for important intellectual content. All authors have given final approval of the version to be published. All authors are fully accountable for the content of the manuscript.

Ethics approval and consent to participate

The registry protocol has been approved by the "Comitato Etico Catania 1" and by local ethics committees at each individual institution and will be performed in accordance with the Declaration of Helsinki and its amendments. All patients included will be required to provide written informed consent.
Study oversight.
Principal investigators.
Jan Baan (Amsterdam, the Netherlands), Marco Barbanti (Catania, Italy), Mark S Spence (Belfast, United Kingdom), Corrado Tamburino (Catania, Italy), Marije Vis (Amsterdam, the Netherlands).
Steering Board.
Jan Baan (Amsterdam, the Netherlands), Marco Barbanti (Catania, Italy), Peter Bramlage (Cloppenburg, Germany), Mark S Spence (Belfast, United Kingdom), Corrado Tamburino (Catania, Italy), Marije Vis (Amsterdam, the Netherlands).
Participating centers.
Italy: Ferrarotto Hospital, Catania (Dr. Barbanti, Dr. Tamburino); "Montevergine" Clinic, Mercogliano (Dr. Iacovelli); Clinica San Gaudenzio,

Novara (Dr. Martinelli); S. Orsola-Malpighi University Hospital (Dr. Saia); University of Bari "Aldo Moro", Bari (Dr. Bortone).
The Netherlands: Academic Medical Center, Amsterdam (Dr. Baan, Dr. Vis); Leiden University Medical Center, Leiden (Dr. van der Kley, Dr. Delgado).
United Kingdom: Royal Victoria Hospital, Belfast (Dr. Spence); The James Cook University Hospital, Middlesbrough (Dr. Muir); Papworth Hospital, Cambridge (Dr. Densem).

Competing interests

Peter Bramlage is the representative of the Institute for Pharmacology and Preventive Medicine, Cloppenburg, Germany. Unrestricted educational research grant provided by Edwards Lifesciences, Nyon, Switzerland to the Sponsor Institute for Pharmacology and Preventive Medicine (Cloppenburg, Germany). Marco Barbanti is consultant for Edwards Lifesciences. Victoria Delgado received speaker fees from Abbott Vascular. The department of Cardiology of the Leiden University Medical Center received unrestricted grants from Edwards Lifesciences, Medtronic, Biotronik and Boston Scientific. Mark S Spence is a proctor for transfemoral transcatheter aortic valve implantation and is a consultant for Edwards Lifesciences. Douglas F Muis is a proctor for Edwards Lifesciences.

Author details

[1]Catania Division of Cardiology, Ferrarotto Hospital, University of Catania, Via Salvatore Citelli 6, Catania, Italy. [2]Department of Cardiology, Academic Medical Center, Amsterdam, The Netherlands. [3]Cardiology Department, Royal Victoria Hospital, Belfast, UK. [4]Interventional Cardiology Service, "Montevergine" Clinic, Mercogliano, Italy. [5]Division of Cardiology, Department of Advanced Biomedical Sciences, University of Naples "Federico II", Naples, Italy. [6]Novara Department of Cardiac Surgery, Clinica San Gaudenzio, Novara, Italy. [7]Cardiovascular and Thoracic Department, S. Orsola-Malpighi University Hospital, Bologna, Italy. [8]Department of Interventional Cardiology, University of Bari "Aldo Moro", Bari, Italy. [9]Department of Cardiology, Leiden University Medical Center, Leiden, The Netherlands. [10]Cardiothoracic Division, The James Cook University Hospital, Middlesbrough, UK. [11]Department of Interventional Cardiology, Papworth Hospital, Cambridge, UK. [12]Edwards Lifesciences, Prague, Czech Republic. [13]Institute for Pharmacology and Preventive Medicine, Cloppenburg, Germany.

References

1. Leon MB, Smith CR, Mack MJ, Makkar RR, Svensson LG, Kodali SK, Thourani VH, Tuzcu EM, Miller DC, Herrmann HC, et al. Transcatheter or surgical aortic-valve replacement in intermediate-risk patients. N Engl J Med. 2016; 374(17):1609–20.
2. Reynolds MR, Magnuson EA, Lei Y, Wang K, Vilain K, Li H, Walczak J, Pinto DS, Thourani VH, Svensson LG, et al. Cost-effectiveness of transcatheter aortic valve replacement compared with surgical aortic valve replacement in high-risk patients with severe aortic stenosis: results of the PARTNER (placement of aortic Transcatheter valves) trial (cohort a). J Am Coll Cardiol. 2012;60(25):2683–92.
3. Ailawadi G, LaPar DJ, Speir AM, Ghanta RK, Yarboro LT, Crosby IK, Lim DS, Quader MA, Rich JB. Contemporary costs associated with transcatheter aortic valve replacement: a propensity-matched cost analysis. Ann Thorac Surg. 2016;101(1):154–60.
4. Wijeysundera HC, Li L, Braga V, Pazhaniappan N, Pardhan AM, Lian D, Leeksma A, Peterson B, Cohen EA, Forsey A, et al. Drivers of healthcare costs associated with the episode of care for surgical aortic valve replacement versus transcatheter aortic valve implantation. Open Heart. 2016;3(2):e000468.
5. Babaliaros V, Devireddy C, Lerakis S, Leonardi R, Iturra SA, Mavromatis K, Leshnower BG, Guyton RA, Kanitkar M, Keegan P, et al. Comparison of transfemoral transcatheter aortic valve replacement performed in the catheterization laboratory (minimalist approach) versus hybrid operating room (standard approach): outcomes and cost analysis. JACC Cardiovasc Interv. 2014;7(8):898–904.
6. Noad RL, Johnston N, McKinley A, Dougherty M, Nzewi OC, Jeganathan R, Manoharan G, Spence MS. A pathway to earlier discharge following TAVI: assessment of safety and resource utilization. Catheter Cardiovasc Interv. 2016;87(1):134–42.
7. Toppen W, Johansen D, Sareh S, Fernandez J, Satou N, Patel KD, Kwon M, Suh W, Aksoy O, Shemin RJ, et al. Improved costs and outcomes with conscious sedation vs general anesthesia in TAVR patients: time to wake up? PLoS One. 2017;12(4):e0173777.

8. Durand E, Eltchaninoff H, Canville A, Bouhzam N, Godin M, Tron C, Rodriguez C, Litzler PY, Bauer F, Cribier A. Feasibility and safety of early discharge after transfemoral transcatheter aortic valve implantation with the Edwards SAPIEN-XT prosthesis. Am J Cardiol. 2015;115(8):1116–22.

9. Landes U, Barsheshet A, Finkelstein A, Guetta V, Assali A, Halkin A, Vaknin-Assa H, Segev A, Bental T, Ben-Shoshan J, et al. Temporal trends in transcatheter aortic valve implantation, 2008–2014: patient characteristics, procedural issues, and clinical outcome. Clin Cardiol. 2017;40(2):82–8.

10. Serletis-Bizios A, Durand E, Cellier G, Tron C, Bauer F, Glinel B, Dacher JN, Cribier A, Eltchaninoff H. A prospective analysis of early discharge after transfemoral transcatheter aortic valve implantation. Am J Cardiol. 2016; 118(6):866–72.

11. Lauck SB, Wood DA, Baumbusch J, Kwon JY, Stub D, Achtem L, Blanke P, Boone RH, Cheung A, Dvir D, et al. Vancouver transcatheter aortic valve replacement clinical pathway: minimalist approach, standardized care, and discharge criteria to reduce length of stay. Circ Cardiovasc Qual Outcomes. 2016;9(3):312–21.

12. Barbanti M, Capranzano P, Ohno Y, Attizzani GF, Gulino S, Imme S, Cannata S, Aruta P, Bottari V, Patane M, et al. Early discharge after transfemoral transcatheter aortic valve implantation. Heart. 2015;101(18):1485–90.

13. Kappetein AP, Head SJ, Genereux P, Piazza N, van Mieghem NM, Blackstone EH, Brott TG, Cohen DJ, Cutlip DE, van Es GA, et al. Updated standardized endpoint definitions for transcatheter aortic valve implantation: the valve academic research Consortium-2 consensus document (VARC-2). Eur J Cardiorac Surg. 2012;42(5):S45–60.

14. Franzone A, Pilgrim T, Arnold N, Heg D, Langhammer B, Piccolo R, Roost E, Praz F, Räber L, Valgimigli M, et al. Rates and predictors of hospital readmission after transcatheter aortic valve implantation. Eur Heart J. 2017; 38:2211–17.

15. Kolte D, Khera S, Sardar MR, Gheewala N, Gupta T, Chatterjee S, Goldsweig A, Aronow WS, Fonarow GC, Bhatt DL, et al. Thirty-day readmissions after transcatheter aortic valve replacement in the United States: insights from the nationwide readmissions database. Circ Cardiovasc Interv. 2017;10(1). doi:10.1161/CIRCINTERVENTIONS.116.004472.

16. Olsen SJ, Fridlund B, Eide LS, Hufthammer KO, Kuiper KK, Nordrehaug JE, Skaar E, Norekval TM. Changes in self-reported health and quality of life in octogenarian patients one month after transcatheter aortic valve implantation. Eur J Cardiovasc Nurs. 2017;16(1):79–87.

17. Krane M, Deutsch MA, Piazza N, Muhtarova T, Elhmidi Y, Mazzitelli D, Voss B, Ruge H, Badiu CC, Kornek M, et al. One-year results of health-related quality of life among patients undergoing transcatheter aortic valve implantation. Am J Cardiol. 2012;109(12):1774–81.

18. Reynolds MR, Magnuson EA, Lei Y, Leon MB, Smith CR, Svensson LG, Webb JG, Babaliaros VC, Bowers BS, Fearon WF, et al. Health-related quality of life after transcatheter aortic valve replacement in inoperable patients with severe aortic stenosis. Circulation. 2011;124(18):1964–72.

Violation of prophylactic vancomycin administration timing is a potential risk factor for rate of surgical site infections in cardiac surgery patients

Paolo Cotogni[1]*, Cristina Barbero[2], Roberto Passera[3], Lucina Fossati[4], Giorgio Olivero[5] and Mauro Rinaldi[2]

Abstract

Background: Intensivists and cardiothoracic surgeons are commonly worried about surgical site infections (SSIs) due to increasing length of stay (LOS), costs and mortality. The antimicrobial prophylaxis is one of the most important tools in the prevention of SSIs. The objective of this study was to investigate the relationship between the timing of antimicrobial prophylaxis administration and the rate of SSIs.

Methods: A prospective cohort study was carried out over 1-year period in all consecutive adult patients undergoing elective cardiac surgery. The population was stratified in patients whose antimicrobial prophylaxis administration violated or not the vancomycin timing protocol (i.e., when the first skin incision was performed before the end of vancomycin infusion). To compare SSI rates, the cohort was further stratified in patients at low and high risk of developing SSIs.

Results: Over the study period, 1020 consecutive adult patients underwent cardiac surgery and according to study inclusion criteria, 741 patients were prospectively enrolled. A total of 60 SSIs were identified for an overall infection rate of 8.1%. Vancomycin prophylaxis timing protocol was violated in 305 (41%) out of 741 enrolled patients. SSIs were observed in 3% of patients without violation of the antimicrobial prophylaxis protocol (13/436) compared with 15.4% of patients with a violation of the timing protocol (47/305) ($P < 0.0001$). Patients at low risk with protocol violation had a higher occurrence of SSIs ($P = 0.004$) and mortality ($P = 0.03$) versus patients at low risk without protocol violation. Similarly, patients at high risk with protocol violation had a higher occurrence of SSIs ($P < 0.001$) and mortality ($P < 0.001$) versus patients at high risk without protocol violation. The logistic regression analysis showed that internal mammary artery use ($P = 0.025$), surgical time ($P < 0.001$), intensive care unit (ICU) LOS ($P = 0.002$), high risk of developing SSIs ($P < 0.001$) and protocol violation ($P < 0.001$) were risk factors for SSI occurrence as well as age ($P = 0.003$), logistic EuroSCORE ($P < 0.001$), ICU LOS ($P < 0.001$), mechanical ventilation time ($P < 0.001$) and protocol violation ($P < 0.001$) were risk factors for mortality.

Conclusions: This study showed that violation of the timing of prophylactic vancomycin administration significantly increased the probability of SSIs and mortality from infectious cause in cardiac surgery patients.

Keywords: Antimicrobial prophylaxis, Surgical wound infection, Postoperative infectious complications

* Correspondence: paolo.cotogni@unito.it
[1]Department of Anesthesia and Intensive Care, S. Giovanni Battista Hospital, University of Turin, Via Giovanni Giolitti 9, 10123 Turin, Italy
Full list of author information is available at the end of the article

Background

The incidence of surgical site infections (SSIs) after cardiac surgery ranges differently according to the type of wound infection; specifically, superficial wound infection occurs in 2 to 20% of patients and deep sternal wound infection occurs in 0.25 to 5% [1–6].

Risk factors that have been linked to SSIs include features in the host such as advanced age, the presence of liver or lung dysfunction, cancer, diabetes mellitus and over- or undernutrition [7, 8]. Similarly, several operation characteristics can influence the risk of infection in cardiac surgery: skin antisepsis; length of operation; surgical technique; coronary artery bypass graft (CABG) surgery involving the use of a saphenous vein autograft that can carry bacteria from the harvest site deep into the cardiac operative site; use of the internal mammary artery (IMA) that deprives the sternum of blood supply; the use of prosthetic intracardiac or aortic implants; cardiopulmonary bypass or systemic cooling for myocardial protection; and invasive devices remaining after surgery (chest drains, pacing wires and intravenous catheters) [1, 8, 9]. Recent reports focused on an increasing number of infections caused by resistant Gram-positive pathogens, such as methicillin-resistant Staphylococcus aureus (MRSA) and coagulase-negative staphylococcus [4, 5, 10]. Compared with methicillin-sensitive Staphylococcus aureus mediastinitis, MRSA mediastinitis has up to an 11-fold increased mortality rate [5].

In patients undergoing cardiac surgery, an SSI is associated with increased morbidity, prolonged length of stay and increased costs with an in-hospital mortality rate of 10–20% [1, 6, 11]. Thus, many preventive measures were suggested as effective for reducing the incidence of SSIs, such as preoperative screening for carriage of multiresistant organisms (e.g., MRSA), antimicrobial prophylaxis, preoperative skin preparation, accurate surgical technique, postoperative glycemic control and wound management [9, 12]. Antimicrobial intravenous prophylaxis is routinely administered to patients undergoing cardiac surgery because the benefits of preoperative antibiotic administration in these patients have been clearly demonstrated in placebo-controlled studies [13]. However, the debate over choice, dose, duration and timing of antimicrobial prophylaxis protocol is still all the rage [14].

Seminal literature demonstrated that antimicrobial prophylaxis administered too late or too early reduced the efficacy of the antibiotic and may increase the risk of SSI [7]. The definite timing of administration of the first antibiotic dose has not been assessed in randomized controlled trials; however, there is a strong rationale supporting the need for the timely administration of preoperative antimicrobial prophylaxis [7, 11, 15]. Indeed, the timing of the administration of the prophylactic antibiotic is still an important issue for the cardiac surgical community [16–19], because despite the existence of published guidelines and locally agreed protocols for the antimicrobial prophylaxis administration, often there is a gap between what is recommended and what is practiced [15, 20].

The primary objective of this study was to investigate the relationship between the timing of antimicrobial prophylaxis administration —with respect to surgical incision time— and the rate of SSIs, comparing cardiac surgery patients at low and high risk of infection. This objective was related to a specific exploratory mandate received from our Hospital Infection Control Committee to evaluate our policy of antimicrobial prophylaxis in cardiac surgery.

Methods

Study design

A single-centre prospective cohort study was carried out in the Department of Cardiovascular Surgery of a 1200-bed tertiary care university hospital (S. Giovanni Battista Hospital). Over 1-year period, all consecutive adult patients undergoing cardiac surgery were assessed for eligibility. The exclusion criteria were renal dysfunction (on dialysis or creatinine clearance ≤30 mL/min, estimated by the Cockcroft-Gault formula); infectious diseases that required antibiotic therapy in the previous 2 weeks; heart and lung transplant surgery; solid or hematologic tumours as well as chemotherapy or radiation therapy in the previous 6 months; preoperative stay in intensive care unit (ICU) more than 24 h; allergy to cefazolin or vancomycin; and emergency operations.

The study protocol was reviewed and approved by our Institutional Ethics Committee (No. 0078553) and patients provided written informed consent before their enrolment. The work was conducted in compliance with Institutional Review Board/Human Subjects Research Committee requirements.

Our protocol of antimicrobial prophylaxis was a single 1000 mg cefazolin dose, diluted in 20 mL 0.9% NaCl solution, initiated 30 to 60 min before surgery and administered as a slow intravenous bolus; plus a single 1000 mg vancomycin dose, diluted in 100 mL 0.9% NaCl solution, started within 2 h before surgery and administered over 60 min intravenously infusion to prevent the release of histamine. A further three doses of cefazolin 1000 mg at 8-h intervals were given postoperatively, while no further vancomycin doses were administrated postoperatively. Since 2005, our protocol provides the choice to combine cefazolin with vancomycin for antimicrobial prophylaxis in patients undergoing cardiac surgery. The rationale for using vancomycin was an increased prevalence of MRSA infections, which exceeded 60% hospital-wide and isolates identified in cardiac surgery patients with SSIs. Antimicrobial prophylaxis is started in the preoperative holding area. Vancomycin protocol and timing of administration were chosen based upon recommendations of our Hospital Infection Control Committee according to the Sanford Guide [21] and the Society of Thoracic Surgeons Guidelines [16].

The study population was stratified in patients whose antimicrobial prophylaxis administration violated or not our vancomycin timing protocol. Antimicrobial prophylaxis timing protocol was considered as violated when the first surgical skin incision was performed before the end of the vancomycin infusion. A healthcare provider (i.e., physician, nurse or cardiovascular technician) was required to document the exact time the antibiotic infusion was started, as well anaesthesiologists or cardiac surgeons who recorded the exact time the first skin incision.

To compare SSI rates adequately, the cohort was further stratified in patients at low and high risk of developing SSIs according to the literature [1, 8, 10]. Specifically, patients were included in the high risk group in case of: (i) chronic liver disease (classified as Child-Pugh class B and C); (ii) insulin-dependent diabetes; (iii) body mass index (BMI) <17 or >40 kg/m^2; (iv) steroid or other immunosuppressive drug use; (v) chronic obstructive pulmonary disease; and (vi) extracardiac arteriopathy (i.e., claudication, carotid occlusion or >50% stenosis, amputation for arterial disease and previous or planned intervention on the abdominal aorta, limb arteries or carotids). Thus, cardiac surgery patients were

assigned to four groups according to SSI risk factors and violation of the timing of antimicrobial prophylaxis protocol administration as follows: (i) low risk patients without protocol violation; (ii) low risk patients with protocol violation; (iii) high risk patients without protocol violation; and (iv) high risk patients with protocol violation.

According to Centers for Disease Control and Prevention (CDC) guidelines [8], the definition of an SSI requires that one of the following criteria be met: (i) superficial (infection above the sternum with no bone involvement); (ii) deep (infection involving the sternum and organ/space such as mediastinitis); and (iii) leg donor site infections. Patients with SSI must have positive culture results of surgical sites or drainage from the mediastinal area or evidence of infection during surgical re-exploration or fever, sternal instability and positive blood culture results [8]. Other infectious complications were defined as bloodstream infection (BSI), lower respiratory tract infection (LRTI) and urinary tract infection (UTI) according to CDC guidelines. Perioperative management and skin preparation were standardized in our Department according to CDC guidelines. According to the literature, patients were followed up for 30 days after the surgical procedure [18, 19]. Mortality was defined as death during hospitalization or within 30 days after surgery from infectious cause.

Statistical analysis
The patients' characteristics were analysed by the Fisher's exact test for categorical variables, while by the

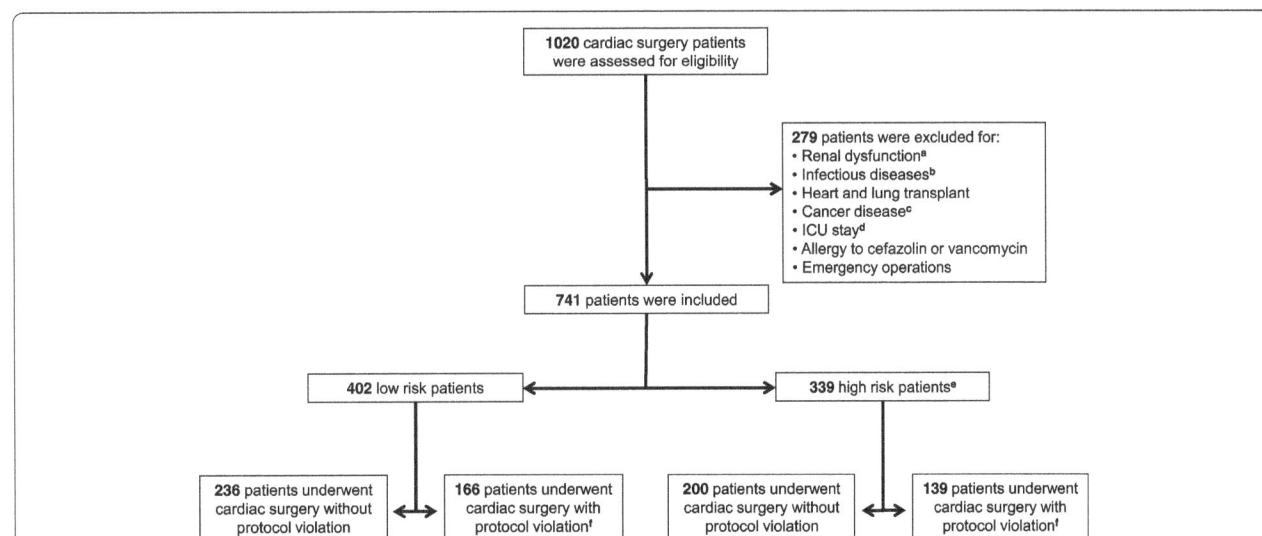

Fig. 1 Study design. [a]Dialysis or creatinine clearance ≤30 mL/min. [b]Infectious diseases that required antibiotic therapy in the previous 2 weeks. [c]Patients with solid or hematologic tumours, as well as patients underwent chemotherapy or radiation therapy in the previous 6 months. [d]Preoperative stay in the intensive care unit (ICU) for more than 24 h. [e]Patients were considered at high risk of developing surgical site infections in case of: chronic liver disease (classified as Child-Pugh class B and C); insulin-dependent diabetes; body mass index <17 or >40 kg/m^2; steroid or other immunosuppressive drug use; chronic obstructive pulmonary disease; and extracardiac arteriopathy (i.e., claudication, carotid occlusion or >50% stenosis, amputation for arterial disease and previous or planned intervention on the abdominal aorta, limb arteries or carotids). [f]Violation of antimicrobial prophylaxis timing protocol

Mann–Whitney test for continuous ones; all results for the latter were expressed as the median (range). Two different independent series of univariate/multivariate binary logistic regression models were used to estimate the odds of SSI occurrence and mortality within 30 days after surgery (dependent variables), evaluating as their risk factors: gender, IMA use, high risk of developing SSIs and protocol violation (independent categorical variables) as well as age, BMI, surgical time, logistic EuroSCORE, mechanical ventilation time and ICU length of stay (LOS) (independent continuous variables). All reported P values were obtained by the two-sided exact method, at the conventional 5% significance level. Data were analysed by R 3.3.2 (R Foundation for Statistical Computing, Vienna-A, http://www.R-project.org).

Results

Over the study period, 1020 consecutive adult patients underwent cardiac surgery. According to study inclusion criteria, 741 patients were prospectively enrolled, while 279 patients were excluded (Fig. 1). Main patients' characteristics are reported in Table 1. According to variables considered as risk factors for infectious complications, 402 patients were considered at low risk of developing SSIs and 339 were considered at high risk. Of the 741 patients included in the study, antimicrobial prophylaxis timing protocol was violated in 305 patients (41.2%); specifically, in these patients the skin incision was performed before the end of the vancomycin infusion. No patients had vancomycin infusion more than 120 min prior to skin incision. No violation regarding cefazolin administration was observed.

Table 2 shows infectious complications. SSIs were 8.1%: two-thirds were superficial wound infections of the chest, deep infections were 25% and few were at a donor site. SSIs were observed in 3% of patients without violation of the antimicrobial prophylaxis protocol (13/436) compared with 15.4% of patients with a violation of the

Table 1 Patients' characteristics

	Low risk (n = 402)			High risk (n = 339)		
	Without protocol violation	With protocol violation	P	Without protocol violation	With protocol violation	P
n	236	166		200	139	
Age, median (range)	70 (25–86)	70 (34–84)	0.51	71 (37–88)	71 (44–88)	0.50
Male gender, n (%)	149 (63)	100 (60.2)	0.63	124 (62)	74 (53.2)	0.13
BMI, kg/m², median (range)	26 (18–40)	26 (18–39)	0.81	28 (17–43)	28 (17–41)	0.84
Diabetes, n (%)	46 (19)[a]	27 (16.3)[a]	0.41	50 (25)[b]	45 (32.4)[b]	0.17
COPD, n (%)	0	0	—	24 (12)	13 (9.3)	0.55
Hypertension, n (%)	151 (64)	108 (65.1)	0.91	132 (66)	99 (71.2)	0.37
Smoke, n (%)	28 (12)	30 (18.1)	0.11	52 (26)	48 (34.5)	0.12
Surgical time, min, median (range)	249 (119–593)	255 (132–495)	0.49	247 (140–442)	243 (152–430)	0.60
Surgical procedure, n (%)			0.08			0.11
CABG	72 (30.5)	58 (34.9)		70 (35)	53 (38.1)	
Valve	113 (47.9)	59 (35.5)		52 (26)	24 (17.3)	
CABG + Valve	34 (14.4)	30 (18.1)		24 (12)	12 (8.6)	
Other[c]	17 (7.2)	19 (11.5)		54 (27)	50 (36)	
Off-pump CABG, n (%)	21 (8.9)	8 (4.8)	0.17	11 (5.5)	9 (6.5)	0.89
Left IMA, n (%)	53 (22.4)	40 (24.1)	0.79	44 (22)	33 (23.7)	0.81
Both IMA, n (%)	17 (7.2)	8 (4.8)	0.44	13 (6.5)	9 (6.5)	>0.99
EuroSCORE additive, median (range)	5 (1–6)	5 (1–6)	0.80	8 (1–16)	8 (1–14)	0.72
EuroSCORE logistic, median (range)	4.8 (1–7.74)	4.6 (1–7.21)	0.41	9.7 (1–44.45)	9.9 (1–61.86)	0.37
Mechanical ventilation, h, median (range)	7 (2–912)	8 (6–415)	0.31	9 (7–816)	9 (8–711)	0.49
ICU stay, d, median (range)	1 (1–24)	1 (1–38)	0.52	1 (1–33)	1 (1–45)	0.30
RBC transfusions, n, median (range)	2 (0–9)	2 (0–6)	0.71	3 (0–11)	2 (0–10)	0.61

BMI body mass index, *COPD* chronic obstructive pulmonary disease, *CABG* coronary artery bypass grafting, *IMA* internal mammary artery, *EuroSCORE* European System for Cardiac Operative Risk Evaluation, *h* hours, *ICU* intensive care unit, *d* days, *RBC* red blood cell
[a]Non-insulin-dependent diabetes
[b]Insulin-dependent diabetes
[c]Aortic, atrial or ventricular septal defect repair, and congenital surgery

Table 2 Infectious complications

| | Low risk (n = 402) | | High risk (n = 339) | | |
	Without protocol violation	With protocol violation	Without protocol violation	With protocol violation	Total
N	236	166	200	139	741
SSI, n (%)	3 (1.3)	12 (7.2)[a]	10 (5)[b]	35 (25.2)[c,d]	60 (8.1)
Superficial, n	1	8	4	25	38 (63.3)
Deep, n	2	2	5	6	15 (25)
Donor site, n	0	2	1	4	7 (11.7)
BSI, n (%)	2 (0.8)	8 (4.8)[e]	12 (6)[b]	49 (35.2)[c,d]	71 (9.6)
LRTI, n (%)	7 (3)	8 (4.8)	25 (12.5)[f]	39 (23.1)[c,d]	79 (10.7)
UTI, n (%)	0	1 (0.6)	3 (1.5)	15 (10.8)[c,d]	19 (2.6)
Mortality[§], n (%)	3 (1.3)	8 (4.8)[g]	9 (4.5)[b]	20 (14.4)[c,h]	40 (5.4)

SSI surgical site infection, BSI bloodstream infection, LRTI lower respiratory trait infection, UTI urinary trait infection
[§]During hospitalization or within 30 days after surgery from infectious cause
[a]P = 0.004 versus low risk group without protocol violation
[b]P = 0.04 versus low risk group without protocol violation
[c]P < 0.001 versus high risk group without protocol violation
[d]P < 0.001 versus low risk group with protocol violation
[e]P = 0.01 versus low risk group without protocol violation
[f]P < 0.001 versus low risk group without protocol violation
[g]P = 0.03 versus low risk group without protocol violation
[h]P = 0.003 versus low risk group with protocol violation

timing protocol (47/305) (P < 0.0001). Patients at low risk with protocol violation had a higher occurrence of SSIs (P = 0.004), BSIs (P = 0.01) and mortality (P = 0.03) versus patients at low risk without protocol violation. Patients at high risk with protocol violation had a higher occurrence of SSIs (P < 0.001), BSIs (P < 0.001), LRTIs (P < 0.001), UTIs (P < 0.001) and mortality (P < 0.001) versus patients at high risk without protocol violation. Patients at high risk without violation of the antimicrobial prophylaxis protocol had a higher occurrence of SSIs (P = 0.0 4), BSIs (P = 0.04), LRTIs (P < 0.001) and mortality (P = 0.04) versus patients at low risk without protocol violation. Patients at high risk with protocol violation had a higher occurrence of SSIs (P < 0.001), BSIs (P < 0.001), LRTIs (P < 0.001), UTIs (P < 0.001) and

mortality (P = 0.003) versus patients at low risk with protocol violation.

The logistic regression analysis showed that IMA use (P = 0.025), surgical time (P < 0.001), ICU LOS (P = 0.002), high risk of developing SSIs (P < 0.001) and protocol violation (P < 0.001) were risk factors for SSI occurrence (Table 3) as well as age (P = 0.003), logistic EuroSCORE (P < 0.001), ICU LOS (P < 0.001), mechanical ventilation time (P < 0.001) and protocol violation (P < 0.001) were risk factors for mortality (Table 4).

Ninety-two pathogens isolated in 60 SSIs are shown in Table 5. Specifically, Gram-positive, Gram-negative and fungi were isolated in 48, 40 and 12%, respectively. Pathogens isolated in SSIs by groups are depicted in Table 6. Methicillin-resistant Staphylococci (aureus, coagulase-

Table 3 Risk factors for surgical site infections (SSIs)

| | Logistic regression Univariate models | | | Logistic regression Multivariate model | | |
	Odds ratio	95% CI	P	Odds ratio	95% CI	P
Body mass index	1.07	1.02-1.13	0.007	1.01	0.94-1.08	0.781
Internal mammary artery use	1.85	1.08-3.17	0.026	2.11	1.10-4.04	0.025
Surgical time	1.01	1.01-1.02	<0.001	1.01	1.01-1.02	<0.001
Intensive care unit LOS	1.12	1.09-1.16	<0.001	1.06	1.02-1.10	0.002
High risk[a]	3.95	2.16-7.22	<0.001	4.70	2.32-9.53	<0.001
Protocol violation[b]	5.93	3.15-11.17	<0.001	7.03	3.41-14.52	<0.001

CI Confidence interval, LOS length of stay
[a]High risk of developing SSIs according to the literature [1, 8, 10]; in case of: (i) chronic liver disease (classified as Child-Pugh class B and C); (ii) insulin-dependent diabetes; (iii) body mass index <17 or >40 kg/m2; (iv) steroid or other immunosuppressive drug use; (v) chronic obstructive pulmonary disease; and (vi) extracardiac arteriopathy (i.e.,claudication, carotid occlusion or >50% stenosis, amputation for arterial disease and previous or planned intervention on the abdominal aorta, limb arteries or carotids)
[b]Antimicrobial prophylaxis timing protocol was considered as violated when the first surgical skin incision was performed before the end of the vancomycin infusion

Table 4 Risk factors for mortality[a]

	Logistic regression Univariate models			Logistic regression Multivariate model		
	Odds ratio	95% CI	P	Odds ratio	95% CI	P
Age	1.13	1.07-1.19	<0.001	1.15	1.05-1.26	0.003
EuroSCORE logistic	1.24	1.17-1.31	<0.001	1.21	1.11-1.33	<0.001
Intensive care unit LOS	1.25	1.20-1.31	<0.001	1.14	1.07-1.21	<0.001
Mechanical ventilation time	1.34	1.24-1.45	<0.001	1.18	1.08-1.29	<0.001
Protocol violation[b]	3.57	1.79-7.14	<0.001	10.16	2.48-41.58	<0.001

CI Confidence interval, *LOS* length of stay
[a]During hospitalization or within 30 days after surgery from infectious cause
[b]Antimicrobial prophylaxis timing protocol was considered as violated when the first surgical skin incision was performed before the end of the vancomycin infusion

negative and *hominis*) accounted for 28% of pathogens. When we studied methicillin-resistance or vancomycin susceptibility of Gram-positive isolates according to the timing of antimicrobial prophylaxis none of the differences between groups in the rate of such resistances reached statistical significance. No clusters of any specific pathogen were noted during the study period.

Discussion

In this study, cardiac surgery population was divided in patients at high risk of developing infections because of well-known risk factors and patients at low risk. As expected, patients at high risk (i.e., patients with severe comorbidities, immunosuppressive therapy, severe obesity or malnutrition) had a significant higher occurrence of SSIs as well as of BSIs, LRTIs and mortality compared with patients at low risk, independently of violation of the antimicrobial prophylaxis protocol. This finding reflects a population of patients who were more severely ill and therefore at higher risk for postoperative infectious complications.

The Society of Thoracic Surgeons Practice Guidelines on antibiotic prophylaxis in cardiac surgery recommended that in the setting of the institutional presence of a 'high incidence' of MRSA, it would be reasonable to combine a β-lactam (cefazolin) with a glycopeptide (vancomycin) for prophylaxis (Class IIB recommendation, Level of Evidence C) [16]. Optimal dosage regimens

Table 5 Pathogens isolated in 60 surgical site infections

Pathogens, n	92
Gram-positive organisms, n (%)	44 (48)
Staphylococcus aureus, n	23
Coagulase-negative staphylococci, n	11
Enterococcus spp, n	9
Streptococci, n	1
Gram-negative organisms, n (%)	37 (40)
Fungi, n (%)	11 (12)

of vancomycin and protocol of administration still remain controversial [16, 22]. The Society of Thoracic Surgeons Guidelines mentioned that any of the following doses and durations may be used: 1000 mg, 1500 mg, or 15 mg/kg; and 24 h versus 48 h or 1 dose versus 2 doses [16, 22]. Specifically, guidelines for appropriate dosing of prophylactic antibiotics stated that 'In patients for whom vancomycin is an appropriate prophylactic antibiotic for cardiac surgery, a dose of 1 to 1.5 g or a weight-adjusted dose of 15 mg/kg administered intravenously slowly over 1 h, with completion within 1 h of the skin incision, is recommended' (Class I, Level of Evidence A) [16]. Similarly, the 2011 American College of Cardiology/American Heart Association guideline for CABG surgery recommended that 'Antibiotic prophylaxis should be initiated 30 to 60 min before surgery, usually at the time of anaesthetic induction, except for vancomycin, which should be started 2 h before surgery and infused slowly' [6]. Finally, the Scottish Intercollegiate Guidelines Network, updated April 2014, stated that 'Vancomycin should be given by intravenous infusion starting 90 min prior to skin incision' (Class B recommendation) [9].

Several studies investigated the association between measure(s) applied for reducing the rate of SSIs and their occurrence [23, 24]. Our study focused on the timing of antimicrobial prophylaxis; specifically, on the relationship between the first skin incision and the end of vancomycin infusion. We found that the initial surgical incision was performed before the vancomycin infusion had been completed in nearly 40% of patients. Generally, the reason for the violation of the antimicrobial prophylaxis protocol was due to our policy to start antimicrobial prophylaxis in the preoperative holding area under supervision of anaesthesiologists. This policy was adopted in our Cardiovascular Surgery Unit following the occurrence of some relevant adverse drug reactions due to vancomycin administration (i.e., mainly hypotension; occasionally, red man syndrome) [23, 24].

Differently, in the Garey's study [25] cardiac surgery patients were assigned to five groups on the basis of the

Table 6 Pathogens isolated in surgical site infections by groups

	Low risk (n = 402)		High risk (n = 339)		Total
	Without protocol violation	With protocol violation	Without protocol violation	With protocol violation	
SSI, n (%)	3/236 (1.3)	12/166 (7.2)	10/200 (5)	35/139 (25.2)	60/741 (8.1)
Pathogen, n	3	24	12	53	92
Gram-positive, n (%)	1 (33)	11 (46)	5 (42)	27 (51)	44 (48)
Methicillin-sensitive, n	1	3	2	12	18
Methicillin-resistant, n	0	8	3	15	26
Vancomycin susceptibility					
MIC ≤1, n	1	9	3	17	30
MIC =2, n	0	2	1	9	12
MIC ≥4, n	0	0	1	1	2
Gram-negative, n (%)	1 (33)	12 (50)	4 (33)	20 (38)	37 (40)
Fungi, n (%)	1 (33)	1 (4)	3 (25)	6 (11)	11 (12)

Multiple pathogens were identified in some patients; therefore, total pathogens identified do not add up to the total number of SSIs. *SSI* Surgical Site Infection, *MIC* minimum inhibitory concentration

relation between the start time of the vancomycin infusion and the time of the initial surgical incision. In this study, antibiotic prophylaxis was started in the preoperative holding area only for the first surgical case of the day and in admission unit for all subsequent cases immediately prior to transferring the patient to the preoperative holding area. These Authors reported that of the 2048 patients in the study, 0.7% received vancomycin 0–15 min before incision, 8.6% 16–60 min before incision, 43.4% 61–120 min before incision, 34.2% 121–180 min before incision and 13.1% >180 min before incision.

The relationship between the timing of antimicrobial prophylaxis and the occurrence of SSIs has been studied with conflicting results. The Surgical Care Improvement Project measure assesses compliance for antimicrobial prophylaxis administration initiated within 60 min (or 120 min for vancomycin) prior to surgical incision [11]. The choice of the preincision 60-min window for antimicrobial prophylaxis was based on two types of evidence: pharmacokinetics of the antibiotics and one large cohort study analyzing the association between timing of antibiotic administration and SSIs in several types of surgical procedures [11].

However, following studies investigating this relationship did not clearly demonstrate the superiority of the 60-min window [17–20]; in particular, some studies showed lower risk of SSI with shorter times between antibiotic administration and skin incision. Garey et al. reported that SSI developed in 26.7% of cardiac surgery patients who received vancomycin 0–15 min before incision, 3.4% of patients between 16 and 60 min before incision, 7.7% of patients between 61 and 120 min before incision, 6.9% of patients between 121 and 180 min before incision and 7.8% of patients >180 min before incision [25]. Steinberg et al. in an observational study (43.6% were cardiac patients) found a

trend toward lower risk of SSI occurring when antimicrobial prophylaxis with vancomycin or cephalosporins were given within 60 and 30 min prior to incision, respectively [18]. Hawn et al. in a retrospective study in noncardiac surgery patients found that the SSI risk was not significantly associated with prophylactic antibiotic timing [19].

SSIs are still among the most severe complications in cardiac surgery patients. The overall SSI rate observed in our study was 8.1%, which was similar or lower to that previously reported [1–3]. The main finding of our study was that violation of the timing of vancomycin prophylaxis protocol was a significant risk factor for development of SSI in patients undergoing cardiac surgery. Specifically, when the first surgical skin incision was performed before the end of the vancomycin infusion, we observed a 5-fold increased rate of SSIs both in low and high risk patients.

Nosocomial infections occur in 10 to 20% of cardiac surgery patients [6]; however, while SSIs incur significant morbidity and costs but rarely lead to death, conversely, postoperative LRTI, BSI and endocarditis are more frequently correlated with mortality [15]. In our study, we also found a consistent relationship between violation of vancomycin prophylaxis timing protocol and rates of postoperative infectious complications as well as mortality from infectious cause. Specifically, BSIs and mortality were increased 6-fold and more than 3-fold, respectively both in low and high risk patients. Moreover, LRTIs and UTIs were increased 2-fold and 7-fold, respectively in high risk patients. Also for mortality, violation of the timing of vancomycin prophylaxis protocol was a significant risk factor.

Actually, before starting this study we did not suspect that the timing of vancomycin prophylaxis administration was being violated at this rate as well as that this violation was associated with a significantly increased rate of SSIs, postoperative infectious complications and mortality from infectious cause. However, the overall SSI rate and mortality observed in our study were similar or lower to those previously reported in other studies in cardiac surgery patients [1–6].

Policies and practices aimed at reducing the risk of SSIs include performing surveillance for SSIs as well as measuring and providing feedback to healthcare providers on the rates of compliance with process measures, including antimicrobial prophylaxis [7, 12]. This study let us to discover that the violation of the protocol was due to the start of antimicrobial prophylaxis in the preoperative holding area. Indeed, the information obtained in this study was reported to our healthcare providers and has altered practice patterns for avoiding the persistent risk of violation of prophylactic vancomycin administration timing.

Strengths and limitations of the study

If compared with previous studies, our study has some relevant features: (1) it was a prospective study; (2) data were collected through a clinical study and not from a database or registry; (3) antibiotic timing data were collected in 'real-time' in the operating room and not from the patient chart; (4) only cardiac surgery patients were enrolled; (5) all patients received the same prophylactic administration of antibiotics; (6) the rate of BSIs, LRTIs, UTIs and mortality from infectious cause were also investigated; (7) it was concluded in only 12 months and (8) no patient was lost to follow-up. Moreover, to the best of our knowledge, this is the first study investigating the relationship between the rate of SSIs in cardiac surgery patients and the presence or absence of violation of the timing of antimicrobial prophylaxis administration, comparing patients at low and high risk of infections.

The study presented several limitations. First, it was a single-centre study. Second, neither a calculation was made on the number of subjects required nor an interim analysis was conducted since the study was designed by our statistician to be continuous over one year. Specifically, the duration of a year was necessary to enrol an adequate number of patients (i.e., 741) to obtain statistically significant differences among the groups. As a matter of fact, the earlier studies enrolled a number of patients ranging among 2048 and 4472 [18, 25].

Moreover, being an observational study, there was no randomization of patients to the two groups (with and without protocol violation), although the characteristics of patients in the two groups turned out not to be statistically different. Finally, in the study period patients were not screened for S. *aureus* colonization prior to surgery.

Conclusions

The variability in antimicrobial prophylaxis timing significance among results reported in the literature suggests that the association between timing and SSIs is greatly related to the surgical population, the antibiotic(s) and the timing intervals investigated.

Despite some limitations, our study showed that violation of the timing of prophylactic vancomycin administration significantly increased the probability of SSIs and mortality from infectious cause in patients undergoing cardiac surgery.

Abbreviations

BMI: Body mass index; BSI: Bloodstream infection; CABG: Coronary artery bypass graft surgery; CDC: Centers for Disease Control and Prevention; EuroSCORE: European system for cardiac operative risk evaluation; ICU: Intensive care unit; IMA: Internal mammary artery; LOS: Length of stay; LRTI: Lower respiratory tract infection; MRSA: Methicillin-resistant Staphylococcus aureus; SSI: Surgical site infection; UTI: Urinary tract infection

Acknowledgements

We thank all anaesthesiologists, cardiac surgeons, nurses and cardiovascular perfusionists of the Cardiovascular Surgery for their continuous support during the study.

Funding

This work was partially supported by the Regione Piemonte (Italy) (grant No. 2472/DA2001 to PC).

Authors' contributions

PC designed the study and drafted the manuscript. CB participated in the study design, carried out the study and helped to draft the manuscript. RP participated in the study design and performed the statistical analysis. LF participated in the study design and performed the microbiological analysis. GO participated in the study design and revised it critically for important intellectual content. MR participated in the study design and coordination and revised it critically for important intellectual content. All authors read and approved the final manuscript.

Competing interests

The authors declare that they have no competing interests.

Author details

[1]Department of Anesthesia and Intensive Care, S. Giovanni Battista Hospital, University of Turin, Via Giovanni Giolitti 9, 10123 Turin, Italy. [2]Department of Cardiovascular Surgery, S. Giovanni Battista Hospital, University of Turin, Turin, Italy. [3]Nuclear Medicine Unit, S. Giovanni Battista Hospital, University of Turin, Turin, Italy. [4]Microbiology and Virology Laboratory, S. Giovanni Battista Hospital, University of Turin, Turin, Italy. [5]Department of Surgical Sciences, S. Giovanni Battista Hospital, University of Turin, Turin, Italy.

References

1. Ridderstolpe L, Gill H, Granfeldt H, Ahlfeldt H, Rutberg H. Superficial and deep sternal wound complications: incidence, risk factors and mortality. Eur J Cardiothorac Surg. 2001;20:1168–75.
2. Salehi Omran A, Karimi A, Ahmadi SH, Davoodi S, Marzban M, Movahedi N, et al. Superficial and deep sternal wound infection after more than 9000 coronary artery bypass graft (CABG): incidence, risk factors and mortality. BMC Infect Dis. 2007;7:112.
3. Filsoufi F, Castillo JG, Rahmanian PB, Broumand SR, Silvay G, Carpentier A, et al. Epidemiology of deep sternal wound infection in cardiac surgery. J Cardiothorac Vasc Anesth. 2009;23:488–94.
4. Kanafani ZA, Arduino JM, Muhlbaier LH, Kaye KS, Allen KB, Carmeli Y, et al. Incidence of and preoperative risk factors for Staphylococcus aureus

bacteremia and chest wound infection after cardiac surgery. Infect Control Hosp Epidemiol. 2009;30:242–8.

5. Tom TS, Kruse MW, Reichman RT. Update: Methicillin-resistant Staphylococcus aureus screening and decolonization in cardiac surgery. Ann Thorac Surg. 2009;88:695–702.

6. Hillis LD, JL SPKa, Bittl JA, Bridges CR, Byrne JG, et al. 2011 ACCF/AHA guideline for coronary artery bypass graft surgery. A report of the American College of Cardiology Foundation/American Heart Association Task Force on Practice Guidelines. Developed in collaboration with the American Association for Thoracic Surgery, Society of Cardiovascular Anesthesiologists and Society of Thoracic Surgeons. J Am Coll Cardiol. 2011;58:123–210.

7. Classen DC, Evans RS, Pestotnik SL, Horn SD, Menlove RL, Burke JP. The timing of prophylactic administration of antibiotics and the risk of surgical-wound infection. N Engl J Med. 1992;326:281–6.

8. Mangram AJ, Horan TC, Pearson ML, Silver LC, Jarvis WR. Guideline for prevention of surgical site infection, 1999. Centers for disease control and prevention (CDC) hospital infection control practices advisory committee. Am J Infect Control. 1999;27:97–132.

9. Scottish Intercollegiate Guidelines Network. Antibiotic Prophylaxis in Surgery: A National Clinical Guideline. July 2008, updated April 2014. http://www.sign.ac.uk/pdf/sign104.pdf. Accessed 1 Dec 2015.

10. Harbarth S, Huttner B, Gervaz P, Fankhauser C, Chraiti MN, Schrenzel J, et al. Risk factors for methicillin-resistant Staphylococcus aureus surgical site infection. Infect Control Hosp Epidemiol. 2008;29:890–3.

11. Bratzler DW, Hunt DR. The surgical infection prevention and surgical care improvement projects: national initiatives to improve outcomes for patients having surgery. Clin Infect Dis. 2006;43:322–30.

12. Yokoe DS, Mermel LA, Anderson DJ, Arias KM, Burstin H, Calfee DP, et al. A compendium of strategies to prevent healthcare-associated infections in acute care hospitals. Infect Control Hosp Epidemiol. 2008;29:S12–21.

13. Kreter B, Woods M. Antibiotic prophylaxis for cardiothoracic operations. Meta-analysis of thirty years of clinical trials. J Thorac Cardiovasc Surg. 1992;104:590–9.

14. Cotogni P, Barbero C, Rinaldi M. Deep sternal wound infection after cardiac surgery: evidences and controversies. World J Crit Care Med. 2015;4:265–73.

15. Lador A, Nasir H, Mansur N, Sharoni E, Biderman P, Leibovici L, et al. Antibiotic prophylaxis in cardiac surgery: systematic review and meta-analysis. J Antimicrob Chemother. 2012;67:541–50.

16. Engelman RM, Shahian D, Shemin R, Guy TS, Bratzler D, Edwards F, et al. The Society of Thoracic Surgeons practice guideline series: antibiotic prophylaxis in cardiac surgery, part II: antibiotic choice. Ann Thorac Surg. 2007;83:1569–76.

17. Weber WP, Marti WR, Zwahlen M, Misteli H, Rosenthal R, Reck S, et al. The timing of surgical antimicrobial prophylaxis. Ann Surg. 2008;247:918–26.

18. Steinberg JP, Braun BI, Hellinger WC, Kusek L, Bozikis MR, Bush AJ, et al. Timing of antimicrobial prophylaxis and the risk of surgical site infections: results from the trial to reduce antimicrobial prophylaxis errors. Ann Surg. 2009;250:10–6.

19. Hawn MT, Richman JS, Vick CC, Deierhoi RJ, Graham LA, Henderson WG, et al. Timing of surgical antibiotic prophylaxis and the risk of surgical site infection. JAMA Surg. 2013;148:649–57.

20. Miliani K, L'Heriteau F, Astagneau P, INCISO Network Study Group. Non-compliance with recommendations for the practice of antibiotic prophylaxis and risk of surgical site infection: results of a multilevel analysis from the INCISO Surveillance Network. J Antimicrob Chemother. 2009;64:1307–15.

21. Gilbert DN, Moellering RC, Eliopoulos GM, Sande MA. The Sanford guide to antimicrobial therapy. 37th ed. Sperryville: Antimicrobial Therapy, Inc; 2007. p. 160.

22. Edwards FH, Engelman RM, Houck P, Shahian DM, Bridges CR, Society of Thoracic Surgeons. The Society of Thoracic Surgeons practice guideline series: antibiotic prophylaxis in cardiac surgery, part I: duration. Ann Thorac Surg. 2006;81:397–404.

23. Cotogni P, Passera R, Barbero C, Gariboldi A, Moscato D, Izzo G, et al. Intraoperative vancomycin pharmacokinetics in cardiac surgery with or without cardiopulmonary bypass. Ann Pharmacother. 2013;47:455–63.

24. Kritchevsky SB, Braun BI, Bush AJ, Bozikis MR, Kusel L, Burke JP, et al. The effect of a quality improvement collaborative to improve antimicrobial prophylaxis in surgical patients: a randomized trial. Ann Intern Med. 2008;149:472–80.

25. Garey KW, Dao T, Chen H, Amrutkar P, Kumar N, Reiter M, et al. Timing of vancomycin prophylaxis for cardiac surgery patients and the risk of surgical site infections. J Antimicrob Chemother. 2006;58:645–50.

9

Predicting operative mortality in octogenarians for isolated coronary artery bypass grafting surgery

Jessica G. Y. Luc[1], Michelle M. Graham[2,3], Colleen M. Norris[1,2,3], Sadek Al Shouli[1,2], Yugmel S. Nijjar[1] and Steven R. Meyer[1,2*]

Abstract

Background: Available cardiac surgery risk scores have not been validated in octogenarians. Our objective was to compare the predictive ability of the Society of Thoracic Surgeons (STS) score, EuroSCORE I, and EuroSCORE II in elderly patients undergoing isolated coronary artery bypass grafting surgery (CABG).

Methods: All patients who underwent isolated CABG (2002 – 2008) were identified from the Alberta Provincial Project for Outcomes Assessment in Coronary Heart Disease (APPROACH) registry. All patients aged 80 and older ($n = 304$) were then matched 1:2 with a randomly selected control group of patients under age 80 ($n = 608$ of 4732). Risk scores were calculated. Discriminatory accuracy of the risk models was assessed by plotting the areas under the receiver operator characteristic (AUC) and comparing the observed to predicted operative mortality.

Results: Octogenarians had a significantly higher predicted mortality by STS Score ($3 \pm 2\%$ vs. $1 \pm 1\%$; $p < 0.001$), additive EuroSCORE ($8 \pm 3\%$ vs. $4 \pm 3\%$; $p < 0.001$), logistic EuroSCORE ($15 \pm 14\%$ vs. $5 \pm 6\%$; $p < 0.001$), and EuroSCORE II ($4 \pm 3\%$ vs. $2 \pm 2\%$; $p < 0.001$) compared to patients under age 80 years. Observed mortality was 2% and 1% for patients age 80 and older and under age 80, respectively ($p = 0.323$). AUC revealed areas for STS, additive and logistic EuroSCORE I and EuroSCORE II, respectively, for patients age 80 and older (0.671, 0.709, 0.694, 0.794) and under age 80 (0.829, 0.750, 0.785, 0.845).

Conclusion: All risk prediction models assessed overestimated surgical risk, particularly in octogenarians. EuroSCORE II demonstrated better discriminatory accuracy in this population. Inclusion of new variables into these risk models, such as frailty, may allow for more accurate prediction of true operative risk.

Keywords: Cardiovascular research, Coronary artery disease, Risk prediction, Octogenarians

Classification Codes: Cardiovascular Surgery, Coronary Artery Disease, Risk Stratification

* Correspondence: srmeyer@ualberta.ca
[1]Division of Cardiac Surgery, Department of Surgery, Faculty of Medicine and Dentistry, University of Alberta, Edmonton, Canada
[2]Mazankowski Alberta Heart Institute, Edmonton, Canada
Full list of author information is available at the end of the article

Background

Coronary artery disease is a leading cause of morbidity and mortality in octogenarian patients [1, 2]. Octogenarians represent the fastest growing segment of our population; over 40% of the very elderly manifest cardiovascular disease [3]. The indications for coronary artery bypass grafting (CABG) surgery are well defined and the number of octogenarians being referred for surgical coronary revascularization is increasing [4]. Accurate risk stratification and the prediction of operative mortality is essential as this aids the clinical decision-making process, helps estimate the need for resources, facilitates proper patient counseling, informed consent, and allows for monitoring of surgeon and institution performance through risk-adjusted outcomes.

Risk-scoring algorithms based on both patient history and functional status have been established. The most widely used are the Society of Thoracic Surgeons Predicted Risk of Mortality (STS) score and the European System for Cardiac Operative Risk Evaluation (EuroSCORE) [5, 6]. Despite the acceptance of these risk scores in the context of CABG, there is little data on the performance of the revised EuroSCORE II in comparison to the established STS, additive EuroSCORE and the logistic Euroscore. Furthermore, these scores have not been validated to specifically predict operative mortality in octogenarians.

The aim of the current study was to evaluate and compare the performance of the recently introduced EuroSCORE II with its previous version EuroSCORE (additive and logistic) and the STS score in predicting perioperative mortality in patients age 80 and older undergoing isolated CABG at our institution.

Methods

Patients and procedures

We retrospectively reviewed 304 consecutive patients age 80 and older and a randomly selected cohort of adult patients under age 80 (n = 608 of 4732) who underwent isolated CABG between January 2002 and December 2008 at the University of Alberta. The older group was compared in a 1:2 ratio to the younger group. Patients undergoing concomitant surgery (e.g., valve, vascular, or congenital) were excluded. All non-emergent cardiac surgery cases undergo multidisciplinary review at our institution. These multidisciplinary rounds include cardiac surgeons, interventional cardiologists and cardiologists. A comparison ratio of 1:2 was selected instead of 1:1 as our population of elderly patients is modest; a larger control group of younger patients generates a more normally distributed dataset for analysis.

The Alberta Provincial Project for Outcome Assessment in Coronary Heart Disease (APPROACH) database has been previously described [7]. In brief, APPROACH is a prospective clinical data collection initiative capturing all patients undergoing cardiac catheterization or cardiac surgery in the province of Alberta, Canada since 1995. The registry includes detailed individual patient demographic, medical, angiographic, surgical and postoperative information. Preoperative patient demographic and medical variables including risk factors, comorbidities, cardiac diagnostic and surgical procedural information are entered into the dataset. Patients captured by the registry are longitudinally followed for all cardiac-specific investigations, interventions and outcomes. Mortality is tracked through an Alberta Bureau of Vital Statistics data linkage [8]. The University of Alberta Health Research Ethics Board has approved the waiver of patient consent for this data registry (Pro00042669).

The APPROACH database was queried for pre, intra and postoperative data of the patients in this study. Risk scores were then calculated online using the official websites and calculators (STS score: http://riskcalc.sts.org/stswebriskcalc/ #/calculate; additive and logistic EuroSCORE: http://euro-score.org/calcold.html; EuroSCORE II: http://euroscore.org/ calc.html). The simple additive EuroSCORE and the full logistic EuroSCORE, were included because both have been adopted in clinical practice for reasons of simplicity for the additive model and accuracy for the logistic model [9].

Outcomes of interest

The primary outcome of interest was perioperative mortality, defined as any death that occurred during the initial hospitalization or within 30 days of isolated CABG. The expected 30-day mortality based on the calculated STS score, EuroSCORE (additive and logistic), and EuroSCORE II were compared with the observed 30-day mortality.

Statistical analysis

Continuous variables were described as mean and standard deviation and categorical variables as percentages. Comparisons between continuous data were made with student t-test or Mann-Whitney U test and comparisons between categorical data were made with Chi-square or Fisher's exact test where appropriate. Sensitivity and specificity of expected versus observed mortality were summarized by receiver operator curves and the area under the receiver operator characteristic (AUC). Net reclassification improvement (NRI) analysis was also performed to formally assess the various scores accuracy in predicting risk in both age groups. A p-value of less than 0.05 was considered significant. All statistical analyses were performed using Statistical Package for Social Sciences (SPSS Statistics, version 21, Chicago, Illinois).

Results

From January 1, 2002 to December 31, 2008, a total of 4732 patients underwent isolated CABG at the University of Alberta. Of these, 304 patients were aged 80 years or older. Baseline characteristics are outlined in Table 1. In general, elderly patients had more comorbidities, cardiac risk factors and were more likely to undergo emergency surgery. Use of multiple arterial conduits is rare in Alberta. No patients in this octogenarian cohort received a third arterial graft.

Relative to younger patients, those aged 80 and older had a significantly higher mean predicted mortality by the STS Score (3 ± 2% vs. 1 ± 1%; $p < 0.001$), additive EuroSCORE (8 ± 3% vs. 4 ± 3%; p < 0.001), logistic EuroSCORE (15 ± 14% vs. 5 ± 6%; p < 0.001), and EuroSCORE II (4 ± 3% vs. 2 ± 2%; p < 0.001) (Fig. 1). The total observed perioperative mortality of 2% for patients aged 80 years and older was not significantly different from the observed perioperative mortality of 1% for patients under age 80 ($p = 0.323$).

The receiver operator characteristic (ROC) for both patient groups are shown in Fig. 2a and b respectively. Patient's age 80 and older had an AUC for the STS score of (0.672; $p = 0.151$, 95% confidence interval [CI] 0.459 to 0.883), additive EuroSCORE (0.709; $p = 0.079$, 95% CI 0.523 to 0.896), logistic EuroSCORE (0.694; $p = 0.104$, 95% CI 0.499 to 0.889) and EuroSCORE II (0.794; $p = 0.014$, 95% CI 0.696 to 0.893). Patients under age 80 had an AUC for the STS score of (0.829; $p = 0.003$, 95% CI 0.710 to 0.947), additive EuroSCORE (0.750; $p = 0.023$, 95% CI 0.544 to 0.955), logistic EuroSCORE (0.785; $p = 0.010$, 95% CI 0.585 to 0.985) and EuroSCORE II (0.845; $p = 0.002$, 95% CI 0.709 to 0.980). The p-value under the AUC represents the ability and accuracy of the score in predicting perioperative mortality in patients who undergo CABG surgery. Overall, all scores assessed underperformed patients age 80 and older compared, with EuroSCORE II demonstrating the best predictive ability in this group.

The net reclassification improvement index (NRI) of STS compared to EuroSCORE II was calculated. Area under the curve analysis demonstrates that the areas of the three curves are similar for patients under age 80, but different for patients age 80 and over where EuroSCORE II had the largest area. The Delong test indicates that the difference of the AUC between the three curves is not significant for both groups. However, NRI analysis reveals that EuroSCORE adds 16% reclassification improvement compared to STS for age under 80, and 67% improvement for in those age 80 and older. The 67% improvement results from ability of EuroSCORE II to discriminate all 6 deaths, while STS is able to discriminate only half (3 out of 6) of deaths.

Discussion

We demonstrate in a large series of consecutive octogenarians undergoing isolated CABG that EuroSCORE II had the best performance for risk assessment among the tools available. However, the expected mortality calculated by all four risk scores overestimated perioperative risk for patients of all ages, most particularly in octogenarians.

Our study is unique in that it includes all four risk scores with a focused evaluation of their performance in isolated CABG surgery. This is particularly relevant given that octogenarians represent a growing proportion of patients being referred for CABG surgery [10]. Early studies report cardiac surgery operative mortality rates of up to 11% [11, 12]. Refinements in surgical technique and perioperative management has resulted in

Table 1 Baseline Demographics

Variable	Under Age 80 (n = 608)	Age 80 and Older(n = 304)	P Value
Age	63.8	82.1	<0.001¶
Gender (Female)	92 (15.1)	78 (25.7)	0.001¶
Body Surface Area	1.94 ± 0.17	1.86 ± 0.18	<0.001¶
Weight (kg)	80.7 ± 12.5	74.8 ± 11.9	<0.001¶
Renal Impairment	116 (19.0)	55 (18.0)	0.044¶
Hypertension	452 (74.3)	243 (79.9)	0.062
Hypercholesterolemia	519 (85.4)	211 (69.4)	0.839
Diabetes	204 (33.6)	76 (25.0)	0.008¶
Extracardiac Arteriopathy	48 (7.9)	31 (10.2)	0.244
Reduced Left Ventricular Ejection Fraction	340 (55.9)	137 (45.1)	0.001¶
Cerebrovascular Disease	44 (7.2)	40 (13.2)	<0.001¶
Chronic Obstructive Pulmonary Disease	65 (10.7)	41 (13.5)	<0.001¶
Emergency Surgery	16 (2.6)	12 (3.9)	0.001¶

Continuous data are reported as mean ± standard deviation; categorical data are (%) are presented by frequency. ¶ Indicates significance p <V 0.05

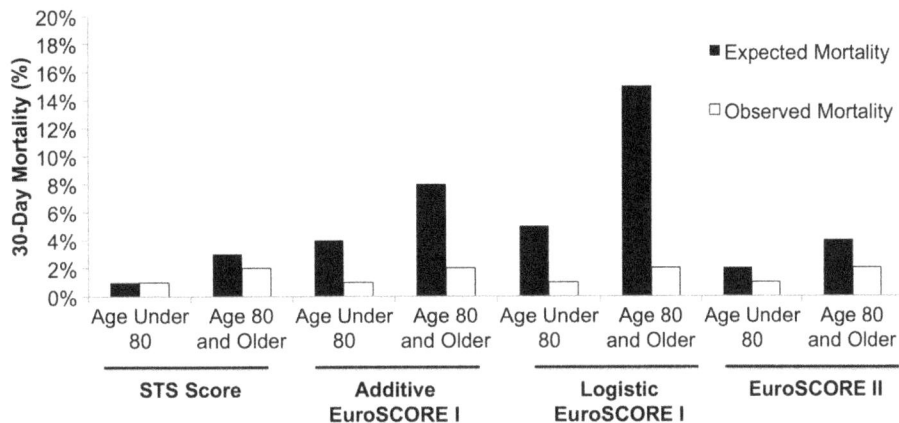

Fig. 1 STS risk score, additive EuroSCORE, logistic EuroSCORE, and EuroSCORE II overestimates operative mortality in patients age 80 and older. Expected 30-day mortality was compared to observed 30-day mortality in patients under the age of 80 and patients age 80 and older who underwent isolated CABG

significantly improved outcomes [13], as well, differences in observed operative mortality in other reports may stem from inherent country or population specific outcomes [14, 15]. We report a low observed perioperative mortality of 2% in patients age 80 and older which is not different from existing contemporary reports [4, 16, 17]. Although elderly patients have worse early outcomes compared to younger patients, long-term outcomes for octogenarians at our institution after CABG are similar to, if not better than, the age-adjusted Canadian population. These are demonstrated by previously published reports on our cohort examining intermediate and long-term survival post-operatively for octogenarians compared to younger subjects [4, 18, 19].

Accurate risk stratification facilitates improved patient selection, prevents complications [20], improves patient quality of life and can justify the cost effectiveness of the procedure [21]. However, risk models, although helpful and objective for operative risk assessment and clinical decision-making, are not without their limitations. The original EuroSCORE and EuroSCORE II were developed with a patient population mean age of 62.5 years and 64.9 years, respectively [13, 22]. Our results show that all scores assessed significantly overestimated operative risk in octogenarians, and were well calibrated in patients under age 80. This identified imprecision in operative risk prediction has important implications for clinical decision making in elderly patients.

Frailty has been shown to be an independent predictor for both postoperative complications and in-hospital mortality after adjusting for age [23]. It is estimated that 20% of octogenarians are frail [24]. Although considered difficult to quantify as compared to the comorbidity-based risk assessment models currently in use, several scores have emerged as an attempt to assess frailty including the Edmonton Frailty Scale, Comprehensive Assessment of Frailty test,

Fried Frailty Scale and others [24–26] These frailty scores are a multidimensional assessment of health and functional status incorporating sociodemographic, biomedical, cognitive capacity, independence with daily activities, social support and mood [27, 28].

Incorporating a quantitative measure of the degree of frailty can introduce objectivity to the assessment of biological status to complement conventional comorbidity risk assessment and improve the accuracy of operative risk assessment in the elderly. This would allow more accurate stratification of risk than current models and aid in selecting the most appropriate modality of intervention to best optimize outcomes for patients. In an age 70 and older population, Prudon et al. [29] demonstrated that the addition of gait speed to logistic EuroSCORE improved the accuracy of the model. Sundermann et al. [24] used a frailty score in addition to conventional risk scores and found frailty to only moderately correlate with STS and EuroSCORE risk models. Other investigators have demonstrated the utility of a frailty score in the preoperative assessment of their patients [24, 30]. Afilalo et al. demonstrate that both frailty and disability (as defined by a 5-m gait speed ≥ 6 seconds and the presence of 3 or more impairments on the Nagi scale) are complementary and additive to existing risk scores where inclusion of them improved the discrimination of the STS score [30]. Thus, incorporation of various risk factors specific to the elderly population as measures of physiological vulnerability may improve the effectiveness of cardiac surgical risk models [31].

Frailty is an emerging concept; collaborative efforts towards defining the optimal method towards measuring frailty and disability deserve further exploration. Multidisciplinary teams involving cardiac surgery, cardiology, geriatric medicine, physiotherapy and occupational therapy may help address the diverse elements

a

ROC Curve – Under Age 80

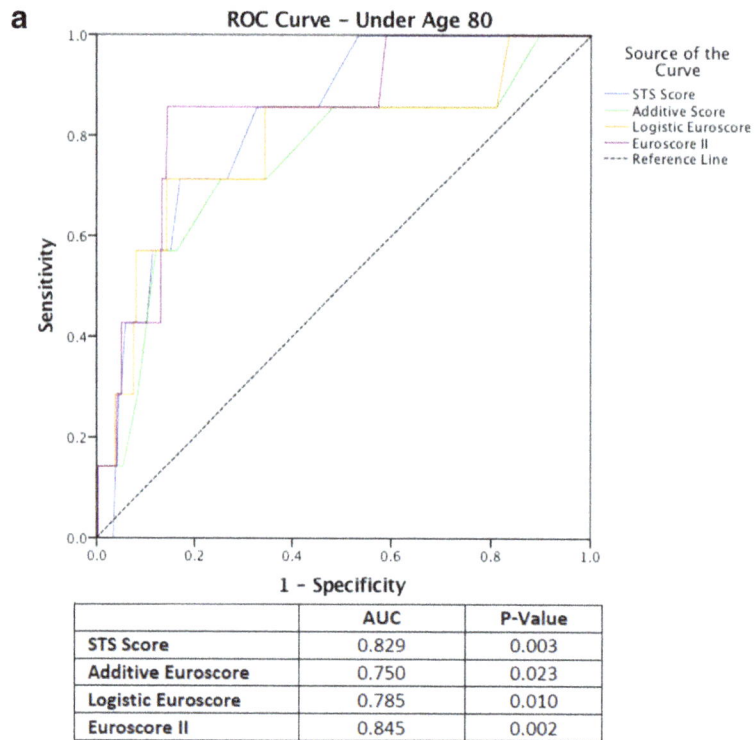

	AUC	P-Value
STS Score	0.829	0.003
Additive Euroscore	0.750	0.023
Logistic Euroscore	0.785	0.010
Euroscore II	0.845	0.002

b

ROC Curve – Age 80 and Older

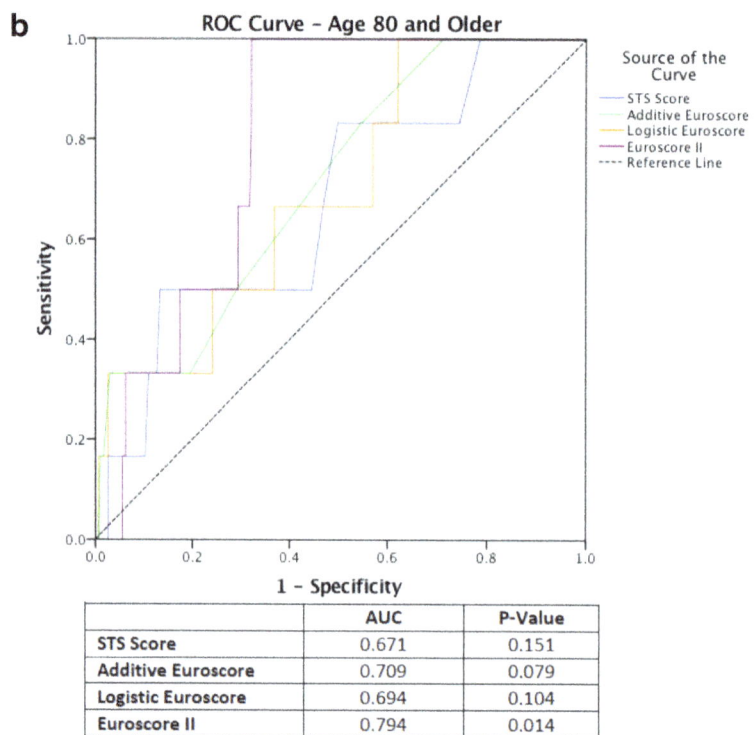

	AUC	P-Value
STS Score	0.671	0.151
Additive Euroscore	0.709	0.079
Logistic Euroscore	0.694	0.104
Euroscore II	0.794	0.014

Fig. 2 EuroSCORE II was superior to STS and EuroSCORE I in predicting operative mortality for both patients under and over the age of 80. Receiver operator characteristic curve for STS, additive EuroSCORE, logistic EuroSCORE and EuroSCORE II predicted risk of operative mortality in patients (**a**) under age 80 and (**b**) age 80 and older

specific to the elderly that contribute to increased risk [32]. A 64-slice-coronary computed tomography shows promise as a non-invasive alternative to the standard coronary angiography to detect CABG graft stenosis [33]. However, in a frail octogenarian population, symptoms and quality of life should be the driver for any further invasive or non-invasive investigations.

Limitations

There are several limitations to this study. First, this is a single institution study, thus our results may not apply to those from other institutions and countries. Second, the present study only included patients undergoing isolated CABG and the results cannot be extrapolated to patients undergoing other cardiac surgical procedures. Third, EuroSCORE II has introduced two variables, poor mobility and pulmonary artery pressure, which are not consistently recorded in the APPROACH database; therefore all patients were analyzed as not scoring for this risk factor. However, if these risks were present in our entire elderly cohort, the estimated risk of surgery would have further increased. Finally, our intention was neither to develop a new score nor to investigate the impact of individual variables on specific postoperative complications. While the predictive value for mortality differs considerably from that of morbidity for most of the variables included in the risk models [34], our analysis focused on the discriminatory ability of these scores in predicting perioperative mortality – which was what these risk scores were originally designed to achieve.

Conclusion

Currently, all risk prediction models overestimate surgical risk, particularly in octogenarians. The EuroSCORE II demonstrated better discriminatory accuracy for predicting operative mortality than STS, additive and logistic EuroSCORE in this population. Inclusion of new variables into these risk models, such as frailty, that are of particular interest in the elderly, may allow for more accurate prediction of true operative mortality and thus lead to improved decision making in this important group of patients.

Abbreviations
APPROACH: Alberta Provincial Project for Outcomes Assessment in Coronary Heart Disease; AUROC: Areas under the receiver operator characteristic; CABG: Coronary artery bypass grafting; EuroSCORE: European System for Cardiac Operative Risk Evaluation; STS: Society of Thoracic Surgeons

Acknowledgements
None.

Funding
None.

Authors' contributions
JGYL contributed to data collection, data analysis/interpretation, drafting and critical revision of the article. MMG contributed to concept/design, critical revision and approval of the article. CMN contributed to data analysis and statistics. SAS contributed to concept/design, data collection, data analysis/interpretation and drafting of the article. YSN contributed to data collection. SRM contributed to concept/design, data analysis/interpretation, critical revision and approval of the article. All authors read and approved the final manuscript.

Competing interests
The authors declare that they have no competing interests.

Author details
[1]Division of Cardiac Surgery, Department of Surgery, Faculty of Medicine and Dentistry, University of Alberta, Edmonton, Canada. [2]Mazankowski Alberta Heart Institute, Edmonton, Canada. [3]Division of Cardiology, Department of Medicine, Faculty of Medicine and Dentistry, University of Alberta, Edmonton, Canada.

References
1. Graham MM, Ghali WA, Faris PD, Galbraith PD, Norris CM, Knudtson ML. Investigators ftAPPfOAiCHD: survival after coronary revascularization in the elderly. Circulation. 2002;105(20):2378–84.
2. Aziz A, Lee AM, Pasque MK, Lawton JS, Moazami N, Damiano RJ, Moon MR. Evaluation of revascularization subtypes in octogenarians undergoing coronary artery bypass grafting. Circulation. 2009;120(11 suppl 1):S65–9.
3. Kurlansky P. Do octogenarians benefit from coronary artery bypass surgery: a question with a rapidly changing answer? Curr Opin Cardiol. 2012;27(6):611–9.
4. Saxena A, Dinh DT, Yap CH, Reid CM, Billah B, Smith JA, Shardey GC, Newcomb AE. Critical analysis of early and late outcomes after isolated coronary artery bypass surgery in elderly patients. Ann Thorac Surg. 2011; 92(5):1703–11.
5. Nilsson J, Algotsson L, Höglund P, Lührs C, Brandt J. Comparison of 19 preoperative risk stratification models in open-heart surgery. Eur Heart J. 2006; 27(7):867–74.
6. Nashef SAM, Roques F, Hammill BG, Peterson ED, Michel P, Grover FL, Wyse RKH, Ferguson TB. Validation of European system for cardiac operative risk evaluation (EuroSCORE) in north American cardiac surgery. Eur J Cardiothorac Surg. 2002;22(1):101–5.
7. Ghali WAKM. Overview of the Alberta provincial project for outcome assessment in coronary heart disease. On behalf of the APPROACH investigators. Can J Cardiol. 2000;16(10):1225–30.
8. Norris CM, Ghali WA, Knudtson ML, Naylor CD, Saunders LD: Dealing with missing data in observational health care outcome analyses. J Clin Epidemiol 2000, 53(4):377-383.
9. Zingone B, Pappalardo A, Dreas L. Logistic versus additive EuroSCORE. A comparative assessment of the two models in an independent population sample. Eur J Cardiothorac Surg. 2004;26(6):1134–40.
10. Statistics Canada: Annual demographic estimates: Canada, provinces and territories 2012.
11. Ben-Gal Y, Finkelstein A, Banai S, Medalion B, Weisz G, Genereux P, Moshe S, Pevni D, Aviram G, Uretzky G. Surgical myocardial revascularization versus percutaneous coronary intervention with drug-eluting stents in octogenarian patients. Heart Surg Forum. 2012;15(4):E204–9.
12. Ghanta RK, Shekar PS, McGurk S, Rosborough DM, Aranki SF. Nonelective cardiac surgery in the elderly: is it justified? J Thorac Cardiovasc Surg. 2010; 140(1):103–9. 109 e101
13. Drury NENS. Outcomes of cardiac surgery in the elderly. Expert Rev Cardiovasc Ther. 2006;4(4):535–42.
14. Gutacker N, Bloor K, Cookson R, Garcia-Armesto S, Bernal-Delgado E. Comparing hospital performance within and across countries: an illustrative study of coronary artery bypass graft surgery in England and Spain. Eur J Pub Health. 2015;25(Suppl 1):28–34.
15. Rangrass G, Ghaferi AA, Dimick JB. Explaining racial disparities in outcomes after cardiac surgery: the role of hospital quality. JAMA Surg. 2014;149(3):223–7.

16. Nicolini F, Contini GA, Fortuna D, Pacini D, Gabbieri D, Vignali L, Campo G, Manari A, Zussa C, Guastaroba P, et al. Coronary artery surgery versus percutaneous coronary intervention in octogenarians: long-term results. Ann Thorac Surg. 2015;99(2):567–74.

17. Yanagawa B, Algarni KD, Yau TM, Rao V, Brister SJ. Improving results for coronary artery bypass graft surgery in the elderly. Eur J Cardiothorac Surg. 2012;42(3):507–12.

18. Wang W, Bagshaw SM, Norris CM, Zibdawi R, Zibdawi M, MacArthur R. Association between older age and outcome after cardiac surgery: a population-based cohort study. J Cardiothorac Surg. 2014;9(1):177.

19. Baskett RBK, Ghali W, Norris C, Maas T, Maitland A, Ross D, Forgie R, Hirsch G. Outcomes in octogenarians undergoing coronary artery bypass grafting. CMAJ. 2005;127(9):1183–6.

20. Toumpoulis IK, Anagnostopoulos CE, DeRose JJ, Swistel DG. Does EuroSCORE predict length of stay and specific postoperative complications after coronary artery bypass grafting? Int J Cardiol. 2005;105(1):19–25.

21. Pinna Pintor P, Bobbio M, Colangelo S, Veglia F, Marras R, Diena M. Can EuroSCORE predict direct costs of cardiac surgery? Eur J Cardiothorac Surg. 2003;23(4):595–8.

22. Nashef SA, Roques F, Sharples LD, Nilsson J, Smith C, Goldstone AR, Lockowandt U. EuroSCORE II. Eur J Cardiothorac Surg. 2012;41(4):734–44. discussion 744-735

23. Lee DHBK, Martin BJ, Yip AM, Hirsch GM. Frail patients are at increased risk for mortality and prolonged institutional care after cardiac surgery. Circulation. 2010;121(8):973–8.

24. Sundermann S, Dademasch A, Praetorius J, Kempfert J, Dewey T, Falk V, Mohr FW, Walther T. Comprehensive assessment of frailty for elderly high-risk patients undergoing cardiac surgery. Eur J Cardiothorac Surg. 2011;39(1):33–7.

25. Rockwood K, Song X, MacKnight C, Bergman H, Hogan DB, McDowell I, Mitnitski A. A global clinical measure of fitness and frailty in elderly people. CMAJ. 2005;173(5):489–95.

26. Graham MM, Galbraith PD, O'Neill D, Rolfson DB, Dando C, Norris CM. Frailty and outcome in elderly patients with acute coronary syndrome. Can J Cardiol. 2013;29(12):1610–5.

27. Wilson JF. Frailty–and its dangerous effects–might be preventable. Ann Intern Med. 2004;141(6):489–92.

28. Ravaglia G, Forti P, Lucicesare A, Pisacane N, Rietti E, Patterson C. Development of an easy prognostic score for frailty outcomes in the aged. Age Ageing. 2008;37(2):161–6.

29. Prudon I, Noyez L, van Swieten H, Scheffer GJ. Is gait speed improving performance of the EuroSCORE II for prediction of early mortality and major morbidity in elderly? J Cardiovasc Surg. 2014;57(4):592–7.

30. Afilalo J, Mottillo S, Eisenberg MJ, Alexander KP, Noiseux N, Perrault LP, Morin J-F, Langlois Y, Ohayon SM, Monette J, et al. Addition of frailty and disability to cardiac surgery risk scores identifies elderly patients at high risk of mortality or major morbidity. Circulation: Cardiovascular Quality and Outcomes. 2012;5(2):222–8.

31. Dupuis JY. Predicting outcomes in cardiac surgery: risk stratification matters? Curr Opin Cardiol. 2008;23(6):560–7.

32. Teo KK, Cohen E, Buller C, Hassan A, Carere R, Cox JL, Ly H, Fedak PW, Chan K, Legare JF, et al. Canadian cardiovascular society/Canadian Association of Interventional Cardiology/Canadian Society of Cardiac Surgery position statement on revascularization–multivessel coronary artery disease. Can J Cardiol. 2014;30(12):1482–91.

33. Barbero U, Iannaccone M, d'Ascenzo F, Barbero C, Mohamed A, Annone U, Benedetto S, Celentani D, Gagliardi M, Moretti C, et al. 64 slice-coronary computed tomography sensitivity and specificity in the evaluation of coronary artery bypass graft stenosis: a meta-analysis. Int J Cardiol. 2016;216:52–7.

34. Geissler HJ, Holzl P, Marohl S, Kuhn-Regnier F, Mehlhorn U, Sudkamp M, de Vivie ER. Risk stratification in heart surgery: comparison of six score systems. Eur J Cardiothorac Surg. 2000;17(4):400–6.

10

Minimally invasive direct coronary artery bypass grafting with an improved rib spreader and a new-shaped cardiac stabilizer: results of 200 consecutive cases in a single institution

Yunpeng Ling[1*], Liming Bao[2], Wei Yang[3], Yu Chen[3] and Qing Gao[3]

Abstract

Background: Performing minimally invasive direct coronary artery bypass (MIDCAB) grafting via small chest incisions on a beating heart is challenging. We report our experiences of MIDCAB with the utilization of both an improved rib spreader to harvest the left internal mammary artery (LIMA) and a new-shaped cardiac stabilizer to facilitate LIMA-left anterior descending (LAD) coronary anastomosis.

Methods: Between May 2012 and June 2104, a total of 200 patients who were consecutively operated on in this period were enrolled in this study. Data reported included demographic information, preoperative clinical and cardiac status, LIMA harvest time, postoperative in-hospital outcomes, and 30-day mortality.

Results: The average LIMA harvest time was 43 min. The mean age was 62.59 ± 10.19 years, and 45 of the 200 were females. The 30-day mortality was 0.5 % (one patient) due to perioperative myocardial infarction. Duration of mechanical ventilation and length of stay in intensive care unit was 9.27 ± 7.65 and 24.27 ± 17.85 h, respectively. The unit of packed RBC transfusion was 0.79 ± 1.58. Postoperative atrial fibrillation was observed in 14 (7 %) patients. There was no postoperative stroke, renal failure, or incision complication.

Conclusion: Performing MIDCAB with the improved retractor and stabilizer utilized in this study showed favorable outcomes in terms of harvesting the LIMA, postoperative morbidities, and 30-day mortality.

Keywords: Minimally invasive direct coronary artery bypass (MIDCAB), Beating heart, Off-pump coronary artery surgery, Rib spreader, Cardiac stabilizer

Background

Minimally invasive direct coronary artery bypass (MIDCAB) grafting attempts to achieve adequate coronary artery revascularization in a less invasive manner than conventional coronary artery bypass grafting (CABG). Unlike conventional revascularization techniques, which are highly invasive due to the use of a large incision (sternotomy) and cardiopulmonary bypass (CPB), MIDCAB limits invasiveness by employing a small incision (thoracotomy) and by operating on the beating heart to avoid the need for CPB [1]. By limiting invasiveness in these ways, MIDCAB can reduce the risk of complications such as infection and stroke [2]. In comparison to conventional CABG and off-pump CABG (via a sternotomy), MIDCAB can improve early post-operative quality of life [3] and recovery time [4], respectively.

While MIDCAB can lead to favorable outcomes, performing coronary anastomosis via a small chest incision on a beating heart can be challenging [5]. This makes it difficult to accomplish two key aspects of the MIDCAB procedure. The first pertains to obtaining an adequate length of left internal mammary artery (LIMA) [6] and

* Correspondence: micsling@163.com
[1]Department of Cardiac Surgery, Peking University Third Hospital, Beijing, China
Full list of author information is available at the end of the article

the second is in regard to adequately stabilizing the wall of the beating heart, without adversely affecting hemodynamics or injuring the myocardium [7]. To overcome these difficulties, a variety of retractors and cardiac stabilizers have been utilized, but there is interest in improving their design [8].

Recently, we started utilizing a Fehling retractor (Fehling, Germany), a rib spreader, to harvest the LIMA under direct vision. Compared to existing retractors, this improved retractor allows for an expanded field of vision and enhances LIMA exposure [9]. Additionally, we started using a newly developed stabilizer during MIDCAB. Compared to existing stabilizers, this stabilizer has a better shape to facilitate anastomosing the deeply located left anterior descending (LAD) coronary artery, and can be applied with light pressure, thereby reducing the risk of adverse hemodynamic effects and myocardial injury. In theory, these new and improved devices might lead to improved patient outcomes during MIDCAB, but empirical data are needed to fully assess this issue. Accordingly, the present study reported outcomes in patients who underwent MIDCAB using both the Fehling retractor and the improved cardiac stabilizer.

Methods

This descriptive, non-experimental study included a total of 200 consecutive patients, who were scheduled to undergo a MIDCAB operation at our institution between May 2012 and June 2014. All patients were treated by a single surgeon at the Department of Cardiac Surgery of Peking University People's Hospital. The study was approved by the institutional ethics committee of the Department of Cardiac Surgery of Peking University People's Hospital, and all study patients provided written informed consent prior to surgery.

Surgical procedures and technique

Double-cavity tracheal cannulas were used along with general anesthesia. Patients were placed in the supine position, with the left chest raised by 30°. A 5–6 cm surgical incision was then made in the area of the fourth or fifth rib, and the thoracic cavity was entered. To enable LIMA harvesting, a specialized suspensory internal mammary artery retraction system was utilized (Fig. 1). This retractor offers advantages compared to other retractors in that it can integrally raise the left chest wall, thereby avoiding excessive traction of local ribs while simultaneously providing a good operative field to facilitate obtaining adequate LIMA. LIMA was harvested from the upper segment to the lower segment, and LIMA branches were clipped using a pen titanium clamp.

Beating heart LIMA-LAD anastomosis was facilitated by a heart stabilizer specially designed for MIDCAB procedures (HK, Figs. 2 and 3). This stabilizer is unique in that its presser foot has an "L"-shape, which is particularly

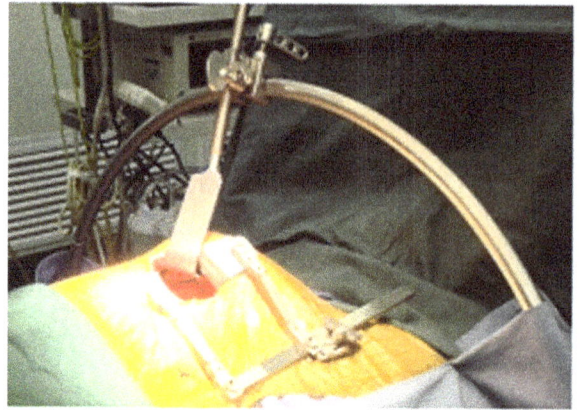
Fig. 1 Suspensory internal mammary artery retraction system

advantageous for procedures performed within a deep space, such as MIDCAB. A second advantage of this stabilizer is that it can be placed on a rib retractor without an external fixator. Because of these two advantages, the stabilizer's presser foot only needs to be in light contact with the epicardium to achieve stability through negative pressure suction. This light contact limits squeezing pressure on the heart, and thereby reduces the risk of circulatory instability. Additionally, the stabilizer has a reduced number of adsorption holes and a reduced adsorption area on the sucker, both of which help to limit the myocardial area that could potentially be damaged by the stabilizer. After incising the coronary artery, routine coronary artery bypass grafting was performed, and 8-0 prolene lines were utilized to perform a continuous suture. All of the 200

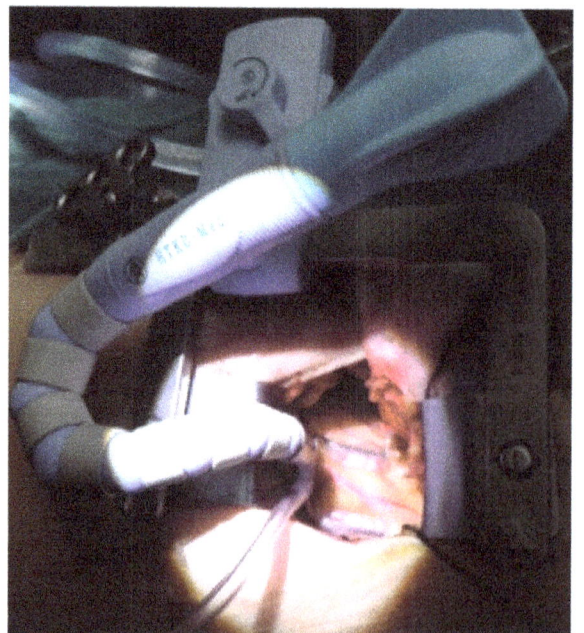
Fig. 2 L-shaped suction stabilizer foot

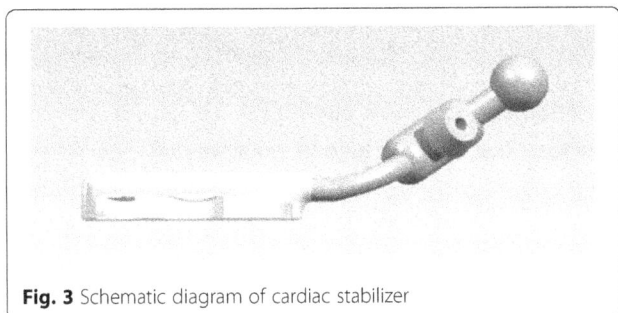

Fig. 3 Schematic diagram of cardiac stabilizer

study subjects underwent LIMA-LAD single bypass during the MIDCAB.

Data collection

Prior to surgery, subjects' height and weight were measured and questionnaires were administered to collect patient's age, gender, history of medical conditions, and history of cardiovascular procedures. Pre-operative measurements were made of each patient's ejection fraction and angiographic status and stored in a hospital database for subsequent access. Study personnel also collected data on procedure duration and other in-hospital outcomes and complications. After the patients were discharged from the hospital, they were followed up as outpatients to obtain the information regarding 30-day mortality. Data were available on all 200 patients. Patient data were examined and presented by descriptive statistics. Setting the Type I error rate at 0.05 and the drop-out rate at 10 %, a power analysis [10] showed that to detect a proportion of 0.07, a sample size of 194 patients would be sufficient to achieve a statistical power of 80 % at a 5 % significance level. This study included a total of 200 patients, which satisfied the required sample based on the post hoc analysis.

Results

The average LIMA harvest time was 43 min. The preoperative characteristics of the patients are displayed in Table 1. The patients included 138 individuals that received MIDCAB alone and 62 individuals that underwent hybrid procedure (MIDCAB for LAD, plus percutaneous coronary intervention (PCI) for other blood vessels). The mean age was 62.59 ± 10.19 years, and 45 of the 200 were females.

Table 2 shows the in-hospital outcomes and 30-day mortality. One (0.5 %) patient died within 30 days due to perioperative myocardial infarction (MI). Duration of mechanical ventilation was 9.27 ± 7.65 h and length of stay in intensive care unit was 24.27 ± 17.85 h. The unit of packed RBC transfusion was 0.79 ± 1.58. Postoperative atrial fibrillation (PAF) was observed in 14 (7 %) patients. No patient had experienced stroke, renal failure, or incision complication.

Table 1 Preoperative patient characteristics (N = 200)

	MIDCAB	Hybrid	Total
	(n = 138)	(n = 62)	(N = 200)
Age, year	63.65 ± 10.48	60.24 ± 9.18	62.59 ± 10.19
Sex, N (%) of female	35 (25.4 %)	10 (16.1 %)	45 (22.5 %)
Height, cm	167.08 ± 7.4	168.3 ± 6.32	167.45 ± 7.1
Weight, kg	70.69 ± 10.53	71.73 ± 9.52	71.01 ± 10.21
Hypertension, N (%)	80 (58.0 %)	26 (41.9 %)	106 (53.0 %)
Diabetes mellitus, N (%)	40 (29.0 %)	27 (43.5 %)	67 (33.5 %)
Smoking, N (%)	63 (45.7 %)	33 (53.2 %)	96 (48.0 %)
Hypercholesterolemia, N (%)	20 (14.5 %)	9 (14.5 %)	29 (14.5 %)
Old MI, N (%)	40 (29.0 %)	17 (27.4 %)	57 (28.5 %)
PCI history, N (%)	17 (12.3 %)	0 (0.0 %)	17 (8.5 %)
Renal insufficiency, N (%)	4 (2.9 %)	0 (0.0 %)	4 (2.0 %)
NYHA grade 1-2, N (%)	120 (87.0 %)	55 (88.7 %)	175 (87.5 %)
NYHA grade 3, N (%)	18 (13.0 %)	7 (11.3 %)	25 (12.5 %)
LVEF, N (%)			
> 55 %	114 (82.6 %)	52 (83.9 %)	166 (83.0 %)
46–55 %	16 (11.6 %)	3 (4.8 %)	19 (9.5 %)
36–45 %	7 (5.1 %)	6 (9.7 %)	13 (6.5 %)
≤ 35 %	1 (0.7 %)	1 (1.6 %)	2 (1.0 %)
LVEDd, mm	50.16 ± 5.96	50.52 ± 5.76	50.27 ± 5.89
Single-vessel disease	89 (64.5 %)	0 (0.0 %)	89 (44.5 %)
Left main or multi-vessel disease	49 (35.5 %)	62 (100.0 %)	111 (55.5 %)

LVEF, left ventricular ejection fractions; LVEDd, left ventricular end diastolic diameter; MI, myocardial infarction; NYHA, New York Heart Association; PCI, Percutaneous coronary intervention

Discussion

In this study of the MIDCAB procedure using an improved retractor and stabilizer, we found the following in-hospital outcomes: an average LIMA harvest time of 43 min, a mean duration of mechanical ventilation of 9 h,

Table 2 In-hospital clinical outcomes and 30-day mortality (N = 200)

	MIDCAB	Hybrid	Total
	(n = 138)	(n = 62)	(N = 200)
30-day mortality, N (%)	1 (0.7 %)	0 (0.0 %)	1 (0.5 %)
Perioperative MI, N (%)	1 (0.7 %)	0 (0.0 %)	1 (0.5 %)
Duration of mechanical ventilation, hour	9.93 ± 8.65	7.79 ± 4.43	9.27 ± 7.65
LOS in ICU, hour	24.17 ± 17.83	24.48 ± 18.03	24.27 ± 17.85
PRBC, units	0.86 ± 1.63	0.61 ± 1.47	0.79 ± 1.58
PAF, N (%)	10 (7.2 %)	4 (6.5 %)	14 (7.0 %)
Stroke, N (%)	0 (0.0 %)	0 (0.0 %)	0 (0.0 %)
Renal failure, N (%)	0 (0.0 %)	0 (0.0 %)	0 (0.0 %)
Incision complications, N (%)	0 (0.0 %)	0 (0.0 %)	0 (0.0 %)

ICU, intensive care unit; LOS, length of stay; MI, myocardial infarction; PAF, postoperative atrial fibrillation; PRBC, packed red blood cell

and a mean ICU stay of 24 h. PAF occurred in only 7 % of the patients, and there was no postoperative stroke, renal failure, or incision complications. The 30-day mortality rate was 0.5 %. Together, these data suggest that performing MIDCAB with the improved retractor and stabilizer used in this study can lead to favorable outcomes.

The MIDCAB procedure was introduced into the surgical literature in 1995 [11]. Subsequently, MIDCAB was adopted by various universities and hospitals in Europe and America [12]. Reports indicate that MIDCAB not only has comparable patency rates with off-pump CABG (via sternotomy) [13] and conventional CABG [14] but leads to favorable outcomes such as shorter hospitalization [4], faster recovery [4], and less need for blood transfusion [15]. Initially, MIDCAB procedures were performed using chest wall retraction under direct vision. However, retraction of the chest wall could lead to postoperative pain and obtaining LIMA under direct vision could be technically challenging. Consequently, some centers started to perform MIDCAB using robotic surgery, yet the robotically assisted approach has a significant learning curve and major costs [11]. As such, MIDCAB using chest wall retraction under direct vision remains a reasonable, affordable approach for developing nations [16, 17] such as China, but concerns remain about pain due to the retraction and about hemodynamic instability and myocardial injury due to the use of cardiac stabilizers.

To address concerns about retraction-associated pain, hemodynamic instability, and myocardial injury, we performed MIDCAB operations during the past two years using an improved retractor and a new-shaped cardiac stabilizer. The retractor is a suspensory internal mammary artery retraction system that facilitates obtaining LIMA under direct vision. In particular, this retractor raises the anterior chest wall integrally, which allows the surgeon to work within a good operative space without having to retract the chest wall excessively. This allows for adequate LIMA harvesting while limiting pain due to retraction. The newly developed stabilizer has an L-shaped presser foot, the shape of which is advantageous for operating within the deep but narrow opening in which MIDCAB procedures take place; furthermore, the stabilizer can be placed on a rib spreader without an external fixator. As such, the stabilizer need only exert light pressure on the epicardium in order to achieve adequate coronary stabilization through negative pressure suction. In this way, the stabilizer reduces the risk of adverse hemodynamic events. Moreover, the stabilizer has a relatively small number of adsorption holes covering a relatively small area on the sucker, and therefore, reduces the area of myocardium that is at risk of damage from stabilizer-induced contact.

Data from our study suggest that MIDCAB procedures performed with the improved retractor and stabilizer

had favorable outcomes. The average time to obtain LIMA was 43 min, which is shorter than in some studies using robotic devices. Fujita et al. successfully performed MIDCAB surgery with robotic LIMA harvesting in 30/33 patients; their average harvest time was 68 min [18]. In another report of robotic endoscopic LIMA harvesting in 100 cases, the reported median harvest time was 48 min; however, there was a significant learning curve so that the harvest time decreased with experience, from 140 min in the first 10 cases to 40 min in the last 10 cases [19]. The harvest time of 43 min in the current study using an improved retractor and stabilizer compares favorably with these two reports using robotic techniques.

Internal mammary artery injuries were not found in any of the patients in the current study. In Fujita's study, 3/33 patients (9 %) had bleeding from the LIMA requiring conversion to a median sternotomy [18]. Additionally, there were 4 cases of LIMA injury in Oehlinger's series, 3 (6 %) during the first half of their experience and 1 (2 %) during the second half. Additionally, one patient required median sternotomy because of LIMA injury during robotic harvesting [19]. Thus, the technique in the current study provided better results in terms of arterial injuries compared with these prior studies using robotic techniques.

Mechanical ventilation is another parameter of concern. A retrospective analysis of 217 patients who underwent MIDCAB in Germany was performed with a focus on fast-track recovery [20]. In that study, extubation was performed immediately after surgery in 182 (83.9 %) patients, only 8 of whom required re-intubation within one hour of arrival in the ICU. Of the remaining 35 patients, 31 required ventilation for <24 h, and 4 patients required >72 h of ventilation [20]. Another group in Germany compared their results for patients undergoing surgery with a full sternotomy (OPCAB, $n = 44$) and those undergoing MIDCAB procedures (n = 58); they generally found that MIDCAB was more challenging and had worse results. For example, although there was no perioperative mortality in either group, time on the ventilator was longer in the MIDCAB compared with the OPCAB group (29 ± 109 h vs 10 ± 6 h, NS) [21]. The time in the ICU was 57 ± 129 h vs 32 ± 14 h for the OPCAB and MIDCAB groups, respectively [21]. Bisbos et al. reported their experience with MIDCAB in 91 patients in Greece; the mean ICU stay was 29 ± 4 h [22]. In the current study, the duration of mechanical ventilation was 9.93 ± 8.65 h, and the length of ICU stay was 24.17 ± 17.83 h, again comparing favorably with prior studies.

In-hospital complications with MIDCAB procedures may include PAF, stroke, renal failure, and incision complications. McGinn et al. reported on the results of 450 minimally invasive coronary artery bypass surgeries at two centers in the US and found the following complications: stroke, $n = 2$ (0.4 %); new-onset atrial fibrillation, $n = 111$ (24.4 %); new-onset renal failure, $n = 12$ (2.9 %); and wound infection, $n = 4$ (0.9 %) [23]. In the current study, the rates of these complications were less: only 7 % of patients developed atrial fibrillation, and no patients developed stroke, renal failure, or incision complications.

Additionally, the 30-day mortality rate was less than 1 % in the current study. In a report of the experience with MIDCAP cases from a single center in the Czech Republic, there was a 30-day mortality rate of 1.3% (2/149 patients) [24]. Similarly, an early (<30 days) mortality rate of 1.3 % (51/4081 patients) was reported in a meta-analysis of 17 studies utilizing MIDCAB grafting [25]. The 30-day mortality rate in the current study compares favorably with these results.

There are several limitations of this study. First, it is observational in nature, with the inherent bias involved in such studies. Also, there was no direct comparison group, so that all comparisons were with the published literature. Since the patients in these prior publications may not be similar populations, firm conclusions cannot be made although the findings in the current study seemed to compare favorably with historical results. Significantly, no patency rates, long-term follow-up or long-term outcomes were available from the current study. Therefore, further studies are needed to better define the full range of outcomes with the new techniques described in the current study.

Conclusions

Taken together, the two devices have the following clinical benefits. The suspensory internal mammary artery retraction system utilized in the current study shortens the LIMA harvest time and minimizes the risk of damaging the internal mammary arteries. In addition, the retractor allows for obtaining the LIMA under direct vision, which facilitates harvesting an adequate length of LIMA via a small surgical incision in the left side of the chest. The newly developed cardiac stabilizer is advantageous in regard to maintaining intraoperative circulatory stability and reducing the risk of injuring the myocardium. Furthermore, this study suggests that performing MIDCAB with the improved retractor and stabilizer can lead to favorable outcomes in terms of postoperative morbidity and 30-day mortality.

Abbreviations
CABG: Coronary artery bypass grafting; CPB: Cardiopulmonary bypass; LAD: LIMA-left anterior descending; LIMA: Left internal mammary artery; MI: Myocardial infarction; MIDCAB: Minimally invasive direct coronary artery bypass; PAF: Postoperative atrial fibrillation; PCI: Percutaneous coronary intervention.

Competing interests
The authors declare that they have no competing interests.

Authors' contributions
We declare that all the listed authors have participated actively in the study and all meet the requirements of the authorship. YL designed the study and wrote the protocol, YL & LB performed research/study, YL & WY contributed important reagents, WY & YC managed the literature searches and analyses, YL & QG undertook the statistical analysis, YL wrote the first draft of the manuscript. All authors read and approved the final manuscript.

Acknowledgements
None declared.

Author details
[1]Department of Cardiac Surgery, Peking University Third Hospital, Beijing, China. [2]Department of Cardiac Surgery, Aero Space Center Hospital, Beijing, China. [3]Department of Cardiac Surgery, Peking University People's Hospital, Beijing, China.

References
1. Greenspun HG, Adourian UA, Fonger JD, Fan JS. Minimally invasive direct coronary artery bypass (MIDCAB): Surgical techniques and anesthetic considerations. J Cardiothorac Vasc Anesth. 1996;10:507–9.
2. Head SJ, Börgermann J, Osnabrugge RL, Kieser TM, Falk V, Taggart DP, Puskas JD, Gummert JF, Kappetein AP. Coronary artery bypass grafting: Part 2—optimizing outcomes and future prospects. Eur Heart J. 2013;34:2873–86.
3. Martens TP, Argenziano M, Oz MC. New technology for surgical coronary revas- cularization. Circulation. 2006;114:606–14.
4. Lapierre H, Chan V, Sohmer B, Mesana TG, Ruel M. Minimally invasive coronary artery bypass grafting via a small thoracotomy versus off-pump: a case-matched study. Eur J Cardiothorac Surg. 2011;40:804–10.
5. Detter C, Reichenspurner H, Boehm DH, Thalhammer M, Schütz A, Reichart B. Single vessel revascularization with beating heart techniques – minithoracotomy or sternotomy? Eur J Cardiothorac Surg. 2001;19:464–70.
6. Halkos ME, Puskas JD. Minimally invasive coronary artery bypass surgery. In: Moorjani N, Ohri SK, Wechsler AS, editors. Cardiac surgery: recent advances and techniques. Boston: CRC press; 2014. p. 1–14.
7. Boodhwani M, Ruel M, Mesana TG, Rubens FD. Minimally invasive direct coronary artery bypass for the treatment of isolated disease of the left anterior descending coronary artery. Can J Surg. 2005;48:307–10.
8. Gummert JF, Opfermann U, Jacobs S, Walther T, Kempfert J, Mohr FW, Falk V. Anastomotic devices for coronary artery bypass grafting: technological options and potential pitfalls. Comput Biol Med. 2007;37:1384–93.
9. Pande S, Agarwal SK, Gupta D, Mohanty S, Kapoor A, Tewari S, Bansal A, Ambesh SP. Early and mid-term results of minimally invasive coronary artery bypass grafting. Indian Heart J. 2014;66:193–6.
10. Faul F, Erdfelder E, Buchner A, Lang AG. Statistical power analyses using G*power 3.1: tests for correlation and regression analysis. Behav Res Methods. 2009;41:1149–60.
11. Iribarne A, Easterwood R, Chan EYH, Yang J, Soni L, Russo MJ, Smith CR, Argenziano M. The golden age of minimally invasive cardiothoracic surgery: current and future perspectives. Future Cardiol. 2011;7:333–46.
12. Hartz RS. Minimally invasive heart surgery. Circulation. 1996;94:2669.
13. Detter C, Reichenspurner H, Boehm DH, Thalhammer M, Raptis P, Schütz A, Reichart B.. Minimally invasive direct coronary artery bypass grafting (MIDCAB) and off-pump coronary artery bypass grafting (OPCAB): Two techniques for beating heart surgery. Heart Surg Forum. 2002;5:157–62.
14. Kofidis T, Emmert MY, Paeschke HG, Emmert LS, Zhang R, Haverich A. Long-term follow-up after minimal invasive direct coronary artery bypass grafting procedure: a multi-factorial retrospective analysis at 1000 patient-years. Interact Cardiovasc Thorac Surg. 2009;9:990–4.
15. Subramanian VA, Patel NU. Current status of MIDCAB procedure. Curr Opin Cardiol. 2001;16:268–70.
16. Hariharan S, Chen D, Merritt-Charles L. Off-pump coronary artery bypass surgery anaesthetic implications and the Trinidad experience. West Indian Med J. 2006;55:298–304.
17. Taggart D, Nir RR, Bolotin G. New technologies in coronary artery surgery. Rambam Maimonides Med J. 2013;4:e0018.

18. Fujita T, Hata H, Shimahara Y, Sato S, Kobayashi J. Initial experience with internal mammary artery harvesting with the da Vinci Surgical System for minimally invasive direct coronary artery bypass. Surg Today. 2014;44:2281–6.

19. Oehlinger A, Bonaros N, Schachner T, Ruetzler E, Friedrich G, Laufer G, Bonatti J. Robotic endoscopic left internal mammary artery harvesting: what have we learned after 100 cases? Ann Thorac Surg. 2007;83:1030–4.

20. Fraund S, Behnke H, Boening A, Cremer J. Immediate postoperative extubation after minimally invasive direct coronary artery surgery (MIDCAB). Interact Cardiovasc Thorac Surg. 2002;1:41–5.

21. Vicol C, Nollert G, Mair H, Samuel V, Lim C, Tiftikidis M, Eifert S, Reichart B. Midterm results of beating heart surgery in 1-vessel disease: minimally invasive direct coronary artery bypass versus off-pump coronary artery bypass with full sternotomy. Heart Surg Forum. 2003;6:341–4.

22. Bisbos AD, Skubas N, Minadakis GN, Smirlis D, Karkanis G, Spanos PK. Surgical revascularization of the left anterior descending artery with the MIDCAB technique. Hellenic J Cardiol. 2002;43:236–41.

23. McGinn Jr JT, Usman S, Lapierre H, Pothula VR, Mesana TG, Ruel M. Minimally invasive coronary artery bypass grafting: dual-center experience in 450 consecutive patients. Circulation. 2009;120 suppl 1:S78–84.

24. Santavy P, Lonsky V, Gwozdziewicz M. Minimally invasive direct coronary artery bypass grafting (MIDCABG) – our experience in Olomouc, Czech Republic. J Cardiothorac Surg. 2013;8 Suppl 1:142.

25. Kettering K. Minimally invasive direct coronary artery bypass grafting: a meta-analysis. J Cardiovasc Surg (Torino). 2008;49:793–800.

11

Clopidogrel discontinuation within the first year after coronary drug-eluting stent implantation

Troels Thim[1], Martin Berg Johansen[2], Gro Egholm Chisholm[1], Morten Schmidt[2], Anne Kaltoft[1], Henrik Toft Sørensen[2], Leif Thuesen[1], Steen Dalby Kristensen[1], Hans Erik Bøtker[2], Lars Romer Krusell[1], Jens Flensted Lassen[1], Per Thayssen[3], Lisette Okkels Jensen[3], Hans-Henrik Tilsted[4] and Michael Maeng[1*]

Abstract

Background: The impact of adherence to the recommended duration of dual antiplatelet therapy after first generation drug-eluting stent implantation is difficult to assess in real-world settings and limited data are available.

Methods: We followed 4,154 patients treated with coronary drug-eluting stents in Western Denmark for 1 year and obtained data on redeemed clopidogrel prescriptions and major adverse cardiovascular events (MACE, *i.e.*, cardiac death, myocardial infarction, or stent thrombosis) from medical databases.

Results: Discontinuation of clopidogrel within the first 3 months after stent implantation was associated with a significantly increased rate of MACE at 1-year follow-up (hazard ratio (HR) 2.06; 95% confidence interval (CI): 1.08-3.93). Discontinuation 3-6 months (HR 1.29; 95% CI: 0.70-2.41) and 6-12 months (HR 1.29; 95% CI: 0.54-3.07) after stent implantation were associated with smaller, not statistically significant, increases in MACE rates. Among patients who discontinued clopidogrel, MACE rates were highest within the first 2 months after discontinuation.

Conclusions: Discontinuation of clopidogrel was associated with an increased rate of MACE among patients treated with drug-eluting stents. The increase was statistically significant within the first 3 months after drug-eluting stent implantation but not after 3 to 12 months.

Keywords: Percutaneous coronary intervention, Dual antiplatelet therapy, Drug-eluting stent, Clopidogrel

Background

Dual antiplatelet therapy (DAPT), *i.e.*, aspirin in combination with a P2Y12 antagonist, has been shown to reduce occurrence of ischemic events after coronary stent implantation in randomized clinical trials [1,2]. In real-world settings, however, the level of adherence to recommended DAPT is difficult to assess and its influence on outcomes is less well known. Moreover, the optimal duration of DAPT after coronary stent implantation is disputed [3].

Twelve months of DAPT after percutaneous coronary intervention (PCI) with coronary stent implantation has been recommended in Denmark since November 2002. This recommendation is based on interpretation of results of existing randomized clinical trials [1,2]. In such trials, we expect adherence to treatment to be high owing to patient selection, trial-related follow-up, and cost-free provision of the platelet inhibitor. Adherence to DAPT in real-world settings is most likely lower than in these randomized trials. Assessment of adherence levels and risks associated with discontinuation of DAPT within the first year after coronary stent implantation is needed in real-world settings.

Danish medical registries allow validated monitoring of coronary interventions, prescription redemption, and clinical outcomes [4-9]. Based on data from these registries, we report rates of discontinuation of clopidogrel treatment after coronary drug-eluting stent (DES) implantation and assess the risk of associated adverse events.

* Correspondence: michael.maeng@ki.au.dk
[1]Department of Cardiology, Aarhus University Hospital, Aarhus, Denmark
Full list of author information is available at the end of the article

Methods

According to the Central Denmark Region Committees on Health Research Ethics, this study could be conducted without an approval from the Committees.

Setting

We conducted this population-based cohort study, retrospectively, using medical registries in Western Denmark, which has approximately three million inhabitants (55% of the Danish population). The Danish National Health Service provides universal tax-supported health care, guaranteeing unfettered access to general practitioners and hospitals. Costs of prescription medications, including clopidogrel, are partially reimbursed. Accurate and unambiguous linkage of data from all registries at the individual level is possible in Denmark using the unique central personal registry number assigned to every Danish citizen at birth or upon immigration [9].

Patients and procedures

We used the Western Denmark Heart Registry (WDHR) [10] to identify all PCI procedures performed between 1 January 2003 and 30 June 2005 [11-13]. For each patient, the first PCI procedure with implantation of one or more coronary DES during the inclusion period was defined as the "index PCI procedure" and the date of that procedure as the "index date". Patients treated with balloon angioplasty without stenting or with bare metal stents alone were excluded. Only first-generation DES, *i.e.*, sirolimus-eluting (SES) (Cypher, Cordis Corp., Johnson & Johnson, Warren, New Jersey) and paclitaxel-eluting stents (PES) (Taxus, Boston Scientific, Nattick, Massachusetts) were in use during the inclusion period.

The cardiac intervention centers in Western Denmark each perform more than 1,200 PCI procedures per year. The interventions were performed according to current standards including selection of interventional strategy (*e.g.*, pre- or post-dilatation, choice of stent, direct stenting, and administration of periprocedural glycoprotein IIb/IIIa inhibitors).

Patient characteristics

We obtained information from Danish National Registry of Patients on potential confounders (diabetes and hypertension) between 1977 and the index date [5]. To ensure complete identification of patients with diabetes, we also searched the Danish National Prescription Database for any use of antidiabetic drugs among study participants since 1994 [14]. From the WDHR, we retrieved procedure data, including date of index PCI, indication for PCI (ST-segment elevation myocardial infarction (MI), non-ST-segment elevation myocardial infarction MI or unstable angina pectoris, or stable angina pectoris), number of treated arteries (1, 2, or 3 or more),

number of implanted stents (1, 2, or 3 or more), lesion type (A, B1, B2, or C), and stent type.

Medication use

We used the Danish National Prescription Database to identify all redeemed prescriptions for clopidogrel [14]. Clopidogrel is available only by prescription in Denmark.

The recommended daily maintenance dose of clopidogrel for secondary prevention of ischemic vascular events is 75 mg (one tablet) daily for 12 months following PCI. Thus, for study purposes, the number of days supplied from a redeemed clopidogrel prescription corresponded to the number of tablets in the package. We computed the number of days exposed by adding 14 days to the number of days supplied. This buffer allowed for a 14-day gap to occur between redeemed prescriptions before a patient was considered to have discontinued clopidogrel. This method is well-established [15-17] and a 14-day gap has been used in previous studies [18].

We also identified redeemed prescriptions for aspirin, other nonselective non-steroidal anti-inflammatory drugs, selective cyclooxygenase-2 inhibitors, proton pump inhibitors, calcium channel blockers, statins, vitamin K antagonists, and systemic glucocorticoids.

Major adverse events

In line with the recommended duration of clopidogrel treatment, we recorded occurrence of major adverse cardiovascular events (MACE) during 12 months after the index date. We defined MACE as the first occurrence of cardiac death, myocardial infarction MI, or definite stent thrombosis (ST). A committee of cardiac specialists, blinded to the history of medication use, reviewed relevant medical records to determine occurrence of definite stent thrombosis ST and cardiac death.

Cardiac death

We obtained data on all-cause mortality from the Danish Civil Registration System [9]. The committee of cardiac specialists reviewed original death certificates obtained from the National Registry of Causes of Deaths [6]. Deaths were classified as either cardiac or non-cardiac based on the underlying cause recorded on the death certificates. We defined cardiac death as known cardiac death, unwitnessed death, or death from unknown causes.

Myocardial infarction (MI)

We used the Danish National Registry of Patients to identify hospital admissions with MI as discharge diagnosis [5].

Stent thrombosis (ST)
Based on review of medical records and angiograms, the committee of cardiac specialists adjudicated the occurrence of definite ST according to Academic Research Consortium definitions [19].

Statistical analysis
We characterized the patients using medical, procedural, and demographic variables and followed all patients from their index date until date of death or completion of 12 months of follow up.

To describe the pattern of clopidogrel compliance, we first calculated the proportion of patients still alive who had prescription coverage for clopidogrel on each day of follow up. We also calculated the mean and median proportion of days within the first year after stent implantation with prescription coverage for clopidogrel among patients not experiencing MACE.

We then estimated the effect of discontinuing clopidogrel treatment. We defined discontinuation as a gap between prescription redemptions of more than 14 days. We estimated the effect separately according to the time of discontinuation, i.e., within the first 3 months (day 1 through 91), 3 to 6 months (day 92 through 182), or 6 to 12 months (day 183 through 365) after the index PCI procedure. We estimated hazard ratios using a Cox proportional hazards regression model. Hazard ratios were adjusted for potential confounders (age, gender, year of index PCI, indication for PCI, comorbidity level (using Charlson Comorbidity Index scores)) and time-varying use (calculated from the number of days exposed) of aspirin, other nonselective non-steroidal anti-inflammatory drugs, and proton pump inhibitors. Patients entered the study at the time of their first clopidogrel prescription redemption after the index date (delayed entry). Patients contributed to time at risk as current users of clopidogrel as long as they had prescription coverage for clopidogrel. From the time point of discontinuation, patients contributed time at risk according to their time window of discontinuation [15-17].

Results
The study included 4,154 patients treated with DES. Of these, 2,570 patients were treated with implantation of SES, 1,525 patients with PES, and 59 patients with SES and PES. Patient and procedure characteristics are shown in Table 1.

Rates of clopidogrel treatment discontinuation
In Figure 1, the proportion of patients with prescription coverage for clopidogrel on each day of follow up is plotted against time since the index PCI procedure date. There was a drop in prescription coverage between 3 and 4 months after the index PCI procedure, and again

Table 1 Patient and procedure characteristics

	N = 4,154*	%
Female	1,127	27.1
Age group (years)		
<60	1,659	39.9
60-70	1,316	31.7
70+	1,179	28.4
Medication use†		
Clopidogrel	3,931	94.6
Proton pump inhibitors	955	23.0
Aspirin	3,718	89.5
Vitamin K antagonists	301	7.2
Nonselective NSAIDs	509	12.3
COX-2 inhibitors	388	9.3
Oral glucocorticoids	309	7.4
Calcium channel blockers	1,153	27.8
Statins	3,606	86.8
Comorbidities‡		
Diabetes	586	14.1
Hypertension	178	4.3
Year of study entry		
2003	847	20.4
2004	1,836	44.2
2005	1,471	35.4
PCI Indication		
STEMI	844	20.3
UAP/NSTEMI	1,277	30.7
SAP	1,902	45.8
Other	131	3.2
Number of treated arteries§		
1	2,877	69.3
2	1,057	25.4
3	212	5.1
Number of Stents§		
1	3,301	79.5
2	631	15.2
3+	208	5.0
Lesion Type§‖		
A	898	21.6
B	2,165	52.1
C	1,091	26.3

*Drug-eluting stents only (n = 3,548) and combination of drug-eluting stents and bare metal stents (n = 606).
†Any prescription redemption during follow up.
‡Registered between 1977 and the index PCI date.
§Data were not available on number of treated arteries for 112 patients, on the number of stents for 62 patients, and on lesion type for 6 patients.
‖Lesion classification: A = non-complicated, length <10 mm; B = irregular, length 10-20 mm; C = irregular, side branch, 90 degrees, chronic occlusion, length 20 mm.
Abbreviations: COX cyclooxygenase, NSAIDs nonsteroidal anti-inflammatory drugs, PCI percutaneous coronary intervention, STEMI ST-segment elevation myocardial infarction, SAP stable angina pectoris, UAP unstable angina pectoris, NSTEMI non-ST-segment elevation myocardial infarction.

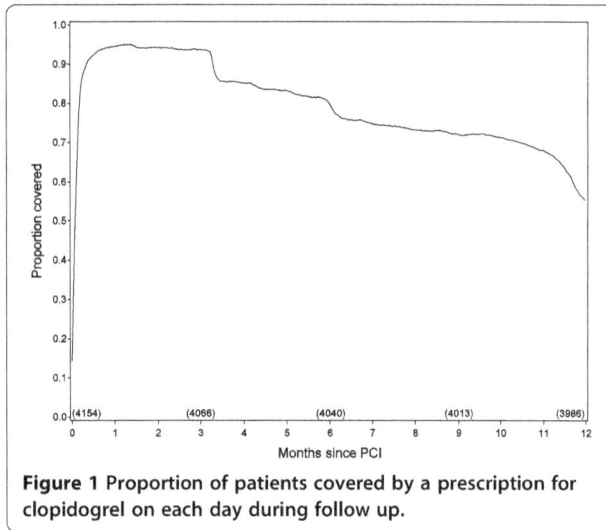

Figure 1 Proportion of patients covered by a prescription for clopidogrel on each day during follow up.

a smaller drop after about 6 months. The percentage of patients who never redeemed a prescription for clopidogrel during follow up was 5.4%. Among the 3,815 event-free survivors, the mean percentage of days covered by a clopidogrel prescription was 81% (median: 96%).

Risk associated with clopidogrel treatment discontinuation

Figure 2 shows the cumulative incidence of MACE during the first year after the index PCI procedure. The risk of MACE increased most within the first 2 weeks following the procedure (approximately 3%) and then increased more gradually during the remainder of the one-year study period (overall 1-year risk was approximately 6%). Figure 3

shows the cumulative incidence of MACE over time starting from the time-point of discontinuation. The increase in cumulative risk of MACE was highest within the first 2 months following discontinuation.

Table 2 shows crude and adjusted hazard ratios for discontinuation of clopidogrel treatment. The 1-year cumulative MACE rate among patients covered by clopidogrel prescriptions for the full year was 3.9%. Discontinuation of clopidogrel within the first 3 months after PCI was associated with an increased rate of MACE (approximately 2-fold) and cardiac death (almost 5-fold). The risk estimates for the individual components of the combined outcome were also increased, with wider confidence intervals due to fewer events. Definite ST as an individual outcome was too rare within the first 3 months to allow for statistical inference. When discontinuation of clopidogrel occurred later than 3 months following PCI, differences in rates were not statistically significant, however, the hazard ratios suggested that risk of MACE was increased by approximately 30%, cardiac death by 80%, and MI by 10% when clopidogrel was discontinued later than 3 months following PCI. ST was rare and clopidogrel discontinuation between 3-6 months was associated with a non-significant 7-fold higher risk of ST, corresponding to an almost 3% risk of ST in this subgroup.

Patients who never redeemed a single clopidogrel prescription were not included in the analyses described above. Among these patients, the cumulative incidence of MACE was 48% within one week, 59% within one month, 61% within 3 months, and 63% within one year following PCI. Thus, these patients experienced very high early MACE rates, but rates after 3 months were

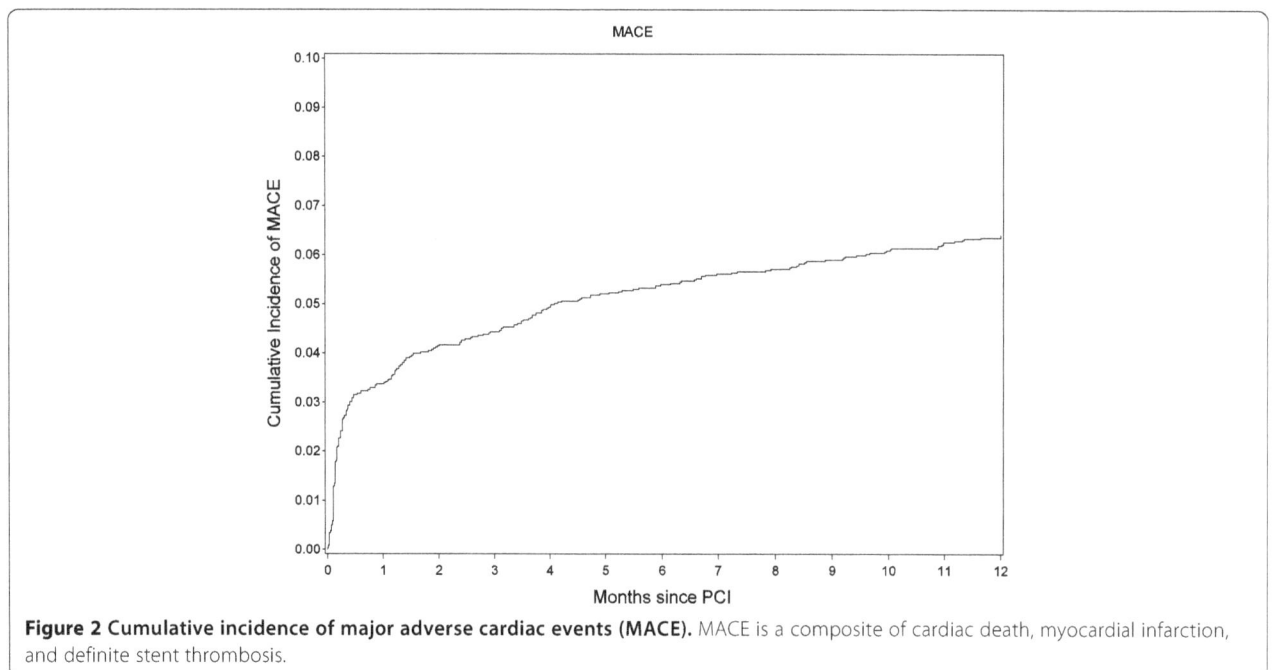

Figure 2 Cumulative incidence of major adverse cardiac events (MACE). MACE is a composite of cardiac death, myocardial infarction, and definite stent thrombosis.

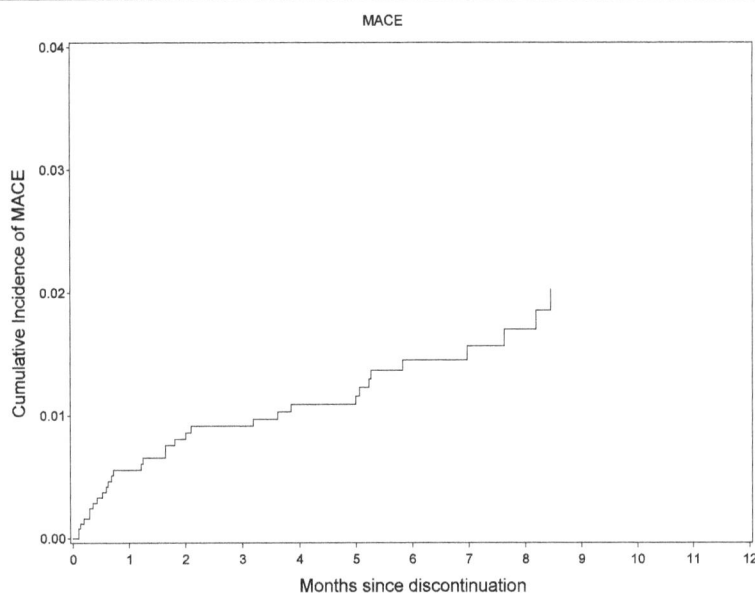

Figure 3 Cumulative incidence of major adverse cardiac events (MACE) following discontinuation of clopidogrel. MACE is a composite of cardiac death, myocardial infarction, and definite stent thrombosis.

comparable to that of the overall patient population, as shown in Figure 2. Early events, such as in-hospital death, may have prevented some of these patients from ever redeeming a clopidogrel prescription.

Discussion

Our main findings from this study of 4,154 consecutive real-world patients treated with first-generation DES are that discontinuation of clopidogrel was common and that discontinuation within the first 3 months after stent implantation was associated with an approximately two-fold increase in risk of MACE and an almost 5-fold increase in risk of cardiac death.

Registry data

In cohort studies, premature clopidogrel discontinuation after DES implantation is fairly common. Data are conflicting on whether discontinuation, at least beyond the first 4-6 months, is associated with adverse events. These conflicting results may reflect major differences among these studies, including data acquisition, study design, and statistical approach.

Clopidogrel treatment is generally recommended for 12 months after DES implantation. Rates of clopidogrel discontinuation within these 12 months have been reported to be 14% within the first month [20], 28% by 6 months [18], and 4%-38% by 12 months [21-26]. The discontinuation rate reported in our study is similar in magnitude to that of most other reports [18,20-22,25,26].

The timing of clopidogrel discontinuation within the first year appears to be of major importance. Patients discontinuing DAPT within 7, 8-30, or >30 days after

PCI due to non-compliance or bleeding had a 7-fold, 2-fold, and 1.3-fold higher risk of MACE, respectively [26]. Among patients with MI, clopidogrel discontinuation within the first month after coronary stent implantation has been associated with a 9-fold increased risk of death by 12 months [20]. Discontinuation within the first year,

Table 2 Hazard ratios (HRs) for discontinuation of clopidogrel treatment

Time following DES implantation		HR (95% CI)	Adjusted HR (95% CI)
MACE	0-3 months	2.48 (1.30-4.71)	2.06 (1.08-3.93)
	3-6 months	1.26 (0.68-2.33)	1.29 (0.70-2.41)
	6-12 months	1.26 (0.53-2.99)	1.29 (0.54-3.07)
Cardiac death	0-3 months	6.84 (3.06-15.3)	4.80 (2.13-10.8)
	3-6 months	1.95 (0.72-5.30)	1.85 (0.68-5.04)
	6-12 months	1.65 (0.42-6.46)	1.74 (0.45-6.78)
Myocardial infarction	0-3 months	2.05 (0.93-4.53)	1.84 (0.83-4.09)
	3-6 months	1.08 (0.51-2.28)	1.14 (0.54-2.43)
	6-12 months	1.09 (0.36-3.35)	1.09 (0.35-3.34)
Definite stent thrombosis	0-3 months	-	-
	3-6 months	6.04 (0.52-70.2)	7.14 (0.61-83.7)
	6-12 months	-	-

MACE is a composite of cardiac death, myocardial infarction, and definite stent thrombosis.
Abbreviations: *HR* hazard ratio, *CI* confidence interval.
Hazard ratios were adjusted for age, gender, year of index PCI, PCI indication, comorbidity level (using Charlson Comorbidity Index scores), and time-varying use (calculated from the number of days exposed) of aspirin, other NSAIDs, and proton pump inhibitors.
0-3 months = day 1 through 91; 3 to 6 months = day 92 through 182; 6 to 12 months = day 183 through 365.

particularly within the first month, has been associated with adverse events [21]. Based on a landmark approach, 3 studies evaluating event-free patients after 4-6-months of follow-up found that continued use of P2Y12 antagonists did not reduce the risk of adverse events [22,27,28], while 2 other studies showed that it reduced the risk [21,29]. Regional differences, particularly socio-economic factors affecting compliance, may explain this discrepancy in part. In addition, the landmark approach is limited by the healthy survivor effect. Further, in all the studies described above, information about clopidogrel adherence relied on self-reports by patients or their relatives during visits or telephone interviews. Such contacts likely influenced clopidogrel compliance positively, making the data subject to non-differential misclassification bias.

A unique feature of the current study is the linkage of Danish national registries, thereby avoiding the misclassification bias associated with self-reporting. Only a single study previously linked data from a national prescription registry with clinical outcomes to assess the impact of premature clopidogrel discontinuation after DES implantation [18]. Similar to our findings, 28% of study patients discontinued clopidogrel within 6 months after their PCI procedure, and patients who discontinued clopidogrel within the first 6 months had a 2-fold higher risk of death at 12 months. In contrast to this earlier study, the current study included patients younger than 65 years, examined occurrence of MI and ST, and assessed the risk of discontinuing clopidogrel for 3 time intervals.

Individual variation in platelet response to clopidogrel is a subject of debate, providing some of the rationale behind development of newer and currently more expensive platelet inhibitors, such as ticagrelor and prasugrel [30,31]. While the clinical benefits of the newer platelet inhibitors are small compared to clopidogrel, they become significant in large populations of patients with acute coronary syndromes. At the same time, the impact of compliance to DAPT, at least within the first 3 months after PCI, is major. Therefore, approaches to decrease rates of early DAPT discontinuation should be a major focus of future research and daily clinical practice.

Randomized trial data
Results from 2 on-going clinical trials are awaited [32,33]. Recently, it was reported that 3 months was non-inferior to 12 months of of DAPT after stent implantation [34]. The balance between reduction of ischemic events and the risk of bleeding may favor DAPT for 3 to 6 months after DES implantation and extending DAPT further might be associated with a risk of bleeding outweighing the benefit [35,36]. However, it has been found that DAPT for 1 year was superior to a 1-month

regimen [2]. Recently, 4 randomized studies have been conducted, in which event-free patients were randomized to 3 [37], 6 [38,39] or 12 [40] months versus prolonged DAPT following PCI. All 4 trials reported no benefit of prolonged clopidogrel treatment [35,37-40]. Importantly, these randomized data, agree with our registry data based on consecutive real-world patients.

Limitations
The strength of this study lies in its use of population-based registries with complete follow-up. However, a number of limitations should be acknowledged. First, some patients may have redeemed their prescriptions without taking all or any of the tablets. Moreover, temporary discontinuations < 14 days were not detected. However, others have shown that such short discontinuations do not affect outcomes [24]. Second, aspirin use could not be completely assessed in this study, as aspirin is available without a prescription. This limitation may be relevant at least for ST [22]. However, low-dose aspirin used for secondary prevention of cardiovascular disease generally is prescribed by physicians because prescription costs are partly reimbursed through the national health insurance program. Third, despite adjustment for comorbidities, we cannot exclude residual confounding. Fourth, it has been reported that the positive effect of compliance with medication regimens is lower than estimated from observational studies [41]. The true protective effect of clopidogrel in routine clinical care patients thus may be lower than estimated here. Fifth, the decline in adherence to clopidogrel treatment after 3-4 months and 6 months after the index PCI procedure was likely caused by a combination of medical decisions for discontinuation and patients' lack of compliance [20,23,26]. Sixth, the results obtained are limited to the 2 first-generation DES. As newer DES are considered safer than the first generation DES [42], the impact of discontinuation of prolonged DAPT is likely to be lower with newer stents.

Conclusion
Discontinuation of clopidogrel was associated with an increased rate of MACE among patients treated with DES. The increase was statistically significant within the first 3 months after DES implantation but not after 3 to 12 months.

Abbreviations
CI: Confidence interval; HR: Hazard ratio; MACE: Major adverse cardiovascular events; PCI: Percutaneous coronary intervention; WDHR: Western Denmark Heart Registry.

Competing interests
TT: Teaching honorarium from AstraZeneca. Travel grants from St. Jude Medical and The Medicines Company. MBJ, GEC, MS, HTS, LT, HEB, LRK, JFL, PT: None. SDK: Lecture fees from AstraZeneca, BMS, Eli Lilly, and The

Medicines Company. AKK: Speakers fee from Cordis and St Jude Medical. Travel grants from Abbott, Biotronik, Cordis, Medtronic, Terumo, The Medicines Company, and St. Jude Medical. LOJ: Unrestricted grant from Terumo and honoraria from AstraZeneca. HHT: None. MM: Travel grants from Abbott, St. Jude Medical, Medtronic, Biotronik, and Terumo.

Authors' contributions

TT conception and design, data quisition, analysis and interpretation of data, and drafting of manuscript. MBJ: analysis and interpretation of data, and drafting of manuscript. GEC, MS, LT, HEB, SDK, LRK, AKK, JFL, PT, LOJ, HHT data quisition and review of manuscript. HTS conception and design and review of manuscript. MM conception and design, data quisition, analysis and interpretation of data, drafting and review of manuscript. All authors read and approved the final manuscript.

Acknowledgements

This is an academic study financed by the Departments of Cardiology and Clinical Epidemiology, Aarhus University Hospital, Denmark.

Author details

[1]Department of Cardiology, Aarhus University Hospital, Aarhus, Denmark. [2]Department of Clinical Epidemiology, Aarhus University Hospital, Brendstrupgaardsvej 100, Aarhus, N 8200, Denmark. [3]Department of Cardiology, Odense University Hospital, Odense, Denmark. [4]Department of Cardiology, Aalborg University Hospital, Aalborg, Denmark.

References

1. Mehta SR, Yusuf S, Peters RJ, Bertrand ME, Lewis BS, Natarajan MK, Malmberg K, Rupprecht H, Zhao F, Chrolavicius S, Copland I, Fox KA, Clopidogrel in Unstable angina to prevent Recurrent Events trial (CURE) Investigators: Effects of pretreatment with clopidogrel and aspirin followed by long-term therapy in patients undergoing percutaneous coronary intervention: the PCI-CURE study. Lancet 2001, 358:527–533.
2. Steinhubl SR, Berger PB, Mann JT III, Fry ET, DeLago A, Wilmer C, Topol EJ: Early and sustained dual oral antiplatelet therapy following percutaneous coronary intervention: a randomized controlled trial. JAMA 2002, 288:2411–2420.
3. Kleiman NS: Grabbing the horns of a dilemma: the duration of dual antiplatelet therapy after stent implantation. Circulation 2012, 125:1967–1970.
4. Sørensen HT: Regional administrative health registries as a resource in clinical epidemiology. Int J Risk Saf Med 1997, 10:1–22.
5. Andersen TF, Madsen M, Jorgensen J, Mellemkjoer L, Olsen JH: The Danish National Hospital Register. A valuable source of data for modern health sciences. Dan Med Bull 1999, 46:263–268.
6. Juel K, Helweg-Larsen K: The Danish registers of causes of death. Dan Med Bull 1999, 46:354–357.
7. Frank L: Epidemiology. When an entire country is a cohort. Science 2000, 287:2398–2399.
8. Madsen M, Davidsen M, Rasmussen S, Abildstrom SZ, Osler M: The validity of the diagnosis of acute myocardial infarction in routine statistics: a comparison of mortality and hospital discharge data with the Danish MONICA registry. J Clin Epidemiol 2003, 56:124–130.
9. Pedersen CB, Gotzsche H, Moller JO, Mortensen PB: The Danish Civil Registration System. A cohort of eight million persons. Dan Med Bull 2006, 53:441–449.
10. Schmidt M, Maeng M, Jakobsen CJ, Madsen M, Thuesen L, Nielsen PH, Botker HE, Sorensen HT: Existing data sources for clinical epidemiology: the Western Denmark Heart Registry. Clin Epidemiol 2010, 2:137–144.
11. Jensen LO, Tilsted HH, Thayssen P, Kaltoft A, Maeng M, Lassen JF, Hansen KN, Madsen M, Ravkilde J, Johnsen SP, Sørensen HT, Thuesen L: Paclitaxel and sirolimus eluting stents versus bare metal stents: long-term risk of stent thrombosis and other outcomes. From the Western Denmark Heart Registry. EuroIntervention 2010, 5:898–905.
12. Kaltoft A, Jensen LO, Maeng M, Tilsted HH, Thayssen P, Bottcher M, Lassen JF, Krusell LR, Rasmussen K, Hansen KN, Pedersen L, Johnsen SP, Sørensen HT, Thuesen L: 2-year clinical outcomes after implantation of sirolimus-eluting, paclitaxel-eluting, and bare-metal coronary stents: results from the WDHR (Western Denmark Heart Registry). J Am Coll Cardiol 2009, 53:658–664.
13. Jensen LO, Maeng M, Kaltoft A, Thayssen P, Hansen HH, Bottcher M, Lassen JF, Krussel LR, Rasmussen K, Hansen KN, Pedersen L, Johnsen SP, Soerensen HT, Thuesen L: Stent thrombosis, myocardial infarction, and death after drug-eluting and bare-metal stent coronary interventions. J Am Coll Cardiol 2007, 50:463–470.
14. Wallach Kildemoes H, Toft Sørensen H, Hallas J: The Danish National Prescription Registry. Scand J Public Health 2011, 39:38–41.
15. Schmidt M, Johansen MB, Robertson DJ, Maeng M, Kaltoft A, Jensen LO, Tilsted HH, Botker HE, Sorensen HT, Baron JA: Use of clopidogrel and calcium channel blockers and risk of major adverse cardiovascular events. Eur J Clin Invest 2012, 42:266–274.
16. Schmidt M, Johansen MB, Robertson DJ, Maeng M, Kaltoft A, Jensen LO, Tilsted HH, Botker HE, Sorensen HT, Baron JA: Concomitant use of clopidogrel and proton pump inhibitors is not associated with major adverse cardiovascular events following coronary stent implantation. Aliment Pharmacol Ther 2012, 35:165–174.
17. Schmidt M, Johansen MB, Maeng M, Kaltoft A, Jensen LO, Tilsted HH, Botker HE, Baron JA, Sorensen HT: Concomitant use of clopidogrel and statins and risk of major adverse cardiovascular events following coronary stent implantation. Br J Clin Pharmacol 2012, 74:161–170.
18. Ko DT, Chiu M, Guo H, Austin PC, Marquis JF, Tu JV: Patterns of use of thienopyridine therapy after percutaneous coronary interventions with drug-eluting stents and bare-metal stents. Am Heart J 2009, 158:592–598.
19. Cutlip DE, Windecker S, Mehran R, Boam A, Cohen DJ, van Es GA, Steg PG, Morel MA, Mauri L, Vranckx P, McFadden E, Lansky A, Hamon M, Krucoff MW, Serruys PW, Academic Research Consortium: Clinical end points in coronary stent trials: a case for standardized definitions. Circulation 2007, 115:2344–2351.
20. Spertus JA, Kettelkamp R, Vance C, Decker C, Jones PG, Rumsfeld JS, Messenger JC, Khanal S, Peterson ED, Bach RG, Krumholz HM, Cohen DJ: Prevalence, predictors, and outcomes of premature discontinuation of thienopyridine therapy after drug-eluting stent placement: results from the PREMIER registry. Circulation 2006, 113:2803–2809.
21. Rossini R, Capodanno D, Lettieri C, Musumeci G, Nijaradze T, Romano M, Lortkipanidze N, Cicorella N, Biondi ZG, Sirbu V, Izzo A, Guagliumi G, Valsecchi O, Gavazzi A, Angiolillo DJ: Prevalence, predictors, and long-term prognosis of premature discontinuation of oral antiplatelet therapy after drug eluting stent implantation. Am J Cardiol 2011, 107:186–194.
22. Kimura T, Morimoto T, Nakagawa Y, Tamura T, Kadota K, Yasumoto H, Nishikawa H, Hiasa Y, Muramatsu T, Meguro T, Inoue N, Honda H, Hayashi Y, Miyazaki S, Oshima S, Honda T, Shiode N, Namura M, Sone T, Nobuyoshi M, Kita T, Mitsudo K, j-Cypher Registry Investigators: Antiplatelet therapy and stent thrombosis after sirolimus-eluting stent implantation. Circulation 2009, 119:987–995.
23. Ferreira-Gonzalez I, Marsal JR, Ribera A, Permanyer-Miralda G, Garcia-Del BB, Marti G, Cascant P, Martin-Yuste V, Brugaletta S, Sabate M, Alfonso F, Capote ML, De La Torre JM, Ruíz-Lera M, Sanmiguel D, Cárdenas M, Pujol B, Baz JA, Iñiguez A, Trillo R, González-Béjar O, Casanova J, Sánchez-Gila J, García-Dorado D: Background, incidence, and predictors of antiplatelet therapy discontinuation during the first year after drug-eluting stent implantation. Circulation 2010, 122:1017–1025.
24. Ferreira-Gonzalez I, Marsal JR, Ribera A, Permanyer-Miralda G, Garcia-Del BB, Marti G, Cascant P, Masotti-Centol M, Carrillo X, Mauri J, Batalla N, Larrousse E, Martín E, Serra A, Rumoroso JR, Ruiz-Salmerón R, de la Torre JM, Cequier A, Gómez-Hospital JA, Alfonso F, Martín-Yuste V, Sabatè M, García-Dorado D: Double antiplatelet therapy after drug-eluting stent implantation: risk associated with discontinuation within the first year. J Am Coll Cardiol 2012, 60:1333–1339.
25. Roy P, Bonello L, Torguson R, Okabe T, Pinto Slottow TL, Steinberg DH, Kaneshige K, Xue Z, Satler LF, Kent KM, Suddath WO, Pichard AD, Lindsay J, Waksman R: Temporal relation between Clopidogrel cessation and stent thrombosis after drug-eluting stent implantation. Am J Cardiol 2009, 103:801–805.
26. Mehran R, Baber U, Steg PG, Ariti C, Weisz G, Witzenbichler B, Henry TD, Kini AS, Stuckey T, Cohen DJ, Berger PB, Iakovou I, Dangas G, Waksman R, Antoniucci D, Sartori S, Krucoff MW, Hermiller JB, Shawl F, Gibson CM, Chieffo A, Alu M, Moliterno DJ, Colombo A, Pocock S: Cessation of dual antiplatelet treatment and cardiac events after percutaneous coronary intervention (PARIS): 2 year results from a prospective observational study. Lancet 2013, 382:1714–1722.

27. Shin DH, Chae IH, Youn TJ, Cho SI, Kwon DA, Suh JW, Chang HJ, Cho YS, Chung WY, Choi YJ, Gwon HC, Han KR, Choi DJ: **Reasonable duration of Clopidogrel use after drug-eluting stent implantation in Korean patients.** *Am J Cardiol* 2009, **104**:1668–1673.

28. Tada T, Natsuaki M, Morimoto T, Furukawa Y, Nakagawa Y, Byrne RA, Kastrati A, Kadota K, Iwabuchi M, Shizuta S, Tazaki J, Shiomi H, Abe M, Ehara N, Mizoguchi T, Mitsuoka H, Inada T, Araki M, Kaburagi S, Taniguchi R, Eizawa H, Nakano A, Suwa S, Takizawa A, Nohara R, Fujiwara H, Mitsudo K, Nobuyoshi M, Kita T, Kimura T, *et al*: **Duration of dual antiplatelet therapy and long-term clinical outcome after coronary drug-eluting stent implantation: landmark analyses from the CREDO-Kyoto PCI/CABG Registry Cohort-2.** *Circ Cardiovasc Interv* 2012, **5**:381–391.

29. Eisenstein EL, Anstrom KJ, Kong DF, Shaw LK, Tuttle RH, Mark DB, Kramer JM, Harrington RA, Matchar DB, Kandzari DE, Peterson ED, Schulman KA, Califf RM: **Clopidogrel use and long-term clinical outcomes after drug-eluting stent implantation.** *JAMA* 2007, **297**:159–168.

30. Wiviott SD, Braunwald E, McCabe CH, Montalescot G, Ruzyllo W, Gottlieb S, Neumann FJ, Ardissino D, De Servi S, Murphy SA, Riesmeyer J, Weerakkody G, Gibson CM, Antman EM, TRITON-TIMI 38 Investigators: **Prasugrel versus clopidogrel in patients with acute coronary syndromes.** *N Engl J Med* 2007, **357**:2001–2015.

31. Wallentin L, Becker RC, Budaj A, Cannon CP, Emanuelsson H, Held C, Horrow J, Husted S, James S, Katus H, Mahaffey KW, Scirica BM, Skene A, Steg PG, Storey RF, Harrington RA, PLATO Investigators, Freij A, Thorsén M: **Ticagrelor versus clopidogrel in patients with acute coronary syndromes.** *N Engl J Med* 2009, **361**:1045–1057.

32. Mauri L, Kereiakes DJ, Normand SL, Wiviott SD, Cohen DJ, Holmes DR, Bangalore S, Cutlip DE, Pencina M, Massaro JM: **Rationale and design of the dual antiplatelet therapy study, a prospective, multicenter, randomized, double-blind trial to assess the effectiveness and safety of 12 versus 30 months of dual antiplatelet therapy in subjects undergoing percutaneous coronary intervention with either drug-eluting stent or bare metal stent placement for the treatment of coronary artery lesions.** *Am Heart J* 2010, **160**:1035–1041.

33. Byrne RA, Schulz S, Mehilli J, Iijima R, Massberg S, Neumann FJ, ten Berg JM, Schomig A, Kastrati A: **Rationale and design of a randomized, double-blind, placebo-controlled trial of 6 versus 12 months clopidogrel therapy after implantation of a drug-eluting stent: The Intracoronary Stenting and Antithrombotic Regimen: Safety And EFficacy of 6 Months Dual Antiplatelet Therapy After Drug-Eluting Stenting (ISAR-SAFE) study.** *Am Heart J* 2009, **157**:620–624.

34. Feres F, Costa RA, Abizaid A, Leon MB, Marin-Neto JA, Botelho RV, King SB III, Negoita M, Liu M, de Paula JE, Mangione JA, Meireles GX, Castello HJ Jr, Nicolela EL Jr, Perin MA, Devito FS, Labrunie A, Salvadori D Jr, Gusmão M, Staico R, Costa JR Jr, de Castro JP, Abizaid AS, Bhatt DL, OPTIMIZE Trial Investigators: **Three vs twelve months of dual antiplatelet therapy after zotarolimus-eluting stents: the OPTIMIZE randomized trial.** *JAMA* 2013, **310**:2510–2522.

35. Cassese S, Byrne RA, Tada T, King LA, Kastrati A: **Clinical impact of extended dual antiplatelet therapy after percutaneous coronary interventions in the drug-eluting stent era: a meta-analysis of randomized trials.** *Eur Heart J* 2012, **33**:3078–3087.

36. Pandit A, Giri S, Hakim FA, Fortuin FD: **Shorter (</=6 months) versus longer (>/=12 months) duration dual antiplatelet therapy after drug eluting stents: A meta-analysis of randomized clinical trials.** *Catheter Cardiovasc Interv* 2014, 10. doi:10.1002/ccd.25520.

37. Kim BK, Hong MK, Shin DH, Nam CM, Kim JS, Ko YG, Choi D, Kang TS, Park BE, Kang WC, Lee SH, Yoon JH, Hong BK, Kwon HM, Jang Y, RESET Investigators: **A new strategy for discontinuation of dual antiplatelet therapy: the RESET Trial (REal Safety and Efficacy of 3-month dual antiplatelet Therapy following Endeavor zotarolimus-eluting stent implantation).** *J Am Coll Cardiol* 2012, **60**:1340–1348.

38. Valgimigli M, Campo G, Monti M, Vranckx P, Percoco G, Tumscitz C, Castriota F, Colombo F, Tebaldi M, Fuca G, Kubbajeh M, Cangiano E, Minarelli M, Scalone A, Cavazza C, Frangione A, Borghesi M, Marchesini J, Parrinello G, Ferrari R, Prolonging Dual Antiplatelet Treatment After Grading Stent-Induced Intimal Hyperplasia Study (PRODIGY) Investigators: **Short- versus long-term duration of dual antiplatelet therapy after coronary stenting: a randomized multicentre trial.** *Circulation* 2012, **125**:2015–2026.

39. Gwon HC, Hahn JY, Park KW, Song YB, Chae IH, Lim DS, Han KR, Choi JH, Choi SH, Kang HJ, Koo BK, Ahn T, Yoon JH, Jeong MH, Hong TJ, Chung WY, Choi YJ, Hur SH, Kwon HM, Jeon DW, Kim BO, Park SH, Lee NH, Jeon HK, Jang Y, Kim HS: **Six-month versus 12-month dual antiplatelet therapy after implantation of drug-eluting stents: the Efficacy of Xience/Promus Versus Cypher to Reduce Late Loss After Stenting (EXCELLENT) randomized, multicenter study.** *Circulation* 2012, **125**:505–513.

40. Park SJ, Park DW, Kim YH, Kang SJ, Lee SW, Lee CW, Han KH, Park SW, Yun SC, Lee SG, Rha SW, Seong IW, Jeong MH, Hur SH, Lee NH, Yoon J, Yang JY, Lee BK, Choi YJ, Chung WS, Lim DS, Cheong SS, Kim KS, Chae JK, Nah DY, Jeon DS, Seung KB, Jang JS, Park HS, Lee K: **Duration of dual antiplatelet therapy after implantation of drug-eluting stents.** *N Engl J Med* 2010, **362**:1374–1382.

41. LaFleur J, Nelson RE, Sauer BC, Nebeker JR: **Overestimation of the effects of adherence on outcomes: a case study in healthy user bias and hypertension.** *Heart* 2011, **97**:1862–1869.

42. Bangalore S, Kumar S, Fusaro M, Amoroso N, Attubato MJ, Feit F, Bhatt DL, Slater J: **Short- and long-term outcomes with drug-eluting and bare-metal coronary stents: a mixed-treatment comparison analysis of 117 762 patient-years of follow-up from randomized trials.** *Circulation* 2012, **125**:2873–2891.

12

Lower diastolic wall strain is associated with coronary revascularization in patients with stable angina

Jaehuk Choi[1], Min-Kyung Kang[2]* ⓘ, Chaehoon Han[2], Sang Muk Hwang[2], Sung Gu Jung[2], Han-Kyul Kim[2], Kwang Jin Chun[2,3], Seonghoon Choi[2], Jung Rae Cho[2] and Namho Lee[2]

Abstract

Background: Left ventricular (LV) diastolic dysfunction occurs earlier in the ischemic cascade than LV systolic dysfunction and electrocardiographic changes. Diastolic wall strain (DWS) has been proposed as a marker of LV diastolic stiffness. Therefore, the objectives of this study were to define the relationship between DWS and coronary revascularization and to evaluate other echocardiographic parameters in patients with stable angina who were undergoing coronary angiography (CAG).

Methods: Four hundred forty patients [mean age: 61 ± 10; 249 (57%) men] undergoing CAG and with normal left ventricular systolic function without regional wall motion abnormalities were enrolled. Among them, 128 (29%) patients underwent revascularization (percutaneous intervention: 117, bypass surgery: 11). All patients underwent echocardiography before CAG and the DWS was defined using posterior wall thickness (PWT) measurements from standard echocardiographic images [DWS = PWT(systole)-PWT(diastole)/PWT(systole)].

Results: Patients who underwent revascularization had a significantly lower DWS than those who did not (0.26 ± 0.08 vs. 0.38 ± 0.09, $p < 0.001$). Age was comparable between the two groups (61 ± 9 vs. 60 ± 11, $p = 0.337$), but the proportion of males was significantly higher among patients who underwent revascularization (69 vs. 52%, $p = 0.001$). The LV ejection fraction was similar but slightly decreased (60.9 ± 5.7 vs. $62.4 \pm 6.2\%$, $p = 0.019$) and the E/E' ratio was elevated (10.3 ± 4.0 vs. 9.0 ± 3.1, $p < 0.001$) among patients who underwent revascularization. In multiple regression analysis, lower DWS was an independent predictor of revascularization (cut-off value: 0.34; sensitivity: 89%; AUC: 0.870; SE: 0.025; $p < 0.001$).

Conclusion: DWS, a simple parameter that can be calculated from routine 2D echocardiography, is inversely associated with the presence of coronary artery disease and the need for revascularization.

Keywords: Echocardiography, Diastolic wall strain, Coronary revascularization

Background

Conditions causing chest pain or discomfort, such as an acute coronary syndrome or angina, have a potentially poor prognosis, emphasizing the importance of a prompt and accurate diagnosis [1]. For patients with acute coronary syndrome (ACS), 12-lead-electrocardiography (ECG), cardiac biomarkers, and echocardiography are used to confirm the diagnosis in combination with the characteristics of chest pain and conventional risk factors [1, 2]. Echocardiography is a good imaging modality for detecting a new loss of viable myocardium or new regional wall motion abnormality (RWMA) [1]. However, stable angina cannot be diagnosed or excluded by clinical assessment alone, and non-invasive functional imaging for myocardial ischemia, coronary computed tomography (CT) calcium scanning or angiography, and coronary angiography (CAG) are often needed. Non-invasive functional imaging for myocardial ischemia uses myocardial perfusion scintigraphy with single-photon emission computed tomography (MPS with SPECT), stress echocardiography, first-pass

---

* Correspondence: homes78@naver.com
2 Cardiology Division, Kangnam Sacred Heart Hospital, Hallym University Medical Center, Seoul, South Korea
Full list of author information is available at the end of the article

contrast-enhanced magnetic resonance (MR) perfusion or MR imaging for stress-induced wall motion abnormalities [3]. Using research by Genders et al. [4], the ESC 2013 guideline contains a similar table of estimated risk percentages to the NICE 2010 guideline. Those with an estimated risk of <15% should be presumed to not have coronary artery disease (CAD). If the estimated risk is >15%, the patient's left ventricular ejection fraction (LV EF) is a key determinant factor. Therefore, cardiac imaging plays a pivotal role in this type of decision- decision-making through determination of the LV systolic function and subsequent selection of a relevant intervention. However, EF cannot be used as an independent parameter to estimate the probability of the presence of CAD, but it can be used to help choose further studies to detect CAD in combination with clinical assessments. Therefore, routine 2-D echocardiography is less useful in patients with stable angina than in patients with ACS.

An echocardiographic study published in 1972 showed abnormal motion of the LV posterior wall during angina pectoris [5]. Recently, a non-invasive, load-independent, and reproducible estimator of LV stiffness using 2-dimensional (2D) echocardiography, namely, diastolic wall strain (DWS), has been used to assess wall distensibility in the absence of LV systolic dysfunction [6]. Decreased DWS is associated with poor prognosis in patients with heart failure with preserved LV ejection fraction (HFpEF) [7] as well as in those with HF with reduced LVEF (HFrEF) [8] and is associated with adverse LV remodelling even in patients with normal LV systolic and diastolic function [9]. Therefore, the aims of this study were to evaluate the relationship between DWS and coronary revascularization as well as to evaluate echocardiographic and other parameters in patients with stable angina who underwent CAG.

Methods

Study design and participants

Of 2375 patients who underwent CAG from January 2013 to December 2015, 440 patients (57% male, average age = 60 years) who were diagnosed with or suspected to have stable angina were studied retrospectively. Patients were referred for evaluation of chest pain or dyspnoea by their general practitioner or by themselves. The character of the chest pain (typical, atypical, or nonanginal) was evaluated, and we excluded any patient with resting pain or suspected unstable angina. A variety of risk factors were recorded during the clinical assessment. Patients who had a prior history of CAD were excluded from this study regardless of their history of coronary stenting. All patients underwent CAG and pre-procedural EF by transthoracic echocardiography (TTE) and were sorted into two groups – the revascularization group (n = 128) and no

revascularization group (n = 312). Patients with ACS, chronic kidney diseases, LV EF < 50%, regional wall motion abnormalities, arrhythmia, severe valvular heart diseases, pericardial diseases, thyroid disease, moderate to severe pulmonary hypertension, sepsis, or haemodynamic instability were excluded from this study. We also collected participant data regarding demographic, anthropometric, and laboratory parameters including cardiac biomarkers.

Echocardiography

TTE was performed using standard techniques with a 2.5-MHz transducer. Standard 2-D and Doppler echocardiography was performed using a commercially available echocardiographic machine (Vivid 7R GE Medical System, Horten, Norway) with the same setup interfaced and a 2.5-MHz phased-array probe. With the study participants in the partial left decubitus position and breathing normally, the observer obtained images from the parasternal long and short axes as well as from the apical four chamber and two-chamber and long-axis views. The depth setting was optimized to display the LV on the screen as large as possible and the same field depth was kept for both the four and two-chamber apical views. The sector width was reduced to increase the spatial and temporal resolution. The LV end-diastolic dimensions (LV EDD), end-diastolic interventricular septal thickness (IVSTd), and end-diastolic LV posterior wall thickness (PWTd) were measured at end-diastole according to the standards established by the American Society of Echocardiography [10]. LV EF was determined by the biplane Simpson's method. The maximal left atrial (LA) volume was calculated using the Simpson method and indexed to the body surface area. The LV mass was calculated using the Devereux formula: LV mass = $1.04[(LVEDD + IVSTd + PWTd)^3 - (LVEDD)^3] - 13.6$. Thereafter, the LV mass index (LVMI) was calculated and indexed to the body surface area. DWS was calculated as $[(PWTs) - (PWTd)/(PWTs)]$ using M-mode echocardiography [6, 7].

The mitral flow velocities were recorded in the apical four-chamber view. The mitral inflow measurements included the peak early (E) and peak late flow velocities (A) as well as the E/A ratio. The tissue Doppler of the mitral annulus movement was also obtained from the apical four-chamber view. A 1.5-mm sample volume was placed sequentially at the septal annular sites. An analysis was performed for the early diastolic (E') and late diastolic (A') peak tissue velocities. As a noninvasive parameter for LV stiffness, the LV filling index (E/E') was calculated by the ratio of the transmitral flow velocity to the annular velocity. Adequate mitral and tissue Doppler image (TDI) signals were recorded in all patients.

The mean longitudinal global strain (GS) of LV was calculated from the apical 4,3,2-chamber views by speckle-tracking 2D–strain imaging [11].

Carotid ultrasound

A high-resolution B-mode ultrasound (Vivid 7R GE Medical Systems, Horten, Norway) equipped with a 7.5-MHz linear array transducer was used for carotid ultrasonography. In the longitudinal view, the carotid intima-media thickness (IMT) was determined as the distance from the media adventitia interface to the intima lumen interface on the far wall in a region free of plaque [12]. The examiner assessed the presence of carotid plaques, which were defined as focal structures that encroached into the lumen by at least 100% of the surrounding IMT value. The common carotid artery IMT (CCA-IMT) was measured between the origin of the carotid bulb and a point 10 mm proximal to the CCA, and the carotid bulb IMT (CB-IMT) was measured in the carotid bulb region. The CCA-IMT and CB-IMT values were determined as the average of the maximum IMT of the left and right CCA and CB.

Statistical analysis

All of the continuous data are expressed as the mean ± SD, and all of the categorical data are presented as percentages or absolute numbers. Continuous variables were analysed using Student's t-test, and dichotomous variables were analysed using the chi-square test. In addition, multivariate analysis (logistic regression, SPSS for Macintosh, version 10.0.7a, SPSS, Inc., Chicago, Ill., USA) was performed. All

variables that had a p value of 0.05 or less were considered statistically significant. The performance of continuous tests was assessed by receiver-operating-characteristic (ROC) curve.

Results

Clinical parameters of the study population

The clinical characteristics of the patients are shown in Table 1. The study population included 440 patients who underwent CAG (mean age 60 ± 10 years) and 128 patients who underwent coronary revascularization. Patients in the revascularization group were predominantly male (69% vs. 52%), and diabetes (27% vs. 17%) and current smoker status (31% vs. 22%) were more common in these patients. The incidence of coronary revascularization in men was 35% (87/248) and in women was 21% (40/192), which was statistically significantly higher in males ($p = 0.001$).

Echocardiographic parameters of the study population

One hundred twenty-eight patients underwent coronary revascularization (percutaneous intervention: 113; bypass surgery: 14) among the 440 patients who underwent CAG. Echocardiographic measurements of the study population are shown in Table 2. The entire study population had a normal cardiac size and systolic function, but

Table 1 Clinical parameters of the study population

	Revascularization ($n = 128$)	No ($n = 312$)	p
Age (years)	61.1 ± 9.4	60.0 ± 10.5	0.337
Male gender	88 (69%)	161 (52%)	0.001
Systolic blood pressure (mmHg)	123.6 ± 14.2	121.1 ± 15.4	0.126
Diastolic blood pressure	74.4 ± 9.5	73.5 ± 9.9	0.385
Heart rate (bpm)	66.7 ± 11.2	66.4 ± 12.4	0.809
Body mass index (kg/m^2)	24.8 ± 3.4	25.2 ± 3.2	0.226
Hypertension	69 (54%)	140 (45%)	0.093
Diabetes	34 (27%)	54 (17%)	0.035
Stroke	5 (4%)	16 (5%)	0.806
Current smoker	40 (31%)	68 (22%)	0.051
Medications			
RASB	38 (30%)	82 (27%)	0.410
CCB	31 (25%)	74 (24%)	0.902
Statin	40 (32%)	84 (27%)	0.350
Aspirin	36 (29%)	67 (21%)	0.135
Clopidogrel	10 (7%)	14 (5%)	0.167
Diuretics	9 (7%)	28 (9%)	0.704
Beta-blocker	17 (14%)	32 (10%)	0.402
Trimetazidine	14 (11%)	19 (6%)	0.075

Data are mean ± standard deviation (SD) or or n (%)

CHD coronary heart disease, *RASB* Renin-Angiotensin system blocker, *CCB* calcium-channel blocker

Table 2 Echocardiographic parameters of the study population

	Revascularization (n = 128)	No (n = 312)	p
LAVI (ml/m²)	22.7 ± 6.9	22.9 ± 8.1	0.862
LVMI (g/m²)	94.6 ± 18.9	91.1 ± 22.2	0.119
LV SWTd (mm)	9.1 ± 1.4	8.9 ± 1.4	0.147
LV SWTs	13.4 ± 1.7	13.0 ± 1.8	0.033
LV PWTd	9.0 ± 1.3	8.7 ± 1.3	0.045
LV PWTs	12.6 ± 1.4	13.9 ± 1.6	<0.001
DWS	0.26 ± 0.08	0.38 ± 0.09	<0.001
LV EDD (mm)	49.9 ± 3.5	49.7 ± 4.1	0.632
LV ESD	32.4 ± 2.9	31.7 ± 3.6	0.049
LV EF (%)	60.9 ± 5.6	62.4 ± 6.2	0.019
GS (%)	−17.4 ± 2.5	−18.3 ± 2.9	0.016
E (cm/s)	63.6 ± 15.7	63.8 ± 15.6	0.901
A (cm/s)	74.6 ± 21.2	71.5 ± 17.8	0.122
E/A ratio	0.90 ± 0.31	0.93 ± 0.32	0.369
DT (ms)	208.6 ± 44.7	202.0 ± 44.2	0.162
E' (cm/s)	6.7 ± 2.1	7.6 ± 2.5	0.001
A' (cm/s)	9.3 ± 1.8	9.3 ± 1.8	0.970
E'/A'	0.75 ± 0.29	0.85 ± 0.34	0.005
E/E'	10.3 ± 4.0	9.1 ± 3.1	<0.001
S' (cm/s)	7.4 ± 1.5	7.6 ± 1.6	0.221
Diastolic grade			<0.001
normal	22 (19%)	94 (31%)	
Grade 1	83 (70%)	201 (66%)	
Grade 2	14 (11%)	9 (3%)	

Data are represented as mean ± SD or n (%)
LAVI left atrial volume index, *LVMI* left ventricular mass index, *LVEDD and ESD* LV end-diastolic and systolic dimension, *EF* ejection fraction, *GS* global strain, *DT* deceleration time

patients in the revascularization group had a slightly but significantly decreased LV systolic end-dimension, EF, and GS. Patients in the revascularization group also had a lower LV posterior wall thickness during systole and DWS. Figure 1 shows normal (a) vs. decreased DWS (b). Patients who underwent revascularization had a more advanced diastolic dysfunction and poorer diastolic parameters (lower E' velocity and elevated E/E'). In the analysis according to gender, ± 0.09 vs. 8 ± 0.10, p = 0.001). However, the mean DWS was significantly lower in the coronary revascularization group in both men (0.38 ± 0.08 vs. 0.28 ± 0.07, p < 0.001) and women (0.42 ± 0.08 vs. 0.29 ± 0.10, p < 0.001).

Laboratory findings and other parameters

Table 3 shows the laboratory parameters and results from the carotid ultrasound. Serum creatinine was higher in patients in the revascularization group. The mean IMT and maximal plaque thickness were higher in patients in the revascularization group.

The angiography results of 127 patients who underwent coronary revascularization

Table 4 shows the angiography results of 127 patients who underwent coronary revascularization. Fifty-six patients had single vessel disease (VD), and 71 patients had multi-vessel involvement. Most patients underwent one stent implantation, and one or more stent implantations were performed in 32 patients. The left anterior descending artery (LAD) was the most common target lesion, and 26% of patients had multiple lesions. All patients underwent coronary revascularization-confirmed complete revascularization (CR). CR was defined as a final angiography result without coronary stenosis ≥70% in major epicardial vessels or stenosis ≥50% in the left main [13].

Univariate analysis

Univariate analysis showed that several clinical, echocardiographic, and other factors had predictive value for coronary revascularization. A lower DWS, decreased GS, diastolic dysfunction, elevated E' velocity, male gender, diabetes, current smoking, higher IMT and higher maximal plaque thickness were associated with coronary revascularization in patients with clinical suspicion of stable angina in those who underwent CAG (Table 5).

Multivariate analyses

Among the variables found to be correlated with coronary revascularization, a lower DWS (OR: 0.920, CI: 0.862–0.981, p = 0.011) and higher IMT (OR: 12.629, CI: 1.277–124.817, p = 0.030) were found to be independently related to coronary revascularization (Table 5). To better analyse the predictive value of the relationship between DWS and coronary revascularization, we used ROC curve analysis to determine if any threshold value of DWS existed. Inspection of the ROC curve showed that DWS < 0.34 was associated with the need for coronary revascularization (sensitivity of 89% and specificity of 48%, AUC: 0.870, SE: 0.025, p < 0.001, Fig. 2a). Figure 2b presents the proportion of patients who underwent coronary revascularization classified according to DWS (> 0.34 vs. 0.34 or less). There was an absolute increase in the proportion of patients undergoing revascularization at a DWS value of 0.34 or lower.

Discussion

The novel finding of this study is that decreased DWS was associated with coronary revascularization in patients with stable angina. The important clinical implication of this finding is that lower DWS may be helpful to predict the need for coronary revascularization in patients with normal pre-procedural LVEF. This suggests a possible role of echocardiography in the diagnosis of stable angina.

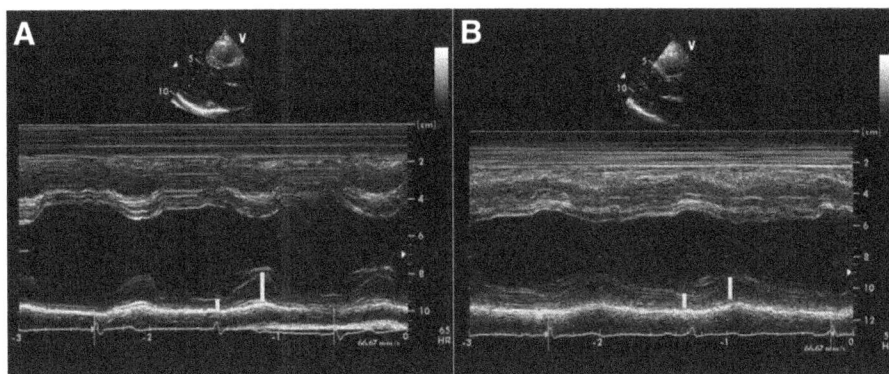

Fig. 1 Echocardiographic images of M-mode from parasternal long-axis view, a patient with normal diastolic wall strain (DWS, **a**) and a patient with decreased DWS (**b**)

Several conditions of either traumatic or atraumatic aetiologies can cause chest pain. To diagnose or exclude ACS, which is a life-threatening condition, prompt evaluation of chest pain using an algorithmic approach is important [2]. The most common causes of chest pain in outpatients are musculoskeletal and gastrointestinal causes; 10% have stable angina, 5% have respiratory conditions, and approximately 2 to 4% have acute myocardial ischaemia [14]. The target population of this study was the 10% of patients with stable angina. Among patients with suspected stable angina according clinical, laboratory, and imaging studies, 29% (128/440) of patients needed coronary revascularization (percutaneous intervention: 113; bypass surgery: 14). However, stable angina could not be ruled out in all patients who did not undergo coronary revascularization. CAG was not an absolute indication in at least 312 study subjects. However, sometimes it is not feasible to perform non-invasive functional tests, such as the treadmill test or imaging tests (MPS with SPECT, stress echocardiography or MR perfusion) [3], in clinical practice. Hence, it is the standard practice at our centre to perform CAG if the suspicion of stable angina is high after clinical, laboratory and imaging studies (chest X-ray, ECG, or echocardiography). If pre-procedural echocardiography in patients with stable angina had some predictable parameters, it

Table 3 Laboratory and other parameters

	Revascularization (n = 128)	No (n = 312)	p
Creatinine (mg/dl)	0.99 ± 1.15	0.81 ± 0.56	0.029
Total cholesterol	167.4 ± 42.7	163.0 ± 36.7	0.301
LDL	100.0 ± 36.2	95.9 ± 32.3	0.278
HDL	42.2 ± 10.8	43.9 ± 11.9	0.187
TG	139.8 ± 74.6	125.2 ± 75.6	0.088
hsCRP	2.49 ± 3.67	2.04 ± 3.11	0.417
BNP	44.1 ± 90.6	32.4 ± 52.8	0.117
CK-MB	6.79 ± 43.42	1.74 ± 2.17	0.196
Troponin I	1.60 ± 10.80	0.11 ± 0.54	0.125
Mean IMT (mm)	0.77 ± 0.24	0.70 ± 0.16	0.009
Carotid plaque (mm)	80 (90%)	166 (81%)	0.125
Max. plaque (mm)	2.36 ± 0.70	2.02 ± 0.57	<0.001
ABI,rt	1.15 ± 0.12	1.17 ± 0.07	0.176
ABI,lt	1.13 ± 0.11	1.16 ± 0.08	0.103

Data are mean ± standard deviation (SD) or or n (%)
CHD coronary heart disease, *LAVI* left atrial volume index, *LV EDD/ESD* left ventricular end-diastolic and systolic dimension, *EF* ejection fraction, *LVMI* left ventricular mass index, *DT* deceleration time, *RVSP* estimated right ventricular systolic pressure

Table 4 The angiography results of 127 patients who performed coronary revascularization

Characteristics	Number of patients (%)
1 Vessel disease (VD)	56 (44%)
2 VD	45 (35%)
3 VD	26 (21%)
Number of stents	
0[a]	19 (15%)
1	76 (60%)
2	26 (20%)
3	5 (4%)
4	1 (1%)
Target lesion	
Involvement of left main	9 (7%)
Left anterior descending artery	46 (36%)
Left circumflex artery	15 (12%)
Right coronary artery	24 (20%)
Multiple	33 (26%)
Proximal	50 (39%)
Mid to distal	44 (35%)
Both (tandem lesion)	33 (26%)

[a]Of the 19 patients who did not undergo stent implantation, 14 patients underwent bypass surgery, 4 patients underwent balloon angioplasty, and 1 patient underwent thrombus suctioning

Table 5 Uni-and multivariate analysis of the determinants of coronary revascularization in patients with stable angina

	Odds ratio	95% CI	p
Univariate analysis			
Diastolic wall strain	0.987	0.984–0.990	< 0.001
Left ventricular EF	0.996	0.958–1.037	0.856
Left ventricular global strain	0.888	0.805–0.979	0.017
E/E'	1.111	1.046–1.179	0.001
Diastolic grading	1.825	1.117–2.8983	0.016
Male gender	2.076	1.344–3.207	0.001
Diabetes	1.721	1.055–2.809	0.030
Current smoking	1.624	1.025–2.574	0.039
Creatinine	1.320	0.973–1.791	0.075
Mean carotid IMT	7.687	1.851–31.926	0.005
Maximal plaque	2.350	1.518–3.636	<0.001
Multivariate analysis			
Diastolic wall strain	0.875	0.806–0.950	0.001
Left ventricular global strain	1.061	0.913–1.232	0.440
E/E'	1.003	0.881–1.143	0.960
Diastolic grading	1.656	0.720–3.811	0.235
Male gender	1.211	0.512–2.864	0.663
Diabetes	0.668	0.281–1.584	0.359
Mean carotid IMT	13.041	1.277–124.827	0.025
Maximal plaque	1.779	0.985–3.215	0.073

EF ejection fraction, *IMT* intima-medial thickness

would be helpful to determine the patients in whom CAG is indicated. Retrospectively, 312 (71%) of our subjects did not require CAG. Non-invasive imaging plays a multifactorial role in patients with a known or suspected myocardial infarction. In particular, the advantages of

echocardiography are to assess the cardiac structure and function and to detect RWMA (myocardial thickness, thickening and motion) [1]. Echocardiographic contrast agents can improve the visualization of the endocardial border and assess myocardial perfusion [15]. Tissue Doppler and strain imaging are very helpful tools for the quantification of global and regional function of LV [11, 15]. However, these modalities have been primarily used in the setting of myocardial infarction. Therefore, we investigated echocardiographic parameters other than LV function or RWMA in the setting of stable angina.

It follows from the concept of the "ischaemic cascade" [16] that exercise or pharmacologic stress tests (ECG, echocardiography, nuclear test, etc.) are the major tests for evaluating coronary artery stenosis with a high accuracy and prognostic value in patients with clinical suspicion of myocardial ischaemia [17–20]. However, performing these tests before deciding to perform CAG is not always possible in clinical practice due to limitations of time and cost or due to contraindications. Considering the ischaemic cascade (the onset of ischaemia is followed by LV diastolic dysfunction, LV systolic dysfunction, ECG changes and angina, in that order) [16], we hypothesized that the evaluation of LV diastolic dysfunction might be helpful in patients with suspected stable angina. Fogelman et al. compared multiple posterior wall echograms taken before, during, immediately after, and 5 min after exercise in normal subjects vs. patients with angina; the angina patients showed not only a significantly decreased resting diastolic posterior wall velocity but also a remarkable slowing of the diastolic posterior wall velocity during angina [5]. DWS, a non-invasive, load-independent, and reproducible estimator of LV stiffness using 2D echocardiography, is used to assess wall distensibility in the absence of LV systolic

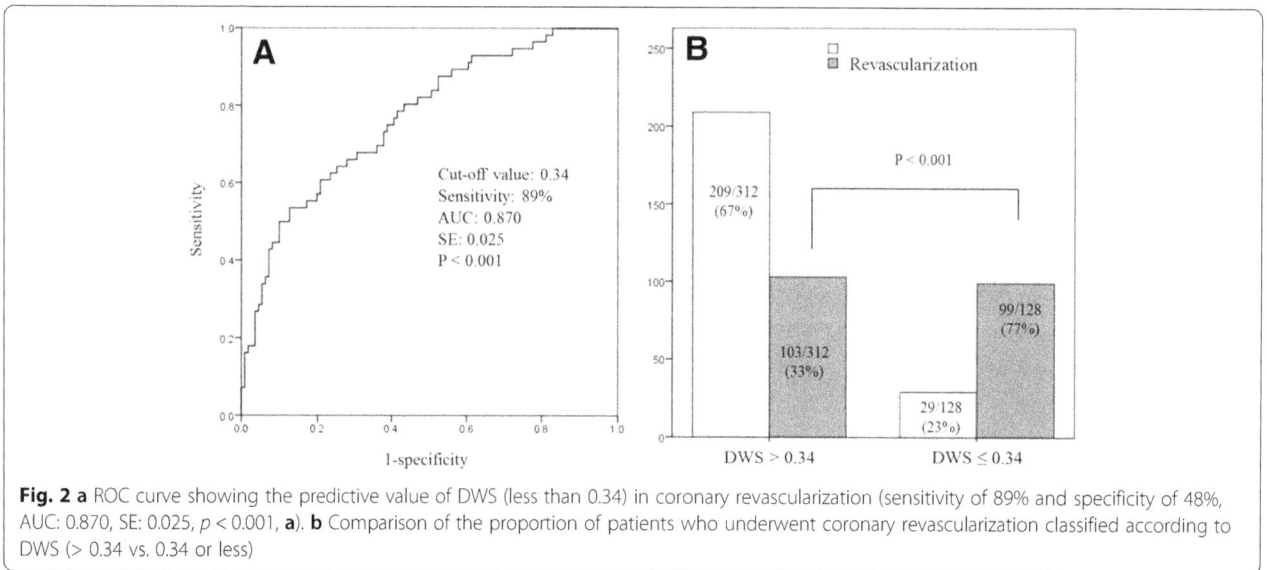

Fig. 2 a ROC curve showing the predictive value of DWS (less than 0.34) in coronary revascularization (sensitivity of 89% and specificity of 48%, AUC: 0.870, SE: 0.025, *p* < 0.001, **a**). **b** Comparison of the proportion of patients who underwent coronary revascularization classified according to DWS (> 0.34 vs. 0.34 or less)

dysfunction [6]. Decreased DWS means increased diastolic myocardial stiffness and is associated with poor prognosis in patients with HFpEF [7] and HFrEF [8]. Hypertension can cause myocardial fibrosis in association with increased deposition of myocardial collagen, and myocardial fibrosis is responsible for myocardial stiffness. Even in patients with treated hypertension, decreased DWS (cut-off value <0.34) is associated with LV diastolic dysfunction [21]. The cut-off value of DWS for predicting coronary revascularization in our study was also 0.34 (sensitivity: 89%). Takagi et al. reported that DWS is inversely correlated with post-exercise E/E' in elderly patients without obvious myocardial ischaemia, and DWS ≤ 0.33 was defined as low DWS [22]. In addition, low DWS (≤ 0.33) is associated with adverse LV remodelling (higher LV end-systolic volume and increased LV mass index) even in patients with normal LV diastolic function [9].

Atrial fibrillation (AF), the most common cardiac arrhythmia, is associated with the LV diastolic dysfunction [23]. Kang et al. observed that diastolic dysfunction (elevated E velocity, E/E') and dys-synchronous LA were associated with the occurrence of stroke in patients with paroxysmal AF, even in those with a similar CHAD (except prior stroke) score [24]. Uetake et al. reported that patients with AF had lower DWS than controls (0.35 vs. 0.41) and that decreased DWS (<0.380) was a strong determinant of the prevalence of AF in patients with paroxysmal AF and structurally normal hearts [25].

Therefore, decreased DWS ≤ 0.33 or 0.34 is definitely associated with increased LV stiffness and diastolic dysfunction in various diseases [7–9, 21, 22, 25] and is associated with poor prognosis in patients with HFpEF, HFrEF [7, 8] and AF [25].

Limitations

This study has a few limitations. First, few patients showed elevated pre-procedural cardiac biomarkers. Suspected ACS patients (typical chest pain, RWMA by echocardiography, ST elevation, or significant ST change in association with elevated cardiac biomarkers) were excluded from this study. Only a few patients who were very stable did not have resting chest pain and showed normal LVEF by echocardiography without discernible RWMA were included. Despite the insensitive and subjective nature of the echocardiographic evaluation of RWMA, the patients included in this study were not high-risk patients. Rarely, cardiac troponin can be elevated if the angina episode is prolonged in patients with chronic stable angina [26]. Second, we evaluated only epicardial coronary obstructions that needed revascularization. Therefore, microvascular angina or coronary spasm was not considered in this study. Third, we did not perform functional studies before CAG in all patients. Finally, the relatively small study population was a major limitation.

Conclusions

In summary, decreased DWS is associated with coronary revascularization in patients with stable angina. The important clinical implication of this finding is that lower DWS may be helpful to predict coronary revascularization in patients with normal pre-procedural LV EF. This implies a possible role of echocardiography in the diagnosis of stable angina.

Abbreviations
ACS: Acute coronary syndrome; CAD: Coronary artery disease; CAG: Coronary angiography; CB: Carotid bulb; CCA: Common carotid artery; CR: Complete revascularization; DWS: Diastolic wall strain; ECG: 12-lead-electrocardiography; EF: Ejection fraction; GS: Global strain; HFpEF: Heart failure with preserved LV ejection fraction; HFrEF: Heart failure with reduced LV ejection fraction; IMT: Intima-media thickness; IVSTd: End-diastolic interventricular septal thickness / PWTd: end-diastolic LV posterior wall thickness; LA: Left atrial; LV EDD: LV end-diastolic dimensions; LV: Left ventricular; LVMI: Left ventricular mass index; MPS with SPECT: Myocardial perfusion scintigraphy with single photon emission computed tomography; MR: Magnetic resonance; ROC: Receiver-operating-characteristic; RWMA: Regional wall motion abnormality; SD: Standard deviation; TDI: Tissue Doppler image; TTE: Transthoracic echocardiography

Acknowledgements
There is nothing to declare with this study.

Funding
This research received no specific grant from any funding agency.

Authors' contributions
JC and MKK designed this study as the first author and corresponding author. CH, SMH, SGJ and HKK made the SPSS data together. KJC, SC, JRC and NL were involved in data acquisition and analysis in this study. All authors read and approved the final manuscript.

Competing interests
The authors declare that they have no competing interests.

Author details
[1]Division of Cardiology, Hangang Sacred Heart Hospital, Hallym University Medical Center, Seoul, South Korea. [2]Cardiology Division, Kangnam Sacred Heart Hospital, Hallym University Medical Center, Seoul, South Korea. [3]Division of Cardiology, Department of Medicine, College of Medicine, Kangwon National University, Chuncheon, South Korea.

References
1. Thygesen K, Alpert JS, Jaffe AS, Simoons ML, Chaitman BR, White HD. Joint ESC/ACCF/AHA/WHF task force for universal definition of myocardial infarction. 3rd universal definition of myocardial infarction. J Am Coll Cardiol. 2012;60:1581–98.
2. Skinner JS, Smeeth L, Kendall JM, Adams PC, Timmis A. Chest pain guideline development group. NICE guidance. Chest pain of recent onset: assessment and diagnosis of recent onset chest pain or discomfort of suspected cardiac origin. Heart. 2010:974–8.
3. Henderson RA, O'Flynn N. Guideline development group. Management of stable angina: summary of NICE guidance. Heart. 2012;98:500–7.
4. Genders TS, Steyerberg EW, Alkadhi H, Leschka S, Desbiolles L, Nieman K, et

al. CAD Consortium. A clinical prediction rule for the diagnosis of coronary artery disease: validation, updating, and extension. Eur Heart J. 2011;32:1316–30.

5. Fogelman AM, Abbasi AS, Pearce ML, Kattus AA. Echocardiographic study of the abnormal motion of the posterior left Ventricular Wall during angina pectoris. Circulation. 1972;46:905–13.

6. Takeda Y, Sakata Y, Higashimori M, Mano T, Nishio M, Ohtani T, et al. Noninvasive assessment of wall distensibility with the evaluation of diastolic epicardial movement. J Card Fail. 2009;15:68–77.

7. Ohtani T, Mohammed SF, Yamamoto K, Dunlay SM, Weston SA, Sakata Y, et al. Diastolic stiffness as assessed by diastolic wall strain is associated with adverse remodelling and poor outcomes in heart failure with preserved ejection fraction. Eur Heart J. 2012;33:1742–9.

8. Soyama Y, Mano T, Goda A, Sugahara M, Masai K, Masuyama T. Prognostic value of diastolic wall strain in patients with chronic heart failure with reduced ejection fraction. Heart Vessel. 2017;32:68–75.

9. Kang MK, Ju S, Mun HS, Choi S, Cho JR, Lee N. Decreased diastolic wall strain is associated with adverse left ventricular remodeling even in patients with normal left ventricular diastolic function. J Echocardiogr. 2015;13:35–42.

10. Lang RM, Badano LP, Mor-Avi V, Afilalo J, Armstrong A, Ernande L, et al. Recommendations for cardiac chamber quantification by echocardiography in adults: an update from the American Society of Echocardiography and the European Association of Cardiovascular Imaging. J Am Soc Echocardiogr. 2015;28:1–39.

11. Dandel M, Lehmkuhl H, Knosalla C, Suramelashvili N, Hetzer R. Strain and strain rate imaging by echocardiography - basic concepts and clinical applicability. Curr Cardiol Rev. 2009;5:133–48.

12. Touboul PJ, Hennerici MG, Meairs S, Adams H, Amarenco P, Bornstein N, et al. Mannheim carotid intima-media thickness and plaque consensus (2004-2006-2011). An update on behalf of the advisory board of the 3rd, 4th and 5th watching the risk symposia, at the 13th, 15th and 20th European stroke conferences, Mannheim, Germany, 2004, Brussels, Belgium, 2006, and Hamburg, Germany, 2011. Cerebrovasc Dis. 2012;34:290–6.

13. Quadri G, D'Ascenzo F, Moretti C, D'Amico M, Raposeiras-Roubín S, Abu-Assi E, et al. Complete or incomplete coronary revascularisation in patients with myocardial infarction and multivessel disease: a propensity score analysis from the "real-life" BleeMACS (bleeding complications in a multicenter registry of patients discharged with diagnosis of acute coronary syndrome) registry. Eur Secur. 2017;13:407–14.

14. Ebell MH. Evaluation of chest pain in primary care patients. Am Fam Physician. 2011;83:603–5.

15. Flachskampf FA, Schmid M, Rost C, Achenbach S, deMaria AN, Daniel WG. Cardiac imaging after myocardial infarction. Eur Heart J. 2011;32:272–83.

16. Nesto RW, Kowalchuk GJ. The ischemic cascade: temporal sequence of hemodynamic, electrocardiographic and symptomatic expressions of ischemia. Am J Cardiol. 1987;59:23C–30C.

17. Schinkel AF, Bax JJ, Elhendy A, van Domburg RT, Valkema R, Vourvouri E, et al. Long-term prognostic value of dobutamine stress echocardiography compared with myocardial perfusion scanning in patients unable to perform exercise tests. Am J Med. 2004;117:1–9.

18. Mathias W Jr, Arruda A, Santos FC, Arruda AL, Mattos E, Osorio A, et al. Safety of dobutamine-atropine stress echocardiography: a prospective experience of 4,033 consecutive studies. J Am Soc Echocardiogr. 1999;12:785–91.

19. Gebker R, Jahnke C, Manka R, Hamdan A, Schnackenburg B, Fleck E, Paetsch I. Additional value of myocardial perfusion imaging during dobutamine stress magnetic resonance for the assessment of coronary artery disease. Circ Cardiovasc Imaging. 2008;1:122–30.

20. Ohman EM. CLINICAL PRACTICE. Chronic stable angina. N Engl J Med. 2016; 374:1167–76.

21. Liu YW, Lee WH, Lin CC, Huang YY, Lee WT, Lee CH, et al. Left ventricular diastolic wall strain and myocardial fibrosis in treated hypertension. Int J Cardiol. 2014;172:e304–6.

22. Takagi T, Takagi A, Yoshikawa J. Low diastolic wall strain is associated with raised post-exercise E/E' ratio in elderly patients without obvious myocardial ischemia. J Echocardiogr. 2014;12:106–11.

23. Tsang TS, Gersh BJ, Appleton CP, Tajik AJ, Barnes ME, Bailey KR, et al. Left ventricular diastolic dysfunction as a predictor of the first diagnosed nonvalvular atrial fibrillation in 840 elderly men and women. J AmColl Cardiol. 2002;40:1636–44.

24. Kang MK, Han C, Chun KJ, Choi J, Choi S, Cho JR, Lee N. Factors associated with stroke in patients with paroxysmal atrial fibrillation beyond CHADS2 score. Cardiol. 2016;23:429–36.

25. Uetake S, Maruyama M, Yamamoto T, Kato K, Miyauchi Y, Seino Y, Shimizu W. Left ventricular stiffness estimated by diastolic wall strain is associated with paroxysmal atrial fibrillation in structurally normal hearts. Clin Cardiol. 2016;39:728–32.

26. Thygesen K, Mair J, Katus H, Plebani M, Venge P, Collinson P, et al. study group on biomarkers in cardiology of the ESC working group on acute cardiac care. Recommendations for the use of cardiac troponin measurement in acute cardiac care. Eur Heart J. 2010;31:2197–204.

The effect of tolvaptan on renal excretion of electrolytes and urea nitrogen in patients undergoing coronary artery bypass surgery

Tomoko S. Kato[1*†], Hiroshi Nakamura[1†], Mai Murata[1], Kishio Kuroda[1], Hitoshi Suzuki[2], Yasutaka Yokoyama[1], Akie Shimada[1], Satoshi Matsushita[1], Taira Yamamoto[1] and Atsushi Amano[1]

Abstract

Background: Adequate fluid management is an important component of patient care following cardiac surgery. Our aim in this study was to determine the benefits of tolvaptan, an oral selective vasopressin-2 receptor antagonist that causes electrolyte-free water diuresis, in postoperative fluid management. We prospectively examined the effect of tolvaptan on renal excretion of electrolytes and urea nitrogen in cardiac surgery patients.

Methods: Patients undergoing coronary artery bypass surgery were randomized to receive conventional loop diuretics (Group C, $n = 30$) or conventional loop diuretic therapy plus tolvaptan (Group T, $n = 27$). Fractional excretions of sodium (FENA), potassium (FEK) and urea nitrogen (FEUN) were measured in both groups during post-surgical hospitalization.

Results: Urine output was greater with tolvaptan (Group T) than without it (Group C), and some patients in Group C required intravenous as well as oral loop diuretics. Serum sodium concentrations decreased after surgery in Group C, but were unchanged in Group T (postoperative day [POD] 3, 139.8 ± 3.5 vs. 142.3 ± 2.6 mEq/L, $p = 0.006$). However, postoperative FENA values in Group C did not decrease, and the values were similar in both groups. Serum potassium levels remained lower and FEK values remained higher than the preoperative values, but only in Group C (all $p < 0.05$). BUN increased postoperatively in both groups, but it remained higher than its preoperative value only in Group C (all $p < 0.01$). Group T showed an initial increase in BUN, which peaked and then returned to its preoperative value within a week. The FEUN increased postoperatively in both groups, but the change was more pronounced in Group T (POD7, 52.7 ± 9.3 vs. 58.2 ± 6.5 %, $p = 0.025$).

Conclusions: Renal excretion of sodium and potassium reflects the changes in serum concentration in patients treated with tolvaptan. Patients treated only with loop diuretics showed a continuous excretion of sodium and potassium that led to electrolyte imbalance, whereas the combination of loop diuretics and tolvaptan increased renal urea nitrogen elimination. Tolvaptan therefore appears to be an effective diuretic that minimally affects serum electrolytes while adequately promoting the elimination of urea nitrogen from the kidneys in patients undergoing coronary artery bypass surgery.

Keywords: Coronary artery bypass surgery, Tolvaptan, Renal excretion, Electrolyte, Urea nitrogen

* Correspondence: tokato@juntendo.ac.jp; rinnko@sannet.ne.jp
†Equal contributors
[1]Department of Cardiovascular Surgery, Heart Center, Juntendo University,
2-1-1, Hongo, Bunkyo-ku, Tokyo 113-8421, Japan
Full list of author information is available at the end of the article

Background

Fluid management following cardiac surgery is one of the most important parts of postoperative cardiac patient care [1, 2]. Loop diuretics are commonly administrated postoperatively; however, their continuous usage sometimes leads to electrolyte imbalances, neurohumoral activation, worsening renal failure, and diuretic resistance [3]. Loop diuretics inhibit sodium reabsorption at the thick ascending limb of the loop of Henle and passively increase water excretion. Consequently, loop diuretics cause hyponatremia. However, the efficacy of loop diuretics is reduced under hyponatremia, resulting in a need to increase the dosage. This, in turn, further worsens the hyponatremia, creating a futile cycle [4]. In addition, loop diuretics increase sodium delivery to the distal segment of the distal tubule, which stimulates the aldosterone-sensitive sodium pump to increase sodium reabsorption in exchange for potassium. Volume depletion causes further increases in aldosterone secretion, resulting in excessive urinary potassium secretion and hypokalemia [3, 4]. Hypokalemia, in turn, may provoke both supraventricular and ventricular postoperative cardiac arrhythmias, with adverse effects on myocardial contractility [5]. These adverse effects of loop diuretics emphasize the need for better therapeutics for postoperative fluid management in cardiac patients.

One promising candidate is tolvaptan, an oral selective vasopressin V2-receptor antagonist that causes electrolyte-free water diuresis [6, 7]. Water balance in the early postoperative phase is modulated by the level of plasma arginine vasopressin (AVP), which increases in response to operative stress [8, 9]. AVP plays an important role in water reabsorption at the renal collecting duct and this increase causes an excessive body water imbalance during the early postoperative phase. The use of a vasopressin inhibitor like tolvaptan, which promotes water excretion without changes in renal hemodynamics or sodium and potassium excretion [6], therefore may represent an ideal strategy for maintaining fluid balance in patients undergoing cardiac surgery. Furthermore, tolvaptan may have benefits in reducing blood urea nitrogen (BUN) levels, which are associated with increased cardiovascular mortality and morbidity [10, 11]. Vasopressin promotes reabsorption of urea in the distal nephron, resulting in increased BUN [12]; therefore, vasopressin inhibition by tolvaptan treatment may also be effective for eliminating the excessive BUN associated with surgery-induced protein catabolism.

To the best of our knowledge, no detailed study has yet examined the effect of tolvaptan on renal electrolyte excretion following cardiac surgery. Therefore, we prospectively compared the fractional excretion of electrolytes and urea nitrogen in postoperative cardiac surgery patients following treatment with loop diuretics with or without tolvaptan.

Methods
Study design

Data on the effects of tolvaptan on changes in body weight and other clinical parameters after bypass surgery were collected at Juntendo University Hospital. Seventy patients undergoing off-pump coronary artery bypass surgery were prospectively enrolled in the study and randomized to either the group receiving conventional loop diuretic treatment only (Group C) or the group receiving conventional loop diuretic treatment plus tolvaptan (Group T). Patients in Group T received tolvaptan 7.5 mg once daily on postoperative days 1 and 2, in addition to conventional oral loop diuretics; intravenous loop diuretics were given only if needed. Tolvaptan was administered as needed from postoperative day 3 in Group T patients. Patients in Group C received only conventional loop diuretic therapy. Patients with renal insufficiency, such as those with chronic kidney disease stage 4 or greater, were excluded from the study. Patients requiring emergency surgery, those undergoing cardiopulmonary bypass, and those undergoing concomitant extracardiac/vascular and/or valvular surgery were also excluded. Laboratory values were serially measured after surgery for up to 7 days during hospitalization, and the fractional excretion of sodium (FENA), potassium (FEK), and urea nitrogen (FEUN) were calculated for both groups of patients.

The study was approved by the institutional review board of Juntendo University Hospital (UMIN000011039). All participants received detailed information about the study and provided written informed consent.

Statistical analysis

Data are presented as mean ± SD. Normality was evaluated for each variable from normal distribution plots and histograms. Data obtained at the same time-point were compared between groups using Student's unpaired two-tailed t-test for continuous variables and the chi-square test for categorical variables. Intragroup changes in preoperative vs. postoperative values were assessed with Student's paired t-test. All data were analyzed using the Statistical Analysis Systems software JMP 11.0 (SAS Institute Inc., Cary, NC, USA).

Results
Patient characteristics

A total of 70 patients scheduled to undergo off-pump coronary artery bypass surgery were initially reviewed. Of those, 2 patients were excluded as they required another procedure in addition to bypass surgery. After randomization of patients into Groups T and C, incomplete datasets were collected from 7 patients in Group T and 4 patients in Group C. Therefore, analyzable data were obtained from 27 patients in Group T and 30 patients in Group C (Fig. 1).

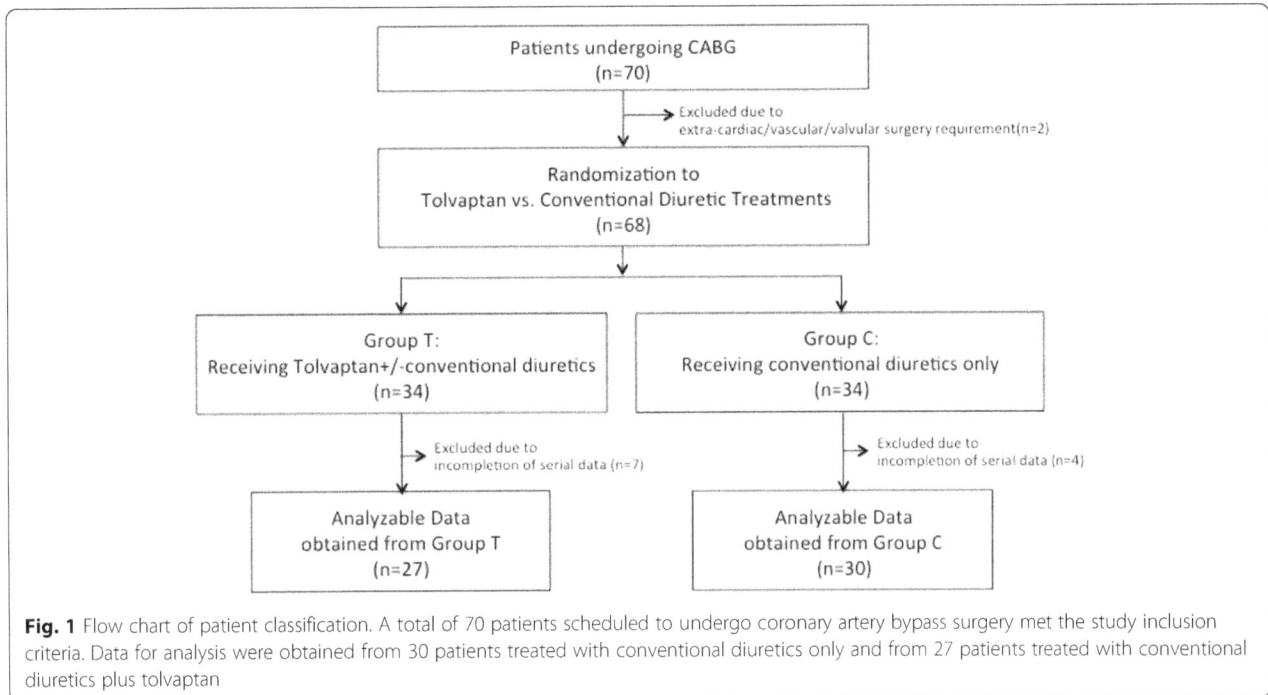

Fig. 1 Flow chart of patient classification. A total of 70 patients scheduled to undergo coronary artery bypass surgery met the study inclusion criteria. Data for analysis were obtained from 30 patients treated with conventional diuretics only and from 27 patients treated with conventional diuretics plus tolvaptan

Patient demographics, laboratory values prior to the surgery, and operative information for both groups are summarized in Table 1. Age, gender distribution, body surface area, and preoperative laboratory values, including the estimated glomerular filtration rate (eGFR), did not differ between the groups. The average operative duration was around 240 min, and the mean number of grafts was 3 in both groups.

Postoperative urinary output

Both groups received loop diuretics after surgery in a routine manner in order to rectify postoperative hypervolemia. In our institution, Lasix® 40 mg per day orally is generally given to patients undergoing coronary bypass surgery. Additional Lasix® is administered intravenously if a patient's hourly urine output is approximately less than 50 mL. In the present study, only some patients in Group C required additional intravenous loop diuretics (Fig. 2). Even so, the amounts of urine after surgery were greater in Group T than in Group C, and the differences were statistically significant on postoperative days 2 and 3. The estimated glomerular filtration rate (eGFR) values were not significantly different between the groups throughout the entire study period (Fig. 2).

Serial changes in serum electrolytes, FENA, and FEK

Figure 3 shows the serial changes in serum sodium concentrations and FENA before and after surgery in both groups. We were unable to obtain values at postoperative days 4 and 6 from some patients; therefore, the data from postoperative days 4 and 6 were omitted from the analysis. Serum sodium concentrations decreased postoperatively in Group C (from pre-surgery to postoperative days 2, 5, and 7, $p = 0.046$, 0.027, and 0.029, respectively), but they remained unchanged in Group T. Comparison of the values between the groups revealed that postoperative

Table 1 Patient characteristics

	Group T (n = 27)	Group C (n = 30)	p value
Age (years)	69.0 ± 10.7	70.1 ± 7.5	0.697
Men	23 (85.2 %)	20 (66.7 %)	0.189
Body surface area (m²)	1.70 ± 0.16	1.60 ± 0.16	0.061
Preoperative laboratory examinations			
Hb (g/dL)	11.9 ± 1.9	12.3 ± 1.2	0.341
Na (mEq/L)	141.5 ± 3.2	140.9 ± 3.1	0.537
K (mEq/L)	4.2 ± 0.2	4.3 ± 0.3	0.225
BUN (mg/dL)	14.3 ± 5.3	14.3 ± 5.5	0.965
Cre (mg/dL)	0.86 ± 0.32	0.80 ± 0.28	0.466
T-Bil (mg/dL)	1.0 ± 0.3	1.1 ± 0.2	0.065
TP (g/dL)	6.3 ± 0.5	6.3 ± 0.4	0.805
Alb (g/dL)	3.6 ± 0.3	3.4 ± 0.5	0.363
eGFR (ml/min./1.73 m²)	77.7 ± 31.0	76.4 ± 25.4	0.871
BNP (pg/mL)	263.1 ± 201.0	276.6 ± 197.5	0.814
Operative information			
Operative duration (minutes)	247.7 ± 54.3	240.1 ± 64.3	0.688
Number of grafts	3.0 ± 1.1	2.9 ± 1.3	0.899

Abbreviations not defined in the text: *Hb* hemoglobin, *Na* sodium, *K* potassium, *Cre* creatinine, *T-Bil* total bilirubin, *TP* total protein, *Alb* albumin, *BNP* brain natriuretic peptide

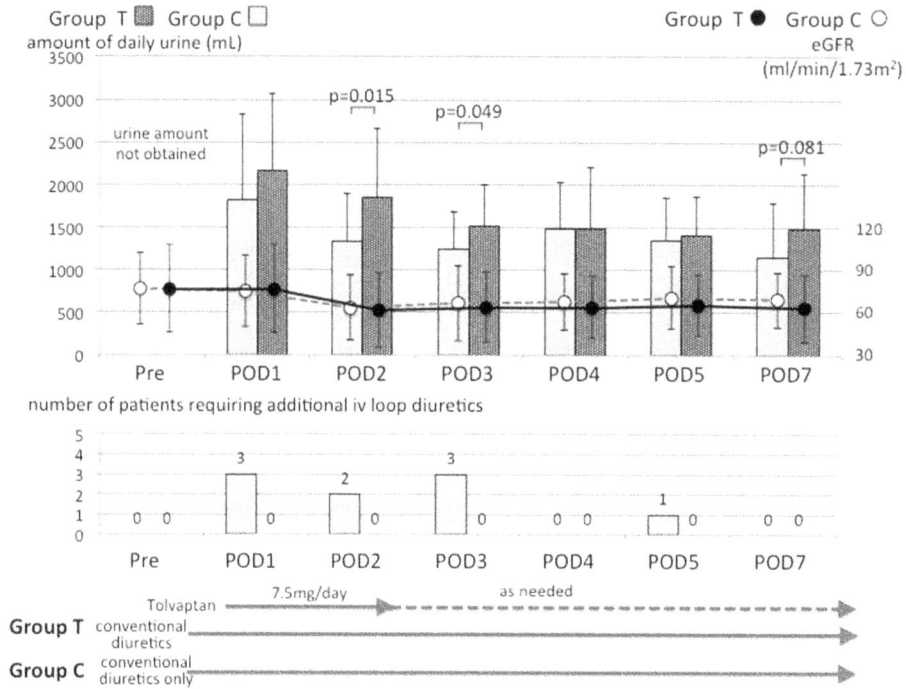

Fig. 2 Serial changes in the amounts of daily urinary output after surgery and eGFR (*upper*), and numbers of patients who required intravenous loop diuretic administration (*lower*). Dark gray spotted bars and black circles indicate values for patients receiving conventional diuretic therapy plus tolvaptan (*Group T*) and gray bars and white circles indicate values for patients receiving conventional diuretic therapy only (*Group C*). POD, postoperative day

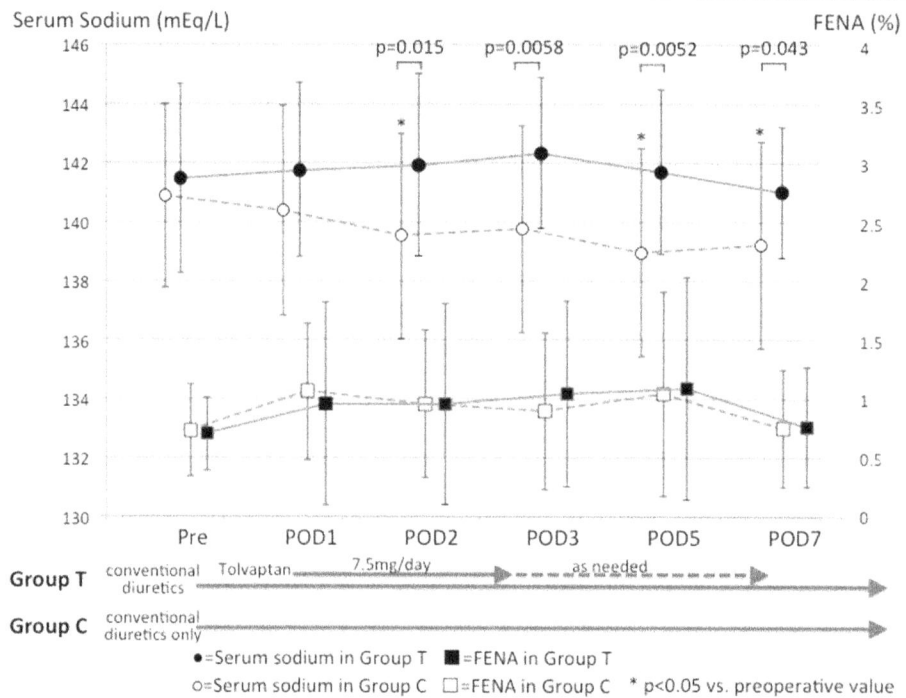

Fig. 3 Serial changes in sodium concentrations (*upper*) and FENA (lower) in patients receiving conventional diuretics plus tolvaptan (*black symbols and solid lines*) or conventional diuretics only (*white symbols and dotted lines*). FENA, fractional excretion of sodium; POD, postoperative day

serum sodium concentrations at postoperative days 2, 3, 5, and 7 were higher in Group T than in Group C. However, even though the serum sodium concentrations decreased postoperatively in Group C, the renal sodium excretion in that group remained constant. In other words, FENA did not decrease in Group C.

Figure 4 shows the serial changes in serum potassium concentrations and FEK before and after surgery. Serum potassium levels in both groups showed a gradual decrease after surgery until postoperative day 3 (from pre-surgery to postoperative day 3: for 4.2 ± 0.2 to 3.9 ± 0.2 mEq/L for Group T and 4.3 ± 0.3 to 3.9 ± 0.3 mEq/L for Group C, both $p < 0.001$). After postoperative day 3, serum potassium levels in Group T returned to the preoperative range, whereas the levels stayed lower in Group C. The FEK values increased from their preoperative value on postoperative day 1 in both groups (both $p < 0.001$). In Group C, the FEK values further increased until postoperative day 3, and they remained higher than the preoperative value (from pre-surgery to postoperative days 2, 3, and 5, all $p < 0.001$). In Group T, the FEK value, which was higher on postoperative day 1 than on the preoperative value, decreased and returned to the preoperative range after postoperative day 2.

Serial changes in blood urea nitrogen (BUN) and FEUN

Figure 5 shows the serial changes in BUN levels and FEUN before and after surgery. BUN increased postoperatively in both groups, but remained higher than its preoperative value until postoperative day 7 in Group C (from presurgery to postoperative day 7, 14.3 ± 5.5 to 21.0 ± 9.9 mg/dL, $p = 0.0003$). In Group T, the increase in BUN peaked on postoperative day 2 and then gradually decreased to its preoperative value.

In both groups, FEUN increased postoperatively and remained higher than the preoperative values. The increase in postoperative FEUN was more pronounced in Group T. Intergroup comparison showed that the FEUN values at postoperative days 2 and 7 were statistically higher in Group T than in Group C ($p = 0.049$ and 0.025, respectively).

Postoperative clinical courses

The postoperative clinical courses in all patients are compared in Table 2. Because some patients were seen at outside community hospitals after discharge, we were unable to gather long-term data, such as laboratory examinations, from all patients. No differences were evident in mortality between the groups up to 2.9 years after the surgery (mean 2.1 years). The occurrence of perioperative adverse events was not statistically different between the groups. None of the patients required renal replacement therapy after the surgery; however, one patient in Group T (3.7 %) and 4 in Group C (13 %) developed RIFLE classification-R (risk) acute kidney injury (AKI) [13].

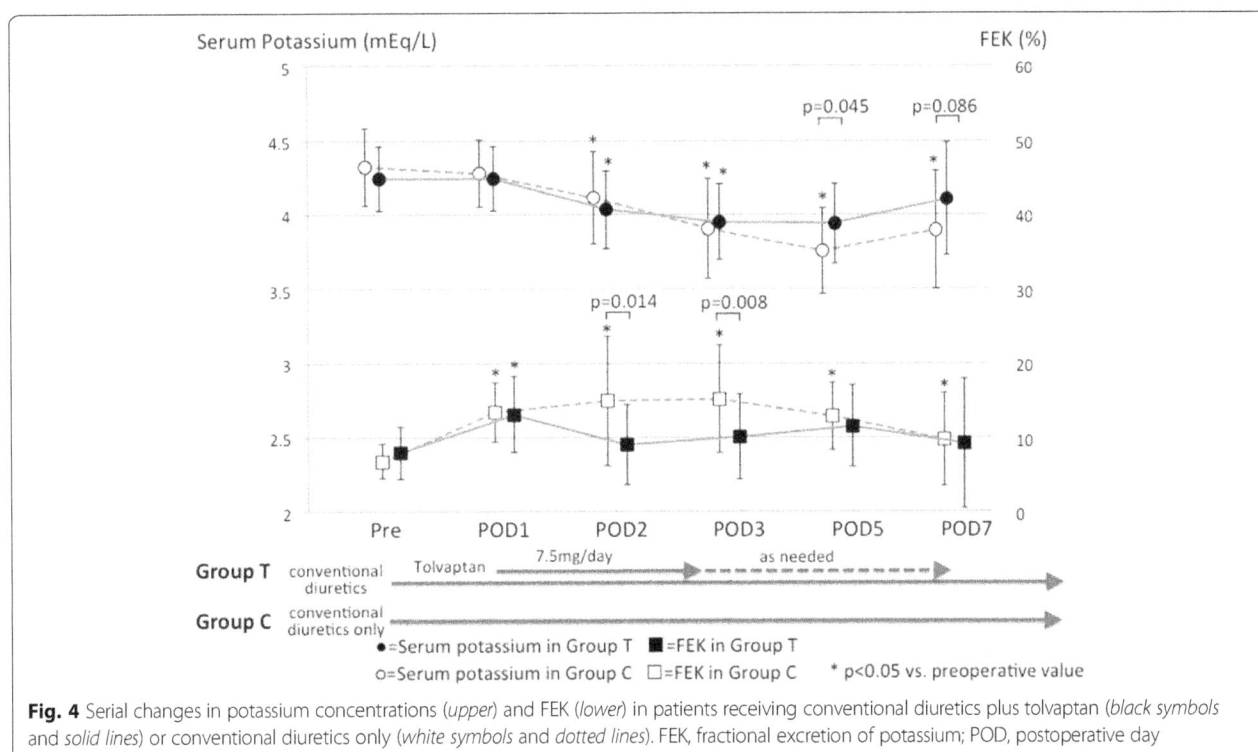

Fig. 4 Serial changes in potassium concentrations (*upper*) and FEK (*lower*) in patients receiving conventional diuretics plus tolvaptan (*black symbols and solid lines*) or conventional diuretics only (*white symbols* and *dotted lines*). FEK, fractional excretion of potassium; POD, postoperative day

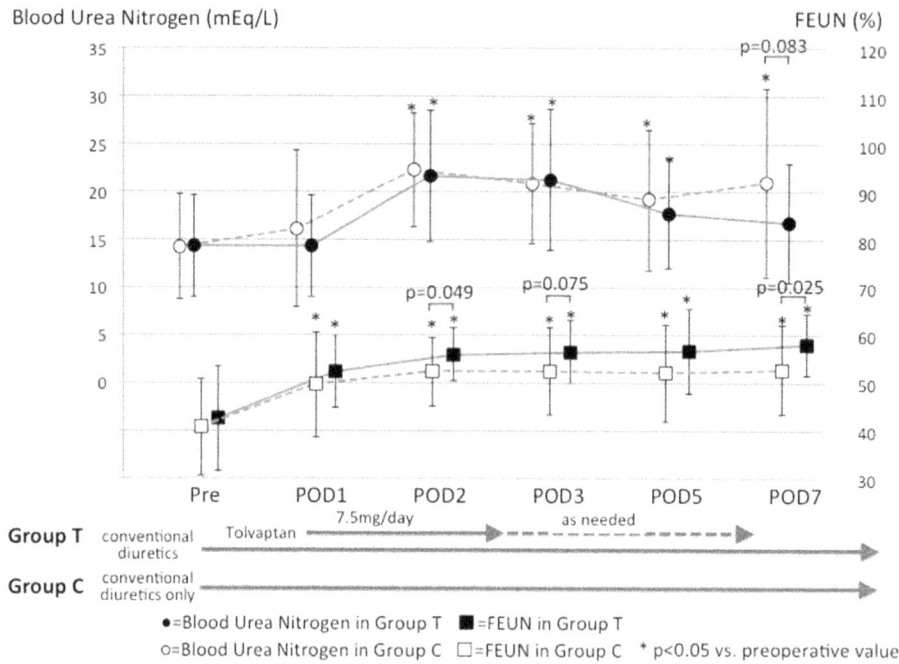

Fig. 5 Serial changes in BUN levels (*upper*) and FEUN (*lower*) in patients receiving conventional diuretics plus tolvaptan (*black symbols* and *solid lines*) or conventional diuretics only (*white symbols* and *dotted lines*). FEUN, fractional excretion of urea nitrogen; POD, postoperative day

Discussion

In the present investigation, both groups of patients received loop diuretics after surgery; therefore, the data did not reflect any independent effect of tolvaptan on renal excretion of electrolytes and urea nitrogen, as these were also influenced by the conventional loop diuretics. Even so, we believe that our detailed observations of the serial daily changes in laboratory values in serum and urine can aid in understanding how tolvaptan affects renal excretion mechanisms in patients undergoing cardiac surgery.

Table 2 Postoperative clinical course

	Group T (n = 27)	Group C (n = 30)	p value
Mortality, n (%)[a]	0 (0 %)	0 (0 %)	-
Duration of intensive care unit stay (days)	1.3 ± 1.9	1.2 ± 1.3	0.816
Bleeding amount (mL)	324.2 ± 273.4	308.4 ± 202.3	0.804
Intubation time (hours)	9.3 ± 5.3	11.2 ± 6.4	0.230
Perioperative adverse events, n (%)			
Neurological complications, n (%)	0 (0 %)	0 (0 %)	-
Arrhythmia, n (%)	6 (22.2 %)	8 (26.7 %)	0.697
Renal replacement therapy, n (%)	0 (0 %)	0 (0 %)	-
RIFLE classification-Risk, n (%)	1 (3.7 %)	4 (13.3 %)	0.467

[a]The observation period for mortality was 2.9 years (mean 2.1 years)

Our data show that (i) the amount of daily urine output was well maintained and somewhat greater with tolvaptan (Group T) than without it (Group C), although some patients in Group C required intravenous loop diuretic administration; (ii) serum sodium concentrations decreased after surgery only in Group C, but the postoperative FENA values were not significantly different with or without tolvaptan; (iii) in the absence of tolvaptan (Group C), postoperative serum potassium concentrations decreased and stayed lower than the preoperative level, with an associated increase in FEK. By contrast, the addition of tolvaptan (Group T) maintained the postoperative serum potassium levels at essentially the preoperative levels; and (iv) both groups showed an increase in BUN and FEUN after surgery, but tolvaptan treatment led to a higher FEUN and a rapid decrease in BUN as time progressed.

We speculate that the similar FENA values with and without tolvaptan after surgery may reflect an enhancement of the effectiveness of loop diuretics by tolvaptan. Previous papers have also noted that concomitant administration of tolvaptan enhances the effects of loop diuretics [14]. Nishizaki et al. showed an enhancement of natriuresis that could be an indirect effect of tolvaptan, and they assumed that tolvaptan relieves renal congestion, thereby enhancing the performance of the loop diuretics [14]. Furthermore, the dose-response curves for the loop diuretics [15] indicate that patients with renal insufficiency and/or heart failure require a higher diuretic dose to achieve the desired FENA. Therefore, our finding that the patients in Group T showed a similar FENA value to patients in Group C under a smaller loop diuretic dosage could be confirmation that tolvaptan enhances loop diuretic-induced natriuresis.

In the current study, both groups of patients were placed on a salt-restricted diet soon after surgery, and the amount of peroral sodium intake did not likely differ between the groups. Therefore, the higher serum sodium concentration seen in Group T, compared to Group C, might have resulted from the effective free-water diuresis induced by tolvaptan in Group T. Indeed, the amount of daily urine volume was larger in Group T soon after surgery (Fig. 2). In addition, the serum albumin levels were substantially higher in Group T than Group C after surgery (e.g., postoperative day 5, 3.3 ± 0.3 vs. 3.5 ± 0.2 mg/dL, $p = 0.024$). Probably because the number of studied patients was too small, we failed to show a tolvaptan effect on eGFR values (Fig. 2); however, there was a tendency for the patients in Group C to develop RIFLE classification-R (risk) AKI more frequently than the patients in Group T. This result may reflect the findings by Shirakabe et al., who reported that early administration of tolvaptan could prevent exacerbation of AKI in heart failure patients [16].

The decrease in serum potassium concentrations and the slight increase in FEK after surgery in Group C are reasonable responses to loop diuretic therapy. Group T patients also received loop diuretics, although the dosage was smaller than in Group C, and the changes in their serum potassium and FEK values soon after surgery showed similar trends to those in Group C.

The increase in BUN just after surgery most likely reflects surgery-induced protein catabolism. Although the operative duration was about 4 h and the peri-operative fasting period was approximately 1 day in both groups, maintenance fluid replacement, together with the fasting, would elicit protein degradation. However, the sustainment of this increase in BUN after surgery may also reflect neurohormonal activation and renal hypoperfusion [10, 11, 17, 18]. Testani et al. reported that excessive neurohormonal activation, as estimated by BUN elevation, can predict potential adverse effects of loop diuretics [19]. Several studies have suggested that BUN is a simple and significant prognostic marker associated with morbidity and mortality in patients with heart failure [10, 11, 17, 18, 20], and increases in BUN appear to be associated with cardiovascular mortality [11, 20]. In patients with heart failure, an increase in renin-angiotensin aldosterone system activity provokes urea reabsorption at the proximal tubule, while sympathetic nervous system activation promotes urea reabsorption at the distal and proximal tubules, and elevation of AVP upregulates urea transporters in the collecting tubule [12, 18]. Our

observations indicate that tolvaptan could reasonably modulate this AVP-associated urea reabsorption, as indicated by the decrease in BUN in Group T.

Operative stress induces neurohormonal activation and increases serum AVP levels [8, 9]. The measurements of serum AVP levels in 239 critically ill patients and 70 healthy volunteers by Jochberger et al. confirmed higher AVP concentrations in patients undergoing cardiac surgery than in patients undergoing noncardiac surgery or who had nonsurgical diseases [21]. Terazawa et al. reported that serum AVP levels increased during and soon after cardiac surgery, and that the increase was larger in patients with more severe conditions [22]. Therefore, patients undergoing cardiac surgery could have a volume overload that could be related to increased plasma AVP due to operative stress. We believe that tolvaptan may be an ideal diuretic for neurohormonal control as well as maintenance of adequate electrolyte balance. Furthermore, tolvaptan may cause excretion of the excessive BUN produced by protein catabolism and operative stress, which may be beneficial for long-term prognoses.

We admit that tolvaptan is a relatively expensive medication; however, it effectively enables diuresis without causing electrolyte imbalance, which is helpful in the management of postsurgical patients who are at high risk for cardiac arrhythmia and for progression to acute kidney injury. Therefore, the high cost of this treatment may be offset by reductions in the lengths of stays in the intensive care unit and further costly postsurgical treatment. Additional studies are needed to analyze the efficacy of tolvaptan on a medical-care cost basis in patients undergoing cardiac surgery. Moreover, elevated BUN and low sodium concentration have well known associations with poor patient prognosis [10, 11, 16], and tolvaptan treatment is expected to improve survival in heart failure patients by normalization of these factors [23]. The present observation that urea nitrogen excretion was enhanced by tolvaptan treatment without affecting sodium concentration supports this expectation. The effect of tolvaptan on long-term prognosis in patients undergoing cardiac surgery should be further investigated.

The present study had several limitations. First, this was a single-center, retrospective, observational analysis with a small number of patients. According to the protocol, tolvaptan was given only on postoperative days 1 and 2 in Group T, and the decision to continue tolvaptan was up to the attending doctor. Therefore, among the Group T patients, some received tolvaptan throughout their hospital stay and some received it for only 2 days. This may have affected the data obtained after postoperative day 3, which complicates the interpretation of our results. In addition, because most of the patients were able to consume fluids orally within a day after surgery, we were unable to estimate the effect of intravenous fluid administration on serum and/or urinary electrolytes. We also did not measure plasma AVP levels or urine Aquaporin-2, which have been reported to be predictive markers of the response to tolvaptan [24, 25]. Other than diuretics, we did not include information on the use of other drugs, such as inotropic agents and beta-blockers. Furthermore, we reviewed only the short-term clinical course and did not review long-term outcomes. Lastly, the objective variables had a relatively larger standard deviation than we initially expected, so the statistical power derived from the present results was not sufficient to draw conclusions. However, this is a preliminary analysis and we would like to enroll greater numbers of patients in more specific studies.

Conclusions

In conclusion, loop diuretics can cause continuous excretion of sodium and potassium, irrespective of their serum concentrations, which may result in electrolyte imbalance. The addition of tolvaptan in the present study prevented the generation of an electrolyte imbalance in the cardiac surgery patients investigated here. Furthermore, tolvaptan seems to enhance the effectiveness of loop diuretics. Tolvaptan also showed potential to promote the excretion of urea nitrogen produced by protein catabolism and in response to operative stress, and it does so more effectively than loop diuretics in patients undergoing coronary artery bypass surgery.

Abbreviations

AVP: Arginine vasopressin; BUN: Blood urea nitrogen; eGFR: Estimated glomerular filtration rate; FEK: Fractional excretion of potassium; FENA: Fractional excretion of sodium; FEUN: Fractional excretion of urea nitrogen; POD: Postoperative day

Funding

The present study was funded partially by Otsuka Pharmaceutical Co. Ltd.

Authors' contributions

TSK, MM, KK, and SM were responsible for data management and linkage. TSK and HS contributed to data analysis, performed the literature search for the systematic review, and helped draft the paper. MM, KK, AS and YY participated in data collection and analysis and helped draft the paper. TSK, HN, HS, TY, and AA conceived of the study and helped review the manuscript. All authors contributed significantly to the completion of the study and the manuscript, including reading and approving of the manuscript in its current form.

Competing interests

The first and fourth authors received lecture fees from Otsuka Pharmaceutical Co. Ltd. in 2015.

Author details

[1]Department of Cardiovascular Surgery, Heart Center, Juntendo University, 2-1-1, Hongo, Bunkyo-ku, Tokyo 113-8421, Japan. [2]Division of Nephrology, Department of Internal Medicine, Juntendo University School of Medicine, Bunkyo-ku, Tokyo, Japan.

References

1. Gandhi A, Husain M, Salhiyyah K, Raja SG. Does perioperative furosemide usage reduce the need for renal replacement therapy in cardiac surgery patients? Interact Cardiovasc Thorac Surg. 2012;15:750–5.
2. Nishi H, Toda K, Miyagawa S, Yoshikawa Y, Fukushima S, Kawamura M, et al. Effects of tolvaptan in the early postoperative stage after heart valve surgery: results of the STAR (Study of Tolvaptan for fluid retention AfteR valve surgery) trial. Surg Today. 2015;45:1542–51.
3. Felker GM. Loop diuretics in heart failure. Heart Fail Rev. 2012;17:305–11.
4. Haller C, Salbach P, Katus H, Kübler W. Refractory oedema in congestive heart failure: a contributory role of loop diuretics? J Intern Med. 1995;237:211–4.
5. Peretto G, Durante A, Limite LR, Cianflone D. Postoperative arrhythmias after cardiac surgery: incidence, risk factors, and therapeutic management. Cardiol Res Pract. 2014;2014:615987. doi:10.1155/2014/615987.
6. Costello-Boerrigter LC, Smith WB, Boerrigter G, Ouyang J, Zimmer CA, Orlandi C, et al. Vasopressin-2-receptor antagonism augments water excretion without changes in renal hemodynamics or sodium and potassium excretion in human heart failure. Am J Physiol Renal Physiol. 2006;290:F273–8.
7. Matsuzaki M, Hori M, Izumi T, Fukunami M. Efficacy and safety of tolvaptan in heart failure patients with volume overload despite the standard treatment with conventional diuretics: a phase III, randomized, double-blind, placebo-controlled study (QUEST study). Cardiovasc Drugs Ther. 2011;25 Suppl 1:S33–45.
8. Woods WG, Forsling ML, Le Quesne LP. Plasma arginine vasopressin levels and arterial pressure during open heart surgery. Br J Surg. 1989;76:29–32.
9. Lee WJ, Choo YE, Song WY, Lee JC, Kim KT, Lee SH. Responses of vasopressin release in patients with cardiopulmonary bypass anesthetized with enflurane and morphine. J Korean Med Sci. 1989;4:71–6.
10. Filippatos G, Rossi J, Lloyd-Jones DM, Stough WG, Ouyang J, Shin DD, et al. Prognostic value of blood urea nitrogen in patients hospitalized with worsening heart failure: insights from the Acute and Chronic Therapeutic Impact of a Vasopressin Antagonist in Chronic Heart Failure (ACTIV in CHF) study. J Card Fail. 2007;13:360–4.
11. Miura M, Sakata Y, Nochioka K, Takahashi J, Takada T, Miyata S, et al. Prognostic impact of blood urea nitrogen changes during hospitalization in patients with acute heart failure syndrome. Circ J. 2013;77:1221–8.
12. Sands JM, Blount MA, Klein JD. Regulation of renal urea transport by vasopressin. Trans Am Clin Climatol Assoc. 2011;122:82–92.
13. Bellomo R, Ronco C, Kellum JA, Mehta RL, Palevsky P. Acute renal failure: Definition, outcome measures, animal models, fluid therapy and information technology needs: The Second International Consensus Conference of the Acute Dialysis Quality Initiative (ADQI) Group. Crit Care. 2004;8:R204–12.
14. Nishizaki Y, Yamagami S, Sesoko M, Yamashita H, Daida H. Successful treatment of congestive heart failure with concomitant administration of tolvaptan to enhance the effects of furosemide. J Cardiol Cases. 2013;8:151–4.
15. Ellison DH. Diuretic therapy and resistance in congestive heart failure. Cardiology. 2001;96:132–43.
16. Shirakabe A, Hata N, Yamamoto M, Kobayashi N, Shinada T, Tomita K, Tsurumi M, Matsushita M, Okazaki H, Yamamoto Y, Yokoyama S, Asai K, Shimizu W. Immediate administration of tolvaptan prevents the exacerbation of acute kidney injury and improves the mid-term prognosis of patients with severely decompensated acute heart failure. Circ J. 2014;78:911–21.
17. Aronson D, Mittleman MA, Burger AJ. Elevated blood urea nitrogen level as a predictor of mortality in patients admitted for decompensated heart failure. Am J Med. 2004;116:466–73.
18. Kazory A. Emergence of blood urea nitrogen as a biomarker of neurohormonal activation in heart failure. Am J Cardiol. 2010;106:694–700.
19. Testani JM, Cappola TP, Brensinger CM, Shannon RP, Kimmel SE. Interaction between loop diuretic-associated mortality and blood urea nitrogen concentration in chronic heart failure. J Am Coll Cardiol. 2011;58:375–82.

20. Lombardi C, Carubelli V, Rovetta R, Castrini AI, Vizzardi E, Bonadei I, et al. Prognostic value of serial measurements of blood urea nitrogen in ambulatory patients with chronic heart failure. Panminerva Med. 2015 Jul 8. [Epub ahead of print]
21. Jochberger S, Mayr VD, Luckner G, Wenzel V, Ulmer H, Schmid S, et al. Serum vasopressin concentrations in critically ill patients. Crit Care Med. 2006;34:293–9.
22. Terazawa E, Dohi S, Akamastsu S, Ohata H, Shimonaka H. Changes in calcitonin gene-related peptide, atrial natriuretic peptide and brain natriuretic peptide in patients undergoing coronary artery bypass grafting. Anaesthesia. 2003;58:223–32.
23. Imamura T, Kinugawa K, Fujino T, Inaba T, Maki H, Hatano M, Yao A, Komuro I. Increased urine aquaporin-2 relative to plasma arginine vasopressin is a novel marker of response to tolvaptan in patients with decompensated heart failure. Circ J. 2014;78:2240–9.
24. Tanaka A, Nakamura T, Sato E, Node K. Aquaporin-2 is a potential biomarker for tolvaptan efficacy in decompensated heart failure complicated by diabetic nephrotic syndrome. Int J Cardiol. 2016;210:1–3.
25. Jensen JM, Mose FH, Kulik AE, Bech JN, Fenton RA, Pedersen EB. Abnormal urinary excretion of NKCC2 and AQP2 in response to hypertonic saline in chronic kidney disease: an intervention study in patients with chronic kidney disease and healthy controls. BMC Nephrol. 2014;15:101.

14

Chronic hyperglycemia is associated with acute kidney injury in patients undergoing CABG surgery

Mehmet Oezkur[1*†], Martin Wagner[2,3,4†], Dirk Weismann[3,5], Jens Holger Krannich[1], Christoph Schimmer[1], Christoph Riegler[2], Victoria Rücker[2], Rainer Leyh[1] and Peter U. Heuschmann[2,3,6]

Abstract

Background: Chronic hyperglycemia (CHG) with HbA1c as an indicator affects postoperative mortality and morbidity after coronary artery bypass grafting surgery (CABG). Acute kidney injury (AKI) is one of the frequent postoperative complications after CABG impacting short-and long-term outcomes. We investigated the association between CHG and postoperative incidence of AKI in CABG patients with and without history of diabetes mellitus (DM).

Methods: This cohort study consecutively enrolled patients undergoing CABG in 2009 at the department for cardiovascular surgery. CHG was defined as HbA1c ≥ 6.0 %. Patients with advanced chronic kidney disease (CKD) were excluded. The incidence of postoperative AKI and its association with CHG was analyzed by univariate and multivariate logistic regression modeling.

Results: Three-hundred-seven patients were analyzed. The incidence of AKI was 48.2 %. Patients with CHG (n = 165) were more likely to be female and had greater waist circumference as well as other comorbid conditions, such as smoking, history of DM, CKD, hypertension, pulmonary hypertension, and chronic obstructive pulmonary disease (all $p \leq 0.05$). Preoperative eGFR, atrial fibrillation (AF), history of DM and CHG were associated with an increased risk of postoperative AKI in univariate analyses. In multivariate modelling, history of DM as well as preoperative eGFR and AF lost significance, while age, CHG and prolonged OP duration ($p < 0.05$) were independently associated with postoperative AKI.

Conclusions: Our results suggest that CHG defined on a single measurement of HbA1c ≥ 6.0 % was associated with the incidence of AKI after CABG. This finding might implicate that treatment decisions, including the selection of operative strategies, could be based on HbA1c measurement rather than on a recorded history of diabetes.

Background

Acute kidney injury (AKI) is a frequent postoperative complication with an incidence ranging from 20 to 40 % in patients undergoing cardiac surgery [1–6]. Even slight changes in creatinine-levels, *e.g.* by 0.3 mg/dl (AKI Stage I [7]), are associated with impaired long-term outcome, such as risk of mortality or development or progression of chronic kidney disease (CKD), as multiple studies have indicated in CABG patients [4–6, 8]. Age, gender, preoperative creatinine, diabetes mellitus (DM), and metabolic syndrome, but also urgent operations and operation duration have been discussed as potential risk factors for AKI [1, 9–13]. Both, chronic and acute hyperglycemias are associated with cardiac dysfunction, susceptibility for infections and endothelial dysfunction [14–18]. These factors are known risk factors of perioperative morbidity and mortality after CABG surgery, in particular of renal dysfunction [1, 9, 11–13, 19–21].

HbA1c is an established parameter for evaluating diabetic control and chronic hyperglycemia (CHG) in patients with DM [22]. Elevated HbA1c levels have been implemented in recent guidelines [22] and can now be used for diagnosis of diabetes. Furthermore, HbA1c has been identified as an important marker for insulin resistance, risk for acute hyperglycemia and endothelial dysfunction and atherosclerosis in diabetic and non-diabetic patients [14, 16].

* Correspondence: Oezkur_m@ukw.de
†Equal contributors
[1]Department of Cardiovascular Surgery, University Hospital Würzburg, Würzburg, Germany
Full list of author information is available at the end of the article

A history of diabetes at baseline clinical assessment is frequently used as a marker of cardiovascular risk of individual patients after cardiac surgery [19–21]. However, information on history of diabetes mellitus is often based on self-reports of patients or from the patient's records and does not reflect current glucose control. Furthermore, even patients without the formal criteria for DM can suffer from hyperglycemia due to pathological glycemic control or pre-DM [22]. It is unknown whether preoperative CHG is associated with the risk of AKI after cardiac surgery.

In the current study, we aimed to investigate the association between CHG and postoperative incidence of AKI in a cohort of CABG patients, independent from potential confounders including history of diabetes.

Methods

The study protocol of this prospective cohort study was approved by the Ethics Committee at the University Hospital of Würzburg. All patients who received cardiac surgery between January 1st and December 31st 2009 were screened for participation. Patients were included if they underwent CABG surgery or combination procedures including CABG. Further inclusion criteria were elective or urgent (start of operation > 6 h after admission) CABG surgery, and HbA1c-level measured on admission. Exclusion criteria were operations in which CABG was not planned preoperatively, age < 18 years, pregnancy and lactation, advanced stages of chronic kidney disease (CKD) with a eGFR <30 ml/min/1.73 m^2 according to the creatinine-based CKD-EPI equation, acute infection (C-reactive protein >4.0 mg/dl, procalcitonin >1.0 µg/l), high-urgent or salvage surgery (preoperative resuscitation, i.v. catecholamine therapy started preoperatively, assist device, operation < 6 h after admission).

The primary endpoint of the present study was defined as the postoperative incidence of any stage of AKI, according to recent KDIGO guideline recommendations [23], similar to the AKIN - and STS criteria [24]. Thus, even a slight creatinine level rise of 0.3 mg/dl compared to baseline within 48 hrs after surgery or Creatinine 1.5 to 1.9-times baseline (stage I) was defined as AKI. Creatinine values of blood-samples drawn at hospital admission were considered as baseline. More severe stages of AKI were a rise in Creatinine 2.0 to 2.9-times baseline (stage II) and ≥3-times baseline, Creatinine ≥4 mg/dl or the need of renal replacement therapy (stage III).

Standard demographic data of patients were collected and comorbidities such as a history of diabetes, hypertension, pulmonary hypertension and smoking were taken from the patient's chart and personal interview. Furthermore, intraoperative data (e.g., operation time, paracorporal bypass time, aortic cross clamping time, etc.) and standard laboratory results of clinical routine including HbA1c measurement at admission were collected. Preoperative

chronic hyperglycemia was defined as an HbA1c ≥ 6.0 % on admission [17, 18, 22]. Postoperative serum glucose (SG) was taken on admission to the ICU after surgery. Postoperative hyperglycemia was defined as fastening serum glucose of ≥126 mg/dl during the postoperative course.

Intraoperative data about relevant time-points were taken from the digital protocol of the heart-lung machine. Metformin was stopped 24 hours before admission. For the purposes of the study, chronic kidney disease (CKD) was defined as eGFR <60 ml/min.

Statistical analyses

Patient demographics are presented as mean and standard deviations, medians and interquartile ranges and number of observations with proportions (%), as appropriate. Differences across group were assessed by t-test, Mann-Whitney-U-Test/ and χ^2-test/Fisher's exact test, respectively. Determinants of the postoperative incidence of AKI which were significant in the univariate analyses (age, history of DM, HbA1c, eGFR, AF, OP duration, COPD, metabolic syndrome and sex) were investigated by logistic regression analysis. In a sensitivity analysis, we tested the robustness of the results in a propensity score approach: age, history of DM, HbA1c, eGFR, AF, OP duration, COPD, metabolic syndrome and sex were included to assess the probability of having a HBA1c level >/< 6.0 % by multivariate logistic regression modelling. These results were included in the multivariate regression analysis, modelling AKI as a covariate.

Results of regression analyses are presented as Odds Ratio with respective 95 % confidence interval (CI). Two-sided p-values of ≤0.05 were considered as statistically significant. Statistical analyses were performed using SPSS Version 21.

Results
Patient population

In 2009, a total of n = 928 adult patients underwent cardiac surgery at the department of cardiovascular surgery at the University Hospital of Würzburg. Of these, 478 received elective or urgent CABG surgery. Thirty-nine patients were excluded because eGFR was less than 30 ml/min, as well as were two patients with acute infection and 75 high urgent/salvage surgery patients. Furthermore, no HbA1c measurement within the clinical routine was available for 55 patients. Therefore the study population consisted of 307 patients.

Patient characteristics of the entire cohort and stratified according to the established HbA1c cutoff <6.0 % and ≥ 6.0 %, respectively) [25], are displayed in Table 1. Patients had a median age of 69 years, 73.9 % were male A history of diabetes was observed in 35 % of patients. Metabolic syndrome according to the definition of WHO (considering DM, hypertension, dyslipidemia and BMI) was detected in 254 (82.3 %) of the patients. Thirty-three (10.7 %) patients were operated with off pump coronary artery bypass

Table 1 Patients characteristics

Variable	All patients (n = 307)	HbA1c < 6.0 % (n = 142)	HbA1c ≥ 6.0 % (n = 165)	P-value
Age, years	69(60-75)	67(57-74)	70(63-75)	0.008
Male, n (%)	227(73.9)	116 (81.7)	111 (67.3)	0.004
Smoking, n (%)	121(39.4)	47(33.1)	74(44.8)	0.046
LV-EF, %	55(45-63)	55(49-65)	55(45-61)	0.048
Waist circumference, cm	103(±11)	102(±10)	105(±12)	0.047
BMI, kg/m²	28(25-30)	27(25-29)	28(96-113)	0.087
Urgent surgery, n (%)	134(42.6)	70(49.3)	64(38.8)	0.066
MI within the last 48 h, n (%)	25(8.1)	15(10.6)	10(6.1)	0.19
Previous cardiac surgery, n (%)	13(4.2)	6(4.2)	7(4.2)	1.00
Metabolic syndrome, n (%)	254(82.7)	107(75.4)	147(89.1)	0.002
COPD, n (%)	57(18.6)	19(13.4)	38(23)	0.039
History of DM, n (%)	106(34.5)	15(10.6)	91(55.2)	<0.001
HbA1c, %	6.0(5.7-6.5)	5.7(5.5-5.8)	6.5(6.2-7.0)	<0.001
FSG, mg/dl	105(97-123)	101(95-106)	116(102-138)	<0.001
Postoperative SG, mg/dl	143(120-179)	136(117-165)	154(125-188)	<0.001
Postop. hyperglycemia, n (%)	209(68.1)	88(42.1)	121(57.9)	0.037
Hypercholesterolemia, n (%)	181(59.0)	80(56.3)	101(61.2)	0.42
Hypertension, n (%)	267(87.0)	122(85.9)	145(87.9)	0.62
Pulmonary Hypertension, n (%)	54(11.3)	16(11.3)	38(23.0)	0.007
AF, n (%)	28(9.1)	8(5.6)	29(12.1)	0.072
TG, mg/dl	128(95-184)	122(89-163)	137(101-205)	0.016
HDL, mg/dl	43(37-53)	44(38-53)	42(35-54)	0.47
LDL, mg/dl	104(82-128)	109(90-135)	98(73-119)	<0.001
Preoperative creatinine, mg/dl	1.0(0.8-1.2)	1.0(0.8-1.2)	1.0(0.8-1.2)	0.55
Preoperative eGFR$_{CKD-EPI}$, ml/min/1.73 m²	74(59-89)	78(62-100)	72(56-86)	0.010
CKD, n (%)	82(26.7)	29(20.4)	53(32.1)	0.028
OP Duration, min	245(219-295)	240(218-291)	250(219-299)	0.91
CPB Time, min	107(88-143)	105(86-137)	115(88-151)	0.07
X-Clamp Time, min	81(61-104)	78(57-95)	83(63-110)	0.05

Data are mean (±SD), number (%) or median (IQR); *LV-EF*: left ventricular ejection fraction; *BMI*: body mass index; *MI*: myocardial infarction; *COPD*: chronic obstructive pulmonary disease; *DM*: diabetes mellitus; *FSG*: fastening serum glucose; *AF*: atrial fibrillation; *HDL*: high density lipoprotein, *LDL*: low density lipoprotein, *eGFR*: estimated glomerular filtration rate; *CKD*: chronic kidney disease; *X-clamp*: aortic cross-clamp; *AKI*: acute kidney injury

(OPCAB), and 2.6 % (n = 8) had an on-pump beating heart procedure. Patients with higher HbA1c levels were more likely to be female and with greater waist circumference. Furthermore, comorbid conditions, such as smoking, history of DM, hypertension, pulmonary hypertension and CKD, were detected more frequently as compared to patients with lower HbA1c levels (all p ≤ 0.05).

All 106 patients with a history of diabetes were treated with some kind of diabetes therapy, with 34 % being on insulin therapy. In only 15 diabetic patients, glucose metabolism was strictly controlled (HbA1c <6.0 %) with a median FSG of 105 mg/dl. Ninety-one diabetic patients had HbA1c >6.0 % (median FSG 140 mg/dl) of which 65 had HbA1c levels greater than 6.5 %. None of the patients without a recorded history of diabetes was treated

with oral antidiabetics or insulin therapy. However, although median FSG in this group was 113 (104 – 123) mg/dl, HbA1c levels >6.0 % were observed in 74 patients, suggesting CHG.

A history of DM was significantly related to postoperative hyperglycemia regardless of HbA1c (OR 1.46 (1.00 – 2.14), $p = 0{,}028$), whereas acute postoperative hyperglycemia was not associated with the incidence of AKI (OR 1.00 (1.00 – 1.01), $p = 0.96$).

Postoperative incidence of AKI

A total of n = 148 patients (49.3 %) experienced AKI (Table 2). Most of the episodes were stage I (n = 125, 41.1 %) with only a slight increase of serum creatinine. In 23 patients (7.5 %) a more severe increase in creatinine was

Table 2 Outcomes

Variable	All patients (n = 307)	HbA1c < 6.0 % (n = 142)	HbA1c ≥ 6.0 % (n = 165)	P-value
AKI, n (%)	148(49.3)	57(41.0)	91(56.5)	0.008
AKI Stage I, n (%)	125(41.1)	49(34.5)	76(46.9)	0.005
AKI Stage II, n (%)	22(7.2)	8(5.6)	14(8.6)	0.028
AKI Stage III, n (%)	1(0.3)	0(0)	1(0.6)	0.31
Creatinine Peak, mg/dl	1.3(1.1-1.7)	1.3(1.0-1.6)	1.4(1.1-1.8)	0.014
Mortality, n (%)	10(3.3)	0	10(6.1)	0.002

Data are number (%) or median (IQR) *AKI*: acute kidney injury

observed and two patients required hemodialysis treatment. Patients with HbA1c ≥ 6.0 % were more likely to develop AKI across all stages, as compared to patients with HbA1c < 6.0 % (Table 2).

Risk factors of AKI

In univariate logistic regression analysis (Table 3), a history of diabetes as well as elevated levels of HbA1c were associated with the incidence of postoperative AKI. Furthermore, older age, impaired kidney function, preoperative atrial fibrillation and prolonged operation time were significantly associated with an increased risk of AKI (all $p < 0.05$). Male gender, FSG and COPD approached significance ($p < 0.10$). In a sensitivity analysis, in which we included the propensity of each patient as presenting with a HbA1c level of >6.0 % in the multivariate regression model for AKI, the results remained largely unchanged, with a HbA1c level >6.0 % being related to a

Table 3 Determinants of postoperative AKI (logistic regression analysis)

Variable	Univariate	Multivariate	
		OR (CI95 %)	p-value
Age	1.08 (1.05-1.11)	1.07 (1.04-1.10)	<0.001
History of DM	1.85 (1.14-3.00)	1.30 (0.72-2.37)	0.39
HbA1c ≥ 6.0 %	1.87 (1.18-2.96)	1.65 (1.00-2.71)	0.049
Preop. eGFR (ml/min)	0.82 (0.72-0.93)	1.00 (0.98-1.01)	0.73
AF	3.05 (1.24-7.49)	2.21 (0.86-5.67)	0.098
OP Duration (min)	1.07 (1.03-1.11)	1.05 (1.01-1.10)	0.013
Sex	1.45 (0.87-2.49)	1.04 (0.58-1.88)	0.89
FSG	1.01 (1.00-1.01)	1.00 (0.99-1.01)	0.73
COPD	1.76 (0.98-3.19)	1.44 (0.76-2.74)	0.26
Post. OP SG	1.00 (1.00-1.01)		
Post. OP HG	1.05 (0.83-1.34)		
Pulm. Hyper.	1.25 (0.68-2.30)	-	-
Smoking	1.02 (0.64-1.62)	-	-
Urgent surgery	0.85 (0.54-1.33)	-	-
BMI	1.00 (0.96-1.07)	-	-

Data are OR (95 % CI); *eGFR*: estimated glomerular filtration rate; *AF*: atrial fibrillation; *FSG*: fastening serum glucose; *BMI*: body mass index; final model based on backward stepwise selection; last OR before elimination shown

higher risk of AKI (OR 1.71, 95 % CI 0.90-3.26, p = 0.10), but this association lost significance (detailed data not shown).

Mortality

During the hospital stay (median 9 days, IQR 8-12), ten patients died (3.3 %), with a median time to death of 6 days (IQR 1-21). Mortality was not significantly associated with the incidence of AKI (OR: 1.62; 95 % CI: 0.40 – 6.67; p = 0.72). However, all patients who died had HbA1c ≥ 6.0 % (p = 0.002) as compared to survivors. Further determinants of mortality in univariate analyses were older age, impaired LV-EF, preoperative eGFR, female gender and pulmonary hypertension ($p < 0.05$).

Discussion

The results of our study suggest that aside from older age and prolonged OP duration, CHG, i.e. elevated HbA1c levels were associated with the postoperative incidence of AKI after CABG surgery. This association was independent from of a history of diabetes, which was only associated with the risk of AKI in univariate analyses. Furthermore, preoperative kidney function lost its univariate association with AKI in multivariate modelling. Even controlling for a multitude of clinical factors employing a propensity score approach suggested an important role of CHG, although this association failed to reach formal statistical significance.

This is of particular interest, as usually a history of diabetes is used in daily clinical practice for clinical decision making including the choice of specific operation strategies as harvesting both mammarial arteries or the extend of the operation. The easy-to-use laboratory marker HbA1c (as compared to the time consuming oGTT) not only provides additional information on the glycemic state of the patient over the last weeks, it is also an indicator for insulin resistance providing information on perioperative incidences of hyperglycemia [14]. Markers of impaired glucose metabolism such as elevated HbA1c levels, history of DM and high levels of FSG were associated with an increased risk of AKI after CABG surgery in univariate analyses. Postoperative glucose control is reported as a risk factor for renal impairment after cardiac surgery [14]. In our cohort, we could not find any strong relation of postoperative hyperglycemia and the development of AKI. The overall incidence of AKI (48 %) was higher than described in recent literature (20 to 40 %) [3, 4, 6, 8, 13]. Compared to these previous studies we used the rigorous definition of AKI as recommended by KDIGO guidelines 2012, of even a slight increase of serum creatinine by 0.3 mg/dl [23]. This definition has also been implements in the recommendations of the STS [24]; although the changes in creatinine are considerably minor, it has been shown that they carry important information predictive for the development of long-term outcome, including aggravated risk of the development of CKD as well as cardiac dysfunction [5, 6]. The preoperative fastening status might have caused hypovolemia which further could have sensitized the kidney for intraoperative stress and thus the development of AKI. However, only few patients experienced severe AKI and only two needed renal replacement therapy. After multivariate modelling, the association of HbA1c ≥ 6.0 % with AKI weakened but stayed statistically significant, suggesting a nearly 1.7-fold increased risk for patients with CHG independent from the history of DM.

In-hospital mortality was comparable to other studies (3.3 %) and was not significantly associated with AKI. In contrast, all patients who died had HbA1c ≥ 6.0 % at admission, as well as they were older, more likely to be of male gender, with previous cardiac surgery and prolonged operation duration in univariate analyses. The overall considerably low mortality-rate did not allow a multivariate analysis of mortality. Our results suggest that the strict criteria for AKI might not have a significant impact on the short-term clinical outcome of patients undergoing CABG surgery, however, due to limited sample size this interpretation needs to be taken with caution.

We also found operation time with respective prolonged duration of CPB and X-Clamp time as another strong and independent risk factor for the incidence of postoperative AKI. Per minute prolonged operation time (including CBP and X-clamp time), the risk of AKI increased by 1 %. Prolonged OP duration potentiates inflammatory processes and the formation of oxidative stress metabolites which are known to affect kidney function, and promote the development of AKI [9, 10, 12]. In our cohort, patients with OPCAB operations showed a high risk for AKI. Most likely treatment bias can be considered as the key issue for that finding – patients were operated OPCAB or beating-heart on-pump when X-clamping or CPB was impossible due to severe calcification of the ascending aorta and aortic arch. We assume that those patients had severe general calcification of their arteries, which might also affect renal arteries and the glomerular convolute. This is also supported by the fact that patients operated OPCAB or beating-heart on-pump had a higher prevalence of hemodynamic stenosis of A. carotis interna (data not shown).

Metabolic syndrome (MS) has been described as a risk factor for AKI in CABG patients [1]. Only 17.7 % of our

cohort did not fulfill the MS criteria according to the definition of WHO. We could not show a statistically signification association of MS and AKI potentially due to the relatively limited number of observations. DM is one of the components of MS and can therefore be seen as an important confounder for the association between MS and AKI described in other studies [26].

We are aware of several limitations of the current study. HbA1c values were not kept blinded to the treating physicians, therefore, specific treatment decisions might have been based on the knowledge of certain HbA1c values (treatment bias). Furthermore, the size of our study sample is relatively limited, although a quite large number of events was observed. Therefore we were not able to assure sufficient statistical power for all our hypotheses as well as for the inclusion of other known risk factors of AKI (e.g. volume management during CPB and medication) in our multivariate models. We refrained from testing too many variables in these models, as we wanted to avoid finding associations by chance (overfitting the model), however, we might have missed "true" associations by chance as well.

Conclusion
Our data suggest that CHG based on a single measurement of HbA1c ≥ 6.0 %, could represent a strong determinant of AKI and mortality after CABG surgery, independent from a recorded history of DM. This finding might implicate that treatment decisions, including the selection of operative strategies, could be based on HbA1c measurement rather than on a recorded history of diabetes. This applies to patients with treated diabetes as well as to those without. Further prospective studies are needed to confirm our findings and to investigate how treatment decisions based on HbA1c levels independent from or in addition to the knowledge of diabetic status of the patient might improve clinical outcomes after cardiac surgery.

Consent
Written informed consent was obtained from the patient for the publication of this report and any accompanying images.

Abbreviations
AKI: Acute kidney injury; BMI: Body mass index; AKIN: Acute kidney injury network; CABG: Coronary artery bypass grafting; CAD: Coronary artery disease; CHG: Chronic hyperglycemia; CKD: Chronic kidney disease; eGFR: Estimated glomerular filtration rate; FSG: Fastening serum glucose; KDIGO: Kidney disease improving global outcome; LV-EF: Left ventricular ejection fraction; MAP: Mean atrial pressure; MS: Metabolic syndrome; OPCAB: Off pump coronary artery bypass; SG: Serum glucose; WHO: World Health Organization.

Competing interests
M Oezkur was supported by a rotational post from the Comprehensive Heart Failure Center Würzburg funded by the German Ministry of Research and Education.
PU Heuschmann receives/received in the recent years research support from the German Ministry of Research and Education (Center for Stroke Research

Berlin; Comprehensive Heart Failure Center Würzburg), the European Union (European Implementation Score Collaboration), the German Stroke Foundation, the Charité–Universitätsmedizin Berlin, the Berlin Chamber of Physicians, and the University Hospital of Würzburg.

This study was supported by the German Ministry of Education and Research (BMBF) within the setting of the Comprehensive Heart Failure Center Wuerzburg (BMBF 01EO1004).

This publication was funded by the German Research Foundation (DFG) and the University of Wuerzburg in the funding program Open Access Publishing.

Authors' contributions

MO and MW concepted, designed, executed the study and had major parts in the statistical analyses. DW substantially contributed to interpretation of the result and design of the manuscript. JHK gave significant input on design of the study and participated in the statistical analyses. CS, RL participated in the design of the study, and gave significant input on the manuscript. CR supported statistical analyses and interpretation of results. VR and CR supported the statistical analyses and revisions significantly. PUH participated in the design of the study, gave significant input on the statistical analyses and on the manuscript. All authors read and approved the final manuscript.

Acknowledgements

We thank all patients providing data to the current study as we as we thank the physicians and study personnel for filling in case report forms for study participant and performing study procedures.

This study was supported by the German Ministry of Education and Research (BMBF) within the setting of the Comprehensive Heart Failure Center Würzburg (BMBF 01EO1004).

Author details

[1]Department of Cardiovascular Surgery, University Hospital Würzburg, Würzburg, Germany. [2]Institute of Clinical Epidemiology and Biometry, University of Würzburg, Würzburg, Germany. [3]Comprehensive Heart Failure Center, University of Würzburg, Würzburg, Germany. [4]Department of Internal Medicine I, Division of Nephrology, University Hospital Würzburg, Würzburg, Germany. [5]Department of Internal Medicine I, Endocrine and Diabetes Unit, University Hospital Würzburg, Würzburg, Germany. [6]Clinical Trial Center Würzburg, University Hospital Würzburg, Würzburg, Germany.

References

1. Hong S, Youn Y-N, Yoo K-J. Metabolic syndrome as a risk factor for postoperative kidney injury after off-pump coronary artery bypass surgery. Circ J. 2010;74(6):1121–6.
2. Yan X, Jia S, Meng X, Dong P, Jia M, Wan J, et al. Acute kidney injury in adult postcardiotomy patients with extracorporeal membrane oxygenation: evaluation of the RIFLE classification and the acute kidney injury network criteria. Eur J Cardiothorac Surg. 2010;37(2):334–8.
3. Englberger L, Suri RM, Li Z, Casey ET, Daly RC, Dearani JA, et al. Clinical accuracy of RIFLE and acute kidney injury network (AKIN) criteria for acute kidney injury in patients undergoing cardiac surgery. Crit Care. 2011;15(1):R16.
4. Li SY, Chen JY, Yang WC, Chuang CL. Acute kidney injury network classification predicts in-hospital and long-term mortality in patients undergoing elective coronary artery bypass grafting surgery. Eur J Cardiothorac Surg. 2011;39(3):323–8.
5. Olsson D, Sartipy U, Braunschweig F, Holzmann MJ. Acute kidney injury following coronary artery bypass surgery and long-term risk of heart failure. Circ Heart Fail. 2013;6(1):83–90.
6. Chawla LS, Amdur RL, Shaw AD, Faselis C, Palant CE, Kimmel PL. Association between AKI and long-term renal and cardiovascular outcomes in United States veterans. Clin J Am Soc Nephrol. 2014;9(3):448–56.
7. Khwaja A. KDIGO clinical practice guidelines for acute kidney injury. Nephron Clin Pract. 2012;120(4):179–84.
8. Wu VC, Wu CH, Huang TM, Wang CY, Lai CF, Shiao CC, et al. Long-term risk of coronary events after AKI. J Am Soc Nephrol. 2014;25(3):595–605.
9. Gaudino M, Luciani N, Giungi S, Caradonna E, Nasso G, Schiavello R, et al. Different profiles of patients who require dialysis after cardiac surgery. Ann Thorac Surg. 2005;79(3):825–9. author reply 829 - 830.
10. Karkouti K, Beattie WS, Wijeysundera DN, Rao V, Chan C, Dattilo KM, et al. Hemodilution during cardiopulmonary bypass is an independent risk factor for acute renal failure in adult cardiac surgery. J Thorac Cardiovasc Surg. 2005;129(2):391–400.
11. Kuitunen A, Vento A, Suojaranta-Ylinen R, Pettila V. Acute renal failure after cardiac surgery: evaluation of the RIFLE classification. Ann Thorac Surg. 2006;81(2):542–6.
12. Aronson S, Fontes ML, Miao Y, Mangano DT, Investigators of the Multicenter Study of Perioperative Ischemia Research G, Ischemia R, et al. Risk index for perioperative renal dysfunction/failure: critical dependence on pulse pressure hypertension. Circulation. 2007;115(6):733–42.
13. Vellinga S, Verbrugghe W, De Paep R, Verpooten GA, Janssen van Doorn K. Identification of modifiable risk factors for acute kidney injury after cardiac surgery. Neth J Med. 2012;70(10):450–4.
14. Sato H, Carvalho G, Sato T, Lattermann R, Matsukawa T, Schricker T. The association of preoperative glycemic control, intraoperative insulin sensitivity, and outcomes after cardiac surgery. J Clin Endocrinol Metab. 2010;95(9):4338–44.
15. Rubin J, Matsushita K, Ballantyne CM, Hoogeveen R, Coresh J, Selvin E. Chronic hyperglycemia and subclinical myocardial injury. J Am Coll Cardiol. 2012;59(5):484–9.
16. Mebazaa A, Gayat E, Lassus J, Meas T, Mueller C, Maggioni A, et al. Association between elevated blood glucose and outcome in acute heart failure: results from an international observational cohort. J Am Coll Cardiol. 2013;61(8):820–9.
17. Abdelmalak BB, Knittel J, Abdelmalak JB, Dalton JE, Christiansen E, Foss J, et al. Preoperative blood glucose concentrations and postoperative outcomes after elective non-cardiac surgery: an observational study. Br J Anaesth. 2014;112(1):79–88.
18. Subramaniam B, Lerner A, Novack V, Khabbaz K, Paryente-Wiesmann M, Hess P, et al. Increased glycemic variability in patients with elevated preoperative HbA1C predicts adverse outcomes following coronary artery bypass grafting surgery. Anesth Analg. 2014;118(2):277–87.
19. Nashef SA, Roques F, Michel P, Gauducheau E, Lemeshow S, Salamon R. European system for cardiac operative risk evaluation (EuroSCORE). Eur J Cardiothorac Surg. 1999;16(1):9–13.
20. Nashef SA, Roques F, Sharples LD, Nilsson J, Smith C, Goldstone AR, et al. EuroSCORE II. Eur J Cardiothorac Surg. 2012;41(4):734–44. discussion 744-735.
21. Qadir I, Salick MM, Perveen S, Sharif H. Mortality from isolated coronary bypass surgery: a comparison of the society of thoracic surgeons and the EuroSCORE risk prediction algorithms. Interact Cardiovasc Thorac Surg. 2012;14(3):258–62.
22. Authors/Task, Force M, Ryden L, Grant PJ, Anker SD, Berne C, et al. ESC Guidelines on diabetes, pre-diabetes, and cardiovascular diseases developed in collaboration with the EASD: the Task Force on diabetes, pre-diabetes, and cardiovascular diseases of the European Society of Cardiology (ESC) and developed in collaboration with the European Association for the Study of Diabetes (EASD). Eur Heart J. 2013;34(39):3035–87.
23. Ad-hoc working group of E, Fliser D, Laville M, Covic A, Fouque D, Vanholder R, et al. A European Renal Best Practice (ERBP) position statement on the Kidney Disease Improving Global Outcomes (KDIGO) clinical practice guidelines on acute kidney injury: part 1: definitions, conservative management and contrast-induced nephropathy. Nephrol Dial Transplant. 2012;27(12):4263–72.
24. Welke KF, Ferguson Jr TB, Coombs LP, Dokholyan RS, Murray CJ, Schrader MA, et al. Validity of the society of thoracic surgeons national adult cardiac surgery database. Ann Thorac Surg. 2004;77(4):1137–9.
25. International Expert C. International expert committee report on the role of the A1C assay in the diagnosis of diabetes. Diabetes Care. 2009;32(7):1327–34.
26. Angeloni E, Melina G, Benedetto U, Refice S, Capuano F, Roscitano A, et al. Metabolic syndrome affects midterm outcome after coronary artery bypass grafting. Ann Thorac Surg. 2012;93(2):537–44.

15

Dynamic changes of paraoxonase 1 activity towards paroxon and phenyl acetate during coronary artery surgery

Anna Wysocka[1,2], Marek Cybulski[3], Henryk Berbeć[3], Andrzej Wysokiński[1], Janusz Stążka[4], Jadwiga Daniluk[2] and Tomasz Zapolski[1*]

Abstract

Background: Serum paraoxonase 1 (PON1), an enzyme associated with high – density lipoproteins (HDL) particles, inhibits the oxidation of serum lipoproteins and cell membranes. PON1 activity is lower in patients with atherosclerosis and in inflammatory diseases. The systemic inflammatory response provoked during cardiopulmonary bypass grafting may contribute to the development of postoperative complications. The aim of the present study was to estimate the dynamic changes in paraoxonase 1 (PON1) activity towards paraoxon and phenyl acetate during and after coronary artery surgery.

Methods: Twenty six patients with coronary heart disease undergoing coronary artery bypass grafting (CABG) were enrolled into the study. Venous blood samples were obtained preoperatively, after aortic clumping, after the end of operation, at 6, 18, 30 and 48 h after operation. Paraoxonase activity was measured spectrophotometrically in 50 mM glycine/NaOH buffer (pH 10.5) containing 1.0 mM paraoxon, and 1.0 mM $CaCl_2$. Arylesterase activity was measured in 20 mM TrisCl buffer (pH 8.0) containing 1 mM phenyl acetate and 1 mM $CaCl_2$.

Results: PON1 activity toward paraoxon and phenyl acetate significantly decreased after aorta cross clumping and increased directly after operation. PON1 activity towards paraoxon in preoperative period and PON1 activity towards phenyl acetate in seventh stage of experiment tended to inversely correlate with the occurrence of postoperative complications.

Conclusion: The paraoxonase 1 plasma activity is markedly reduced during CABG surgery.

Keywords: Coronary artery bypass, Coronary heart disease, Paraoxonase 1

Background

Human serum paraoxonase 1 (PON1), a high density lipoprotein (HDL) associated serum esterase has been shown to be responsible for antioxidative properties of HDL. PON 1 is a 44 kDa, calcium dependent protein that remains associated with apolipoprotein apo-AI and apo-J on the particle of HDL. The enzyme is synthesized in the liver and secreted into the blood [1]. Recent studies have shown that HDL can prevent accumulation of lipid peroxides in LDL and PON1 enzyme is one of the compounds of HDL responsible for this activity. It has been reported that PON1 hydrolyzes the pro – inflammatory lipid peroxides generated by the oxidized low – density lipoprotein (LDL) reducing oxidative stress [2, 3].

PON1 activity is inversely related to atherosclerosis: it is lower in diseases accelerating development of atherosclerosis and it is reduced in inflammatory diseases [4, 5]. Deprivation HDL particles of PON1 as well as modification the biological function of enzyme due genetic recombination makes HDL unable to retard LDL oxidation, whereas returning PON1 to HDL restores its ability to inhibit LDL oxidation [6–8]. Several types of evidence suggest that low levels of PON1 protein raise the risk of development of premature atherosclerosis and low activity of PON1 is a strong independent risk factor for coronary heart

* Correspondence: zapolia@wp.pl
[1]Cardiology Department, Medical University of Lublin, ul. Jaczewskiego 8, 20–954 Lublin, Poland
Full list of author information is available at the end of the article

disease [9–11]. A few studies demonstrate that serum PON1 activity decreases in patients with acute myocardial infarction [12, 13].

During cardiac surgery aorta cross-clumping and cardioplegic cardiac arrest induce global ischaemia, so cardiac surgery can be considered as human model of controlled ischeamia similar to this occurring in myocardial infarction. Moreover, cardiac surgery with cardiopulmonary bypass grafting provokes a systemic inflammatory response [14]. This inflammatory reaction may contribute to the development of postoperative complications including myocardial, renal or neurological dysfunction and respiratory failure.

The aim of the present study was to estimate the dynamic changes in PON1 activity towards paroxon and phenyl acetate during coronary artery surgery.

Methods
Study population
Twenty six unrelated individuals of Caucasian origin (men and women) aged 43–75 with coronary heart disease were included to this study. All patients had been admitted to Cardiosurgery Departament of Medical University in Lublin, for coronary artery by–pass grafting. The study protocol was approved by the local ethics committee (decision of Bioethics Committee of Medical University of Lublin No KE – 0254/76/2002). Written informed consent was obtained from all of the participants. The investigation conforms with the principles outlined in the Declaration of Helsinki.

The demographic data and a clinical history of risk factors were collected including age, gender, hypertension, smoking, diabetes mellitus, hypercholesterolemia and hypertriglicerydemia and family history of coronary heart disease. For each patient body mass index was calculated as body weight (kg) divided by the squared height (m^2). There are also recorded ejection fraction (EF%) measured in echocardiography by the modified biplane Simpson method. Coronary heart disease was confirmed by positive coronary angiogram. Inclusion criteria were >50% narrowing of the lumen of at least one of the major coronary artery. The risk of operation was evaluated according to the Euroscore scale [15]. If the Euroscore was equal 1–2 points the risk of operation was regarded as low, if the Euroscore was equal 3–5 points as intermediate and in the case of score 6–13 points as high.

Surgical technique and sample collection
All patients undergone coronary artery bypass with extracorporeal circulation. After standard general anesthesia a median sternotomy was carried out, followed by routine aortic and right atrial cannulation. Cardiopulmonary bypass was performed using heart –

lung mashine SIII (Stockert) and moderate systemic hypothermia. Myocardial protection was achieved by mild hypothermic blood cardioplegia (32 °C). The degree of normovolemic hemodilution induced by a constant volume of priming (1800 mL) was determined on the basis of haematocrit measurements and body weight. During the procedure heparine was administered and the measured activated clotting time was >400 msek. After the end of the surgery heparin was neutralized with protamine and all patients were followed up in the intensive care unit. Data of aorta clumping and procedure time were collected. Venous blood samples were obtained before and after coronary bypass grafting at the following moments: 1) preoperatively, 2) after aortic clumping, 3) after the end of operation, 4) at 6 h, 5) at 18 h, 6) at 30 h, and 7) at 48 h after operation. Blood samples were anticoagulated with lithium heparin and separated from the cells by centrifugation.

Biochemical analysis
Paraoxonase and arylesterase activities were determined according to Eckerson et al. [16]. PON1 activity towards paraoxon was determined by measuring absorption at 412 nm with using continuously recording spectrophotometer (DU 640; Beckman) after introducing serum to 50 mM glycine/NaOH buffer (pH 10.5) containing 1.0 mM paraoxon, and 1.0 mM $CaCl_2$. Enzyme activity was calculated with a molar extinction coefficient of 18,290 M^{-1} cm^{-1}. One unit of paraoxonase activity produced 1 nmol of p- nitrophenol per minute. PON1 activity towards phenyl acetate was measured in 20 mM TrisCl buffer (pH 8.0) containing 1 mM substrate and 1 mM $CaCl_2$. The absorbance was monitored spectrophotometrically at 270 nm. Enzyme activity was calculated with a molar extinction coefficient of 1310 M^{-1} cm^{-1}. One unit of arylesterase acivity hydrolyzed 1 µmol of phenyl acetate per minute. The concentration of total plasma protein was assayed by biuret method. The relative PON1 activity towards paraoxon and phenyl acetate expressed in U per gram of protein was calculated.

Lipid profile was determined before surgery in blood samples collected through venipuncture in EDTA-coated tubes. Concentration of total cholesterol, triacylglycerols and HDL – cholesterol were tested by specific enzymatic techniques. LDL cholesterol was calculated from Friedwald formula.

Statistical analysis
Data were statistically analyzed using the STATISTICA 9.0 (StatSoft Inc., Tulsa, OK, USA) for Windows software. The Wilcoxon paired test was used to compare mean values at each stage of experiment. The Mann-Whitney test was used to compare the differences of

PON1 activity between groups according to the clinical features. Correlation was calculated using Spearman test. *P* values less than 0.05 were considered significant. Data on plots were presented as median (dot), 25%–75% percentiles (box), and minimum-maximum values (whiskers).

Results

Baseline and operative patients characteristic are reported in Tables 1 and 2. In the early postoperative period (to 48 h after surgery) serious postoperative complications were observed in 6 patients. There were two in-hospital deaths caused by perioperative myocardial infarct and cardiogenic shock and four patients developed left ventricle insufficiency. Paraoxonase activity towards paraoxon and phenyl acetate before, during and after CABG surgery is shown on Figs. 1 and 2. Statistical significance of changes observed in subsequent stages of experiment is reported in Table 3 (*p* values regard each pair of compared PON1 activity levels in previous and next stage of experiment). PON1 activity toward paraoxon in comparison with preoperative values decreased significantly (*p* = 0.014) after aorta cross clumping, increased directly after operation and then the tendency to decreased values in subsequent stages of experiment within 6 to 30 h after operation was observed to achieve the level similar to this one evaluated preoperatively at 48 h after operation. If compared with preoperative values significantly lower PON1 activity towards para-oxon was observed in the second (*p* = 0,014) and sixth (*p* = 0,008) stage of experiment. Comparison of PON1 activity between the next subsequent stages of experiment did not reveals significant differences between subsequent levels except from the tendency (*p* = 0.06) to higher PON1 activity after the end of the operation (third stage of experiment) in comparison with the time after aorta clumping (second stage of experiment). The

Table 1 Patients demographics and clinical data at baseline

Parameter	Value
Men (%)	80,77
Women (%)	19,23
Age (years ±SD)	61,2 ± 9,79
Hypercholesterolemia (%)	50,0
Hypertriglyceridemia (%)	26,92
Obesity (%)	23,08
Overweight (%)	42,31
Smokers (%)	34,62
Hypertensives (%)	57,69
Diabetes (%)	7,69
Family history of CAD (%)	7,69

CAD coronary heart disease

Table 2 Operative patients' characteristics

Parameter	Value
Elective surgery (%)	69,23
Urgent surgery (%)	30,77
Ejection fraction (% ± SD)	53,1 ± 9,78
Patients with EF < 30% (%)	3,85
Patients with 30% ≤ EF <50% (%)	19,23
Operation risk (Euroscore) (±SD)	3,62 ± 2,43
Patients with low risk of operation (%)	26,92
Patients with intermediate risk of operation (%)	50,0
Patients with high risk of operation (%)	23,08
Number of grafts per patient (±SD)	3,5 ± 0,8
Number of arterial grafts per patient	1,0 ± 0,0
Number of venous grafts per patient	2,5 ± 0,7
Patient with implanted	
1 graft (%)	3,85
2 grafts (%)	26,92
3 grafts (%)	50,0
4 or more grafts (%)	19,23
Surgical time (min ± SD)	184,17 ± 51,54
Cross clamping time (min ± SD)	48,12 ± 13,31

tendency (*p* = 0.06) to increasing PON 1 activity towards paraoxon was observed between the sixth and the seventh stage of experiment. Similar differences were found after evaluating PON1 arylesterase activity. In comparison with preoperative period, PON1 activity towards phenyl acetate was significantly lower in all stages of experiment (*p* < 0,05) with exception of stages fifth and sixth, however in these stages the strong tendency to

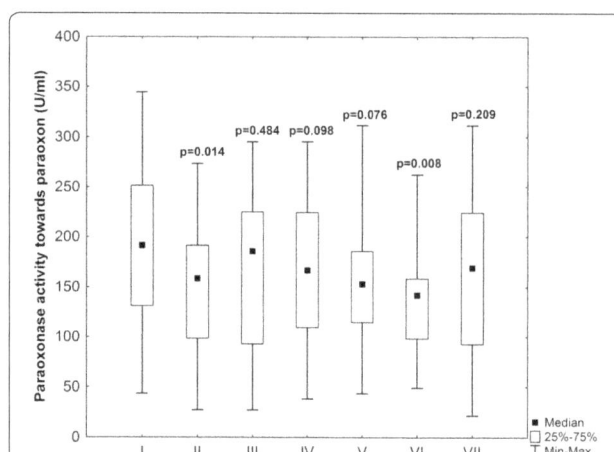

Fig. 1 Paraoxonase activity towards paraoxon (U/ml) in subsequent stages of experiment(1) preoperatively, (2) after aortic clumping, (3) after the end of operation, 4) at 6 h, 5) at 18 h, 6) at 30 h, and 7) at 48 h after operation. *P*-values - preoperative data vs other stages of experiment (Wilcoxon test)

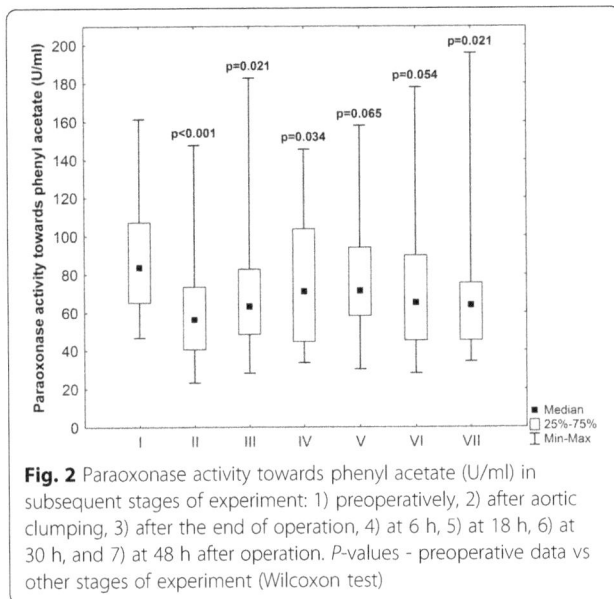

Fig. 2 Paraoxonase activity towards phenyl acetate (U/ml) in subsequent stages of experiment: 1) preoperatively, 2) after aortic clumping, 3) after the end of operation, 4) at 6 h, 5) at 18 h, 6) at 30 h, and 7) at 48 h after operation. P-values - preoperative data vs other stages of experiment (Wilcoxon test)

lower PON1 activities was found (p equal respectively 0.06 and 0.05). Also comparison of PON1 activity towards phenyl acetate between subsequent stages of experiment reveals the significant increase of enzyme activity in the third stage of experiment in comparison with the second stage ($p = 0.01$).

Relative PON1 activity (per gram of total plasma protein) towards paraoxon did not differ significantly in subsequent stages (Table 3). Relative PON1 activity towards phenyl acetate was significantly decreased after aorta clumping ($p = 0.026$) in comparison with preoperative period (Fig. 3) and reached the same value as preoperatively in the third stage of experiment ($p = 0.19$) significantly increasing in the stage third in comparison

with stage two ($p = 0.04$). The PON1 activity towards paraoxon throughout the study was not correlated with PON1 activity towards phenyl acetate ($p > 0.05$, Spearman test, data not shown).

Total protein plasma level significantly decreased ($p < 0.001$) after aorta cross – clumping and remained low ($p < 0.01$) in all stages of the experiment in comparison with preoperative value (Fig. 4). The protein plasma level after the end of operation raised significantly in comparison with the second stage and the tendency to higher values in fourth in comparison with third stage was observed. In other subsequent stages of experiment noted values of protein level did not differ significantly.

PON1 activity towards paraoxon in preoperative period ($R = -0.341$, $p = 0.088$) and PON1 activity towards phenyl acetate in seventh stage of experiment ($R = -409$, $p = 0.056$) tended to inversely correlate with the occurrence of postoperative complications. No correlation between PON1 activity in other stages of experiment and complications was found, although the correlation of protein level in the second stage with occurrence of complications ($R = -0.402$, $p = 0.04$) and similar trend in stage fifth and sixth (respectively $R = -0.383$, $p = 0.05$ and $R = -0.344$, $p = 0.09$) was notified (Table 4). Considering other established risk factors of unfavorable outcome after cardiac surgery, no correlation between PON1 preoperative value and ejection fraction, Euroscore scale, the time of operation and aorta cross clumping time was observed ($p > 0.05$, Spearman test, data not shown). Evaluating relationship of PON1 activity towards both substrates in next stages of experiment inverse correlation between PON1 activity towards phenyl acetate in the stage fourth and Euroscore scale result ($p = 0.01$ for absolute and $p = 0.009$ for relative

Table 3 Comparison of PON 1 activity towards paraoxon and phenyl acetate, relative PON 1 activity in subsequent stages of experiment: (1) preoperatively, (2) after aortic clumping, (3) after the end of operation, 4) at 6 h, 5) at 18 h, 6) at 30 h, and 7) at 48 h after operation

Stage of experiment	Paraoxonase activity towards paraoxon	Relative paraoxonase activity towards paraoxon	Paraoxonase activity towards phenyl acetate	Relative paraoxonase activity towards phenyl acetate	Total plasma protein level (g/dL)
1	188.42 ± 79.28	3057.75 ± 269.58	91.56 ± 32.17	1483.74 ± 516.47	6.17 ± 0,78
2	146.39 ± 64.74 $p = 0.01$	2808.86 ± 1111.34 $p = 0.32$	59.63 ± 29.73 $p < 0.001$	1195.67 ± 663.62 $p = 0.026$	5.03 ± 0.70 $p < 0.001$
3	165.71 ± 77.10 $p = 0.06$	3105.23 ± 1370.27 $p = 0.13$	70.94 ± 36.24 $p = 0.01$	1339.40 ± 653.06 $p = 0.04$	5,28 ± 0.63 $p = 0.02$
4	166.82 ± 68.14 $p = 0.67$	3023.35 ± 1207.66 $p = 0.46$	75.26 ± 32.60 $p = 0.69$	1398.26 ± 693.96 $p = 0.88$	5.59 ± 0.76 $p = 0.06$
5	154.27 ± 66.50 $p = 0.36$	2779.60 ± 1259.10 $p = 0.26$	77.47 ± 29.27 $p = 0.60$	1374.70 ± 539.80 $p = 0.98$	5,69 ± 0.94 $p = 0.67$
6	138.44 ± 55.66 $p = 0.42$	2514.25 ± 1122.20 $p = 0.3$	75.30 ± 40.34 $p = 0.13$	1355.46 ± 708.89 $p = 0.13$	5.62 ± 0.88 $p = 0.70$
7	163.39 ± 82.29 $p = 0.06$	2901.89 ± 1567.51 $p = 0.1$	71.95 ± 40.48 $p = 0.66$	1351.55 ± 815.90 $p = 0.66$	5.65 ± 0.82 $p = 0.34$

Continuous data are reported as mean ± SD. Paraoxonase activities in subsequent stages were pair compared with Mann – Whitney U test. A p value in each stage presents comparison with the previous stage of experiment

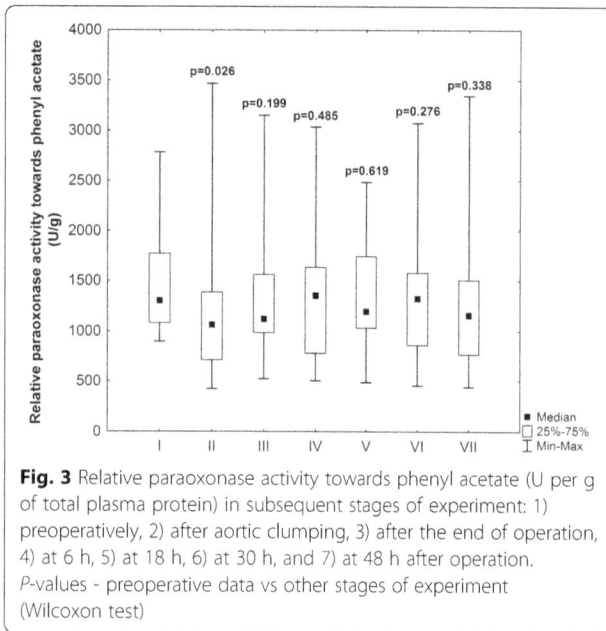

Fig. 3 Relative paraoxonase activity towards phenyl acetate (U per g of total plasma protein) in subsequent stages of experiment: 1) preoperatively, 2) after aortic clumping, 3) after the end of operation, 4) at 6 h, 5) at 18 h, 6) at 30 h, and 7) at 48 h after operation. *P*-values - preoperative data vs other stages of experiment (Wilcoxon test)

activity) was found. The protein level after the end of operation correlate significantly with the time of operation (p = 0.01). Also the correlation between protein level and the time of aorta cross – clumping (p = 0.002 in the second stage, p = 0.04 in the sixth stage and p = 0.02 in the seventh stage) was noted.

Discussion

Our data indicate the significant decrease of PON1 activity after aorta cross clumping during CABG surgery. PON1 activity increased after surgery in comparison with values observed during operation, but the activity towards phenyl acetate remained lower than in

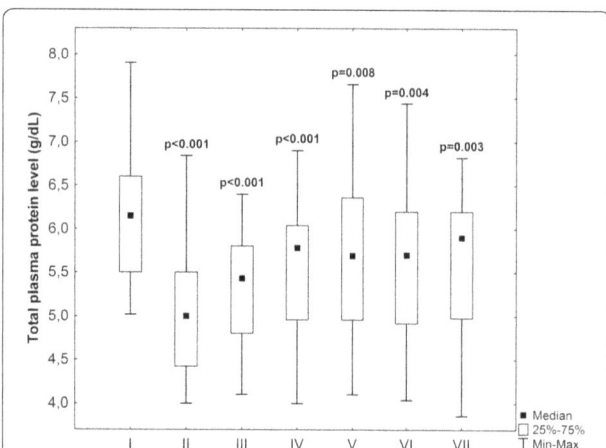

Fig. 4 Total plasma protein level (g/dL) in subsequent stages of experiment: 1) preoperatively, 2) after aortic clumping, 3) after the end of operation, 4) at 6 h, 5) at 18 h, 6) at 30 h, and 7) at 48 h after operation. *P*-values - preoperative data vs other stages of experiment (Wilcoxon test)

preoperative period. Any previous studies evaluating dynamic changes in PON1 activity during cardiac surgery were not presented, yet. Findings achieved in this experiment may be connected with widely discussed processes of oxidative stress and inflammatory reaction associated with cardiac surgery and direct damage of myocardium during CABG. In previously presented data the unfavorable role of extracorporeal circulation (ECC) causing blood contact with non – physiological surface and using of cardioplegia during CABG are underlined, except from the surgical trauma itself.

PON1 hydrolyzes several different compounds including organic phosphates, carboxyl acids arylesters, aromatic carbonates, unsaturated fatty acids esters [17], but in laboratory practice, PON1 activity towards paraoxon (paraoxonase activity) and towards phenyl acetate (arylesterase activity) is usually assessed, as it was done in our study. PON1 activity is related to several genetic polymorphisms localized in coding and promotor region of PON1 gene. There were described two polymorphic forms of coding region of PON1 gene: substitution of glutamine (isoform Q or A) by arginine in position 192 (isoform R or B) and substitution of methionine (M) by leucine (L) in position 55. It was shown that PON1 isoenzymes hydrolyze some substrates in different rates depending on genotype. Hydrolytic activity towards phosphorganic compounds such as paraoxon is higher if the allel 192R is present. Alloenzymes QQ are more efficient in hydrolyzing neurotoxic substances as sarin or soman. Rate of hydrolysis of some substrates including phenyl acetate, naphtyl acetate or diazoxon is independent of genotype in position 192Q/R [18, 19]. In vitro studies have shown that PON1 QQ isoenzymes were more efficient hydrolyzing lipid peroxides in human atherosclerotic plaques derived from coronary and carotic arteries lesions [7]. A lot of studies investigating possible higher risk of CHD in individuals with 192R allel and protective role of 192Q allel were performed, but results were contradictory depending of evaluated population [20–23]. Another authors reported association between 55 M/L polymorphism and PON1 activity. It has been shown that in MM homozygous individuals the PON1 serum activity towards paraoxon is lower in comparison with LL homozygotes [24]. Additionally PON1 gene presents several polymorphism of promotor region: -108/C/ T, –126G/C, –106A/G, –832 A/G and -909G/C [25]. It was proved that PON1 concentration and activity are affected almost exclusively by -108C/T polymorphism [26]. In our previous study [27] evaluating influence of PON1 activity and promotor region polymorphism (–108C/T) on short and long term outcome in 78 patients undergoing CABG we observed lower PON1 activity in the presence of TT genotype in comparison with CT and CC genotypes. Also other authors assessing

Table 4 Correlation between paraoxonase1 activity and total plasma protein level with postoperative complications in patients after CABG in subsequent stages of experiment: (1) preoperatively, (2) after aortic clumping, (3) after the end of operation, 4) at 6 h, 5) at 18 h, 6) at 30 h, and 7) at 48 h after operation (R - correlation ratio and p - p value according to Spearman test)

Stage of experiment	Paraoxonase activity towards paraoxon	Relative paraoxonase activity towards paraoxon	Paraoxonase activity towards phenyl acetate	Relative paraoxonase activity towards phenyl acetate	Total plasma protein level (g/dL)
Stage 1					
R	-0,341	−0,28	-0,073	0,207	−0.219
p	0.088	0.166	0.723	0.31	0.282
Stage 2					
R	-0.313	−0.143	−0.01	0.09	−0.553
p	0.12	0.49	0.95	0.66	0.004
Stage 3					
R	-0.082	−0.164	0.111	0.181	−0.23
p	0.71	0.45	0.60	0.40	0.27
Stage 4					
R	-0.103	0.020	0.083	0.183	−0.401
p	0.61	0.91	0.67	0.37	0.04
Stage 5					
R	-0,317	−0.219	−0.257	−0.111	−0.383
p	0.11	0.28	0.216	0.60	0.05
Stage 6					
R	0,078	0.169	−0.097	0.026	−0.034
p	0.71	0.42	0.64	0.90	0.09
Stage 7					
R	0.049	0.091	−0.409	−0.037	−0.207
p	0.81	0.66	0.06	0.86	0.312

larger group of patients reports that PON1 concentration and activity towards paraoxon were significantly lower in patients with CHD in comparison with healthy control group. In both investigated groups correlation of PON1 activity and -108C/T polymorphism was found with the highest enzyme efficiency in CC homozygotes and the lowest in TT homozygotes. In patients with CHD also relationship with PON1 concentration and −909 GC genotype was revealed [28]. Currently rather PON1 activity than polymorphism are regarded as a factor contributing to CHD occurrence. Thus reported in this paper differences in PON1 activity evaluating both paraoxonase as well as arylesterase activity can minimize the genotype influence on obtained results. Because the PON1 activity towards paraoxon is more affected by the occurrence of coronary heart disease and genetic polymorphism the observed changes in PON1 activity towards phenyl acetate may better express the pathophysiological circumstances of the cardiac surgery itself.

It was previously proved that tissue (also myocardium) ischaemia caused by ECC and blood flow decline are connected with increased level of oxidative stress, but the contribution of different components of oxidative and antioxidative balance (among them PON1) still remains unclear. Under circumstances of intensive oxidative stress plasma antioxidants level becomes lower. During the cardiac surgery using the ECC itself enhances the oxidative stress. Additionally at the time of reperfusion the tissue oxygene supply becomes rapidly restored and free oxygene radicals in amounts exceeding local antioxidative defense are formed. It was proved that in early postoperative period (hours after operation) in patients operated without using the extracorporeal circulation the level of hydroxylipids is significantly higher than in patients operated without using this device [29]. In another study serum concentrations of different oxidative compounds expressed as total antioxidant status, total oxidant status and oxidative stress index during on – pump coronary artery bypass grafting was assessed. Authors found significant increase of oxidative stress measurements after reperfusion. They concluded that oxidative imbalance may be associated with the aortic cross clumping time [30]. Another authors assessing changes in total antioxidant capacity of plasma in patients undergoing CABG found progressive depletion of evaluated values after the beginning of surgery, what remains in concordance with our results regarding PON1 activity towards phenyl acetate [31]. Even in the experiment evaluating influence or potentially less harmful phosphorylcholine – coated extracorporeal circulation system a higher oxidative stress with elevated antioxidant reaction were observed [32]. Also in our study we found a significant decrease of PON1 activity after aorta clumping and then an increase after the end of the operation when cardiopulmonary bypass was not still used, but we did not observed a correlation between PON 1 activity and time of aorta clumping. Our findings support the idea that using of ECC intensifying oxidative stress contributes to exhausting PON1 plasma supply. The reason of this phenomenon may be a result of PON1 gene expression inhibition and decreased protein synthesis in the liver. The decrease in PON1 activity may be concerned as analogy to another antioxidant enzymes depletion – superoxide dysmuthase (SOD) and glutatione peroxidase (GPx) – which activity decrease in enhanced oxidative stress was contributed to their inactivation by free oxygen radicals and products of their disintegration [33], although in the another study strong activation of SOD and GPx during ECC with the maximum level at the end of the cross clamp circulation was observed [34].

PON1 is a negative acute phase protein: PON1 plasma concentration rapidly decreases as a response on systemic inflammatory reaction. Acute phase activation during CABG is triggered by several agents such as surgical trauma itself, blood contact with extracorporeal surface, endotoxemia, tissue ischaemia. Blood contact with non physiological extracorporeal circulation surface leads to complement activation, release of pro – inflammatory cytokines (TNF–α, Il–6, Il-8, Il–13), leukocytes activation and adhesive molecules expression [14]. Pro – inflammatory cytokines unfavorably modify plasma lipid profile deteriorating protective function of HDL. Except from PON1 three other enzymes are responsible for antioxidative activity of HDL: lecithin cholesterol acyl transferase (LCAT), platelet activating factor acetylhydolase (PAF-AH) and above mentioned GPx, but the role of PON1 is considered as crucial. PON1 hydrolyzes peroxidation products contained in LDL particles, arterial walls and macrophages decreasing free radicals formation by NADH oxidase [35]. Modifications ongoing during acute phase reaction in HDL particle involve increase of free cholesterol content, incorporation of serum amyloid A (SAA) and ceruloplasmin and loss of apoJ, apoM and cholesterol esters [36, 37]. It was observed that in patients with septic shock and systemic inflammatory response syndromes apoM concentration significantly decrease and is reversely correlated to acute phase markers [38]. Additionally activity of several proteins attributable to HDL metabolism (LCAT, cholesterol

esters transfer protein—CETP and hepatic lipase) and concentration of proteins responsible for antioxidative function of HDL decrease. Especially enzymatic activity of LCAT is considered as a factor involved in the protection of the formation of atherosclerotic plaques [39], but on the other hand it was shown that in vitro PON1 acts more efficiently than LCAT or PAF – AH protecting LDL against peroxidation [40]. Avian HDL, presenting PAF – AH activity, but devoid of PON1 do not protect human LDL against oxidative modifications [39]. As it was proved HDL particles modified as described above become pro-inflammatory and enhances oxidative stress [2]. It was shown that mentioned processes may occur during acute phase reaction, for example viral infection as well as chronic inflammatory process like atherosclerosis is regarded [41]. In several studies possible relationship between infective factors and acute coronary syndrome occurrence has been reported. It was noted that peridental infections or respiratory system infections increase the risk of myocardial infarction [42, 43]. Van Lenten et al. investigated abilities of HDL isolated from blood of patients 2–3 days after cardiac surgery in comparison with HDL obtained from healthy blood donors. HDL lipoproteins derivative from health persons inhibited LDL oxidative modifications and monocyte adhesion into endothelium cells. HDL from patients after cardiac surgery had pro – inflammatory abilities. In vitro loss of PON1 activity by HDL particles obtained from patients after CABG was proved [44]. During operations different from CABG PON1 activity decline was observed. Kumon et al. proved that PON1 activity decreases in patients after laparoscopic cholecystectomia. Blood samples were taken after 3,6 and 14 days after surgery. Decreased level of PON1 activity in comparison with preoperative period was observed in all stages of experiment despite of an increase of HDL and apo A-I concentration 14 days after operation. Authors suggest that PON1 activity decline maintaining so long may result from prolonging inhibition of PON1 gene expression and unfavorable modifications of HDL accompanied with acute phase reaction. Simultaneously modifying of PON1 activity by other acute phase proteins is also possible [45]. In the recent study it was reported that in a human experimental model of endotoxemia induced with endotoxin (LPS) intravenous administration subject with low HDL cholesterol were more susceptible to an inflammatory challenge. This response was independent of HDL cholesterol level in subject with the highest PON1 activity [46]. The latest phenomenon may contribute to slightly better prognosis in patients with higher PON1 activities, in which we observed postoperative complications less frequent.

Several factors is considered as predictors of worse outcome in patients undergoing CABG, most of them is included into Euroscore scale, but a clinical need to identify new factors that may allow for identification patients of higher risk of operation is underlined. From this reason we try to correlate investigated changes in PON1 activity with early postoperative complications. Poor outcome incidences observed in our study tends to be connected with the preoperative values of PON1 activity towards paroxon and PON1 activity towards phenyl acetate in seventh stage of experiment, but no significant correlation with PON1 activity any other stage of experiment was found. In 4 patients we observed left ventricular insufficiency leading to need of circulation support or low cardiac output syndrome. In 2 patients myocardial infarction confirmed by increase of cardiac troponin >10 times above the normal level was recognized and these patients did not survive. The development of complications affecting cardiac function, as it was observed in our study, is commonly contributed to widely discussed above oxidative stress and inflammatory reaction. The balance between oxygen delivery and consumption in perioperative period is highly unsteady and any unsettling may lead to metabolic acidosis and deterioration of cardiac output [47]. For this reason preoperative low PON1 activity decreasing natural antioxidative defense may lead to imbalance resulting in impairment of cardiac function. As the main source of enhanced oxidative stress and inflammatory response during CABG seems to be ECC using, several studies evaluating influence of on and – off pump operation on outcome were performed and advantages of beating heart techniques was confirmed in terms of early mortality [48]. Providing of on – pump CABG was reported as a predictive factor of low cardiac output syndrome [49] and perioperative myocardial infarct [50], although the results of large randomized trials did not confirm the significant superiority off- pump technique [51]. Also in high operative risk patients treated preventively with intra – aortic balloon pump there was no significant difference in perioperative mortality in comparison with control group [52]. In our study the surgery was performed by conventional on – pump method and postoperative mortality (7.6%) and cardiac insufficiency (23%) did not depart from results of above quoted analyses (respectively 2–8,6% and 14–61% depending on operative risk of assessed population and severity of cardiac insufficiency). In recently published study investigating impact of inflammatory markers on clinical outcome, authors did not confirm differences between on – and off – pump group of patients regarding the occurrence of low cardiac output syndrome, postoperative myocardial infarction and death. Similarly like in our study, quoted authors reported correlation between assessed preoperatively levels of 8-isoprostaglandin $F_{2\alpha}$, asymmetric dimethyloarginine and β- thrombomoduline

and postoperative complications [53]. Observed in our study correlation between total protein level and complications may be considered as being in accordance with the data indicating that in surgical operations including CABG decreased albumin concentration is related with less favorable outcome [54].

Cardiac surgery is reversibly connected with myocardium damage and even is considered as an experimental model of myocardial infarct. Observed in this study dynamic changes of PON1 activity may be compared to PON1 activity changes during myocardial infarct. Ayub et al. found that in patients with myocardial infarct after 2 h from beginning the chest pain occur a significant decrease of PON1 activity. Authors of quoted experiment do not reveal any significant differences of investigating parameters in postinfarctal period (1,2,3 days) [13]. Our data may support hypothesis that PON1 activity changes during myocardial infarct (or its experimental model: cardiac surgery) occur dynamically as a result of processes accompanied with myocardial ischaemia and should not be contributed only to previous decline of PON1 activity associated with atherosclerosis, because we did not find any significant correlation between PON1 activity and clinical (class of angina symptoms) or angiografic (occurrence of left main artery lesions) severity of coronary heart disease.

Discussing reasons of changes of PON1 activity during CABG process of hemodilution should be taken into consideration. Hemodilution is defined as an increase of liquid volume in the blood resulting in increase of plasma volume and decrease of blood red cells mass. During CABG a considerable amounts of liquids are given to supply loosen blood. This process may result in decrease of absolute PON1 activity directly after the heart function arrest and the retardation of the aorta blood flow. Storti et al. described that the level of total plasma protein decreases from 7,3 g/dl before to 4,8 g/dl after CABG. The level of total plasma protein remains decreased to 6 months after surgery [55]. In our study we also found decrease of total plasma protein concentration maintaining in postoperative period. Observed in our study differences of PON1 activity towards phenyl acetate were significant if expressed as PON1 activity per gram of plasma protein. That may indicate that process of hemodilution is not the only reason of changes of PON1 activity.

Limitations

We are aware of several limitations regarding this study. The main is that investigated group of patients was relatively small - from this reason the frequency of noted complications were low, what undoubtedly influence the statistic analysis. We did not divide the group of patients with complications into subgroups according to cause and severity of cardiac insufficiency or used treatment (mechanical or pharmacological support, doses of inotropic drugs) like some other authors did, because statistical analysis of such small number of patients we consider as not valid. Future work should involve the larger group of patients and prolong the follow – up period.

Conclusions

In conclusion our data indicate that PON1 activity is markedly reduced after CABG surgery. These findings support the hypothesis of the role involving oxidative stress and acute phase response in the myocardium damage during cardiac surgery. Informations collected in this study should encourage the development of strategies allowing to protect myocardium and prevent post – ischeamic damage.

Abbreviations

CABG: coronary artery bypass grafting; EDTA: ethylenediaminetetraacetic acid; EF: Ejection fraction; HDL: High density lipoprotein; Il–13: Interleukin-13; Il-6: Intereukin-6; Il-8: Interleukin-8; LDL: Low density lipoprotein; LPS: Lipopolysaccharides; PON1: Serum paraoxonase 1; TNF-α: Tumor necrossi factor-α

Acknowledgements

Not applicable' for that section.

Funding

This study was supported by the grant No 2 P05A 059 30 of the Ministry of Science and Higher Education, Poland.

Authors' contributions

AW have made substantial contributions to conception and design, acquisition of data, analysis of data, performed statistical analysis and interpretation of data, literature search, manuscript preaparation, have been involved in drafting the manuscript and coordinated funding for the project. MC was involved in data collection, HB contributed to the design of the research, AW contributed to the design of the research and coordinated funding for the project, JS was involved in data collection and contributed to the design of the research, JD was involved in data interpretation, TZ conceived the idea of the study, contributed to the design of the research, analyzed the data, performed literature search, manuscript preaparation and coordinated funding for the project, have given final approval of the version to be published. All authors read and approved the final manuscript.

Competing interests

The authors declare that they have no competing interests.

Author details

[1]Cardiology Department, Medical University of Lublin, ul. Jaczewskiego 8, 20–954 Lublin, Poland. [2]Internal Medicine in Nursing Department, Medical University of Lublin, ul. Jaczewskiego 8, 20–954 Lublin, Poland. [3]Biochemistry and Molecular Biology Department, Medical University of Lublin, ul. Chodźki 1, 20-093 Lublin, Poland. [4]Cardiosurgery Department, Medical University of Lublin, ul. Jaczewskiego 8, 20–954 Lublin, Poland.

References

1. Mackness B, Durrington PN, Mackness MI. Human serum paraoxonase. Gen Pharmacol. 1998;31:329 36.

2. Navab M, Berliner JA, Subbanagounder G, et al. HDL and the inflammatory response induced by LDL-derived oxidized phospholipids. Arterioscler Thromb Vasc Biol. 2001;21:481–8.

3. Mackness B, Arrol S, Durrington PN, et al. Paraoxonase prevents accumulation of lipoperoxides in low-density lipoprotein. FEBS Lett. 1991; 286:152–4.

4. Mackness B, Quarck R, Verreth W, et al. Human paraoxonase −1 overexpression inhibits atherosclerosis in a mouse model of a metabolic syndrome. Arteriosc Thromb Vasc Biol. 2006;26:1545–50.

5. Guns PJ, Van Assche T, Verreth W, et al. Paraoxonase 1 gene transfer lower vascular oxidative stress and improves vasomotor function in apolipoprotein E-deficient mice wit preexisting atherosclerosis. Br J Pharmacol. 2008;153:508–16.

6. Shih DM, Gu L, Xia YR, et al. Mice lacking serum paraoxonase are susceptible to organophosphate toxicity and atherosclerosis. Nature. 1998; 394:284–7.

7. Aviram M, Hardak E, Vaya J, et al. Human serum paraoxonase (PON1) Q and R selectively decrease lipid peroxides in human coronary and carotid atherosclerotic lesions. Circulation. 2000;101:2510–7.

8. Bayrak A, Bayrak T, Bodur E, et al. The effect of HDL bound and free PON1 on copper induced LDL oxidation. Chem Biol Interact. 2016;257:141–6.

9. Mackness B, Durrington P, McElduff P, et al. Low paraoxonase1 activity predicts coronary events in the Caerphilly prospective study. Circulation. 2003;107:2775–9.

10. Durmaz T, Keles T, Ayhan H, et al. Diminished serum paraoxonase activity in patients with coronary artery calcification. Kardiol Pol. 2014;72:831–838.

11. Ikeda Y, Inoue M, Suehiro T, et al. Low human paraoxonase predicts cardiovascular events in Japanese patiets with type 2 diabetes. Acta Diabetol. 2009;46:239–42.

12. van Himbergen TM, van der Schouw YT, Voorbij HAM, et al. Paraoxonase1 (PON1) and the risk for coronary heart disease and myocardial infarction in a general population of Dutch women. Atherosclerosis. 2008;198:408–14.

13. Ayub A, Mackness MI, Arrol S, et al. Serum paraoxonase after myocardial infarction. Arterioscler Thromb Vasc Biol. 1999;19:330–5.

14. Paparella D, Yau TM, Young E. Cardiopulmonary bypass induced inflammation: pathophysiology and treatment. An update. Eur J Cardio- th Surg. 2002;21:232–44.

15. Michel P, Roques F, Nashef SA. The Euroscore project group: logistic and additive euro SCORE for high risk patients. Eur J Cardiothorac Surg. 2003;23:684–7.

16. Eckerson H, Romson WJ, Wyte C, La Du B. The human serum paraoxonase polymorphism: identification of phenotypes by their response to salts. Am J Hum Genet. 1983;35:214–27.

17. LaDu BN. Human serum paraoxonase/arylesterase. In: Kalow W, editor. Pharmacogenetics of drug metabolism. New York: Pergamon Press; 1992. p. 51–91.

18. Aviram M, Billecke S, Sorenson R, et al. Paraoxonase active site is required for protection against LDL oxidation involves its free sulfhydryl group and is different from that required for its arylesterase/paraoxonase activities: selective action of human paraoxonase Q and R. Arterioscer Thromb Vasc Biol. 1998;18:1617–24.

19. Davies HG, Richter RJ, Keifer M, et al. The effects of the human serum paraoxonase polymorphism is reversed with diazoxon, soman and sarin. Nat Genet. 1996;14:334–6.

20. Sanghera DK, Saha N, Aston CE, et al. DNA polymorphism in two paraoxonase genes (PON1 and PON2) associated with the risk od coronary heart disease. Am J Hum Genet. 1998;314:410–8.

21. Ombres D, Pannitteri G, Moutali A, et al. The Gln–Arg 192 polymorphism of the human paraoxonase gene is not associated with the coronary heart disease in Italian patients. Arterioscler Thromb Vasc Biol. 1998;18:1611–6.

22. Serrato M, Marian AJ. A variant of human paraoxonase/arylesterase (HUMPONA) gene is a risk factor for coronary heart disease. J Clin Invest. 1995;96:3005–8.

23. Anitkainen M, Muromtki S, Syvnne M, et al. The Gln–Arg 192 polymorphism of the human paraoxonase gene is not associated with the risk of coronary heart disease in Finns. J Clin Invest. 1996;191:883–5.

24. Mackness B, Mackness MI, Arrol S, et al. Effects of the molecular polymorphism of human paraoxonase (PON1) on the rate of hydrolysis of paraoxon. Br J Pharmacol. 1997;122:265–8.

25. Suehiro T, Nakamura T, Inoue M, et al. A polymorphism upstream from the human paraoxonase (PON1) gene and its association with PON1 expression.

Atherosclerosis. 2000;150:295–8.

26. Deakin S, Leviev I, Brulhart Meynet MC, et al. Paraoxonase –1 promoter haplotypes and serum paraoxonase: a predominant role in vivo for polymorphic position –107 implicating the transcription factor Sp1. Biochem J. 2003;372:643–9.

27. Wysocka A, Cybulski M, Berbeć H, et al. Prognostic value of paraoxonase 1 in patients undergoing coronary artery bypass grafting surgery. Med Sci Monit. 2014;20:594–600.

28. Mackness B, Turkie W, Mackness M. Paraoxonase –1 (PON1) promoter region polymorphisms, serum PON1 status and coronary heart disease. Arch Med Sci. 2013;1:8–13.

29. Matata BM, Sosnowski AW, Galinanes M. Off-pump bypass graft operation significantly reduces oxidative stress and inflammation. Ann Thorac Surg. 2000;69:785–91.

30. Mentese U, Dogan OV, Turan I, et al. Oxidant – antioxidant balance during on – pump coronary artery bypass grafting. Sci World J. 2014;2014:263058. doi:10.1155/2014/263058.

31. Kunt AS, Selek S, Celik H, et al. Decrease of total antioxidant capacity during coronary artery bypass surgery. Mt Sinai J Med. 2006;73:777–83.

32. Hatemi AC, Ceviker K, Togut A, et al. Oxidant status following cardiac surgery with phosphorylcholine-coated extracorporeal circulation systems. Oxidative Med Cell Longev. 2016;2016:3932092.

33. Das, Vasisht Nm Das L et al: Correlation between total antioxidant staus and lipid peroxidation in hypercholesterolemia. Current Science. 2000;78:486–487,

34. Luyten CR, van Overveld FJ, De Backer LA, et al. Antioxidant defence during cardiopulmonary bypass surgery. Eur J Cardiothorac Surg. 2005;27:611–6.

35. Maxkness B, Hunt R, Durrington PN. Mackness MI: ncreased immunolocalization of paraoxonase, clusterin, and apolipoprotein A-I in the human artery wall with the progression of atherosclerosis. Arterioscler Thromb Vasc Biol. 1997;17:1233–8.

36. Arrol S, Mackness MI, Durrington PN. High-density lipoprotein associated enzymes and the prevention of low-density lipoprotein oxidation. Eur J Lab Med. 1996;4:33–8.

37. Sato M, Ohkawa R, Yoshimoto A. Effects of serum amyloid a on the structure and antioxidant ability of high density lipoprotein. Biosci Rep. 2016;36 doi:10.1042/BRS20160075.

38. Kumaraswamy SB, Linder A, Akresson P, et al. Decreased plasma concentrations of apolipoprotein M in sepsis and systemic inflammatory response syndromes. Crit Care. 2012;16:R60.

39. Mackness B, Durrington PN, Mackness MI. Lack of protection against oxidative modification of LDL by avian HDL. Biochem Biophys Res Commun. 1998;247:443–6.

40. Kunnen S, Van Eck M. Lecithin: cholesterol acyltransferase: old friend or foe in atheroclerosis? J Lipid Res. 2012;53(1783):1799.

41. Fan J, Watanabe T. Inflammatory reactions in the patogenesis of atherosclerosis. J Atheroscler Thromb. 2003;10:63–71.

42. Mattila KJ, Valtonen VV, Nieminen M, et al. Dental infection and the risk of new coronary events: prospective study of patients with documented coronary artery disease. Clin Infect Dis. 1995;20:588–92.

43. Momiyama Y, Ohmori R, Taniguchi H, et al. Association of Mycoplasma pneumoniae infection with coronary artery disease ant its interaction with chlamydial infection. Atherosclerosis. 2004;176:139–44.

44. Van Lenten BJ, Hama SY, de Beer FC, et al. Anti-inflammatory HDL becomes pro-inflammatory during the acute phase response. Loss of protective effect of HDL against LDL oxidation in aortic wall cell cocultures. J Clin Invest. 1995;96:2758–67.

45. Kumon Y, Nakauchi Y, Kidawara K, et al. A longitudinal analysis of alteration in lecithin-cholesterol acyltransferase and paraoxonase activities following laparoscopic cholecystectomy relative to other parameters of HDL function and the acute phase response. Scand J Immunol. 1998;48:419–24.

46. Levels JHM, Geurts P, Karlsson H, et al. High-density lipoprotein proteome dynamics in human endotoxemia. Proteome Sci. 2011;9:34–48.

47. Masse L, Antonacci M. Low cardiac output syndrome. Identification and management. Crit Care Nurs Clin North Am. 2005;17:375–83.

48. Hussain G, Azam H, Raza Baig MA, et al. Early outcomes of on – pump versus off pump coronary artery bypass grafting. Pak J Med Sci. 2016;32:917–21.

49. WenJun D. Qiang Ji, YunQing Shi et al: predictors of low cardiac out put syndrome after isolated coronary artery bypass grafting. Int Heart J. 2015;56:144–9.

50. Chaudhry UA, Harling L, Sepehripor AH, et al. Beating – heart versus conventional on – pump coronary artery bypass grafting; meta – analysis of clinical outcomes. Ann Thorac Surg. 2015;100:2251–60.

51. Lamy A, Devereaux PJ, Prabhakran D, et al. Off – pump or on pump coronary – artery bypass graffting at 30 days. N Engl J Med. 2012;366:1489–97.

52. Zhang J, Lang Y, Guo L, et al. Preventive use of intra-aortic baloon pump in patients undergoing high risk coronary artery bypass grafting: a retrospective study. Med Sci Monit. 2015;21:855–60.

53. Plicner D, Stoliński J, Wąsowicz M, et al. Preoperative values of inflammatory markers predicts clinical outcomes in patients after CABG regardless of the use of cardiopulmonary bypass. Indian Heart J. 2016;68:S10–5.

54. Bhamidipati CM, LaPar DJ, Mehta GV, et al. Albumin is a better predictor of outcomes than body mass index following coronary artery bypass grafting. Surgery. 2011;150:626–34.

55. Storti S, Cerillo AG, Rizza A, et al. Coronary artery bypass grafting surgery is associated with a marked reduction in serum homocysteine and folate levels in the early postoperative period. Eur J Cardiothorac Surg. 2004;26:682–6.

16

Serum S-100β and NSE levels after off-pump versus on-pump coronary artery bypass graft surgery

Lei Zheng, Qing-Ming Fan[*] and Zhen-Yu Wei

Abstract

Background: We aimed to evaluate serum levels of S-100 beta (S-100β) and neuron specific enolase (NSE) in patients with coronary heart disease (CHD) after off-pump versus on-pump coronary artery bypass graft (CABG) surgery.

Methods: The PubMed (~2013) and the Chinese Biomedical Database (CBM) (1982 ~ 2013) were searched without language restrictions. After extraction of relevant data from selected studies, meta-analyses were conducted using STATA software (Version 12.0, Stata Corporation, College Station, Texas USA). Possible sources of heterogeneity were examined through univariate and multivariate meta-regression analyses and verified by Monte Carlo Simulation.

Results: Eleven studies with a total of 411 CHD patients met the inclusion criteria. Our meta-analysis showed no significant difference in serum S-100β and NSE levels between the on-pump group and the off-pump group before surgery. In the on-pump group, there was a significant difference in serum S-100β levels of CHD patients between before and after surgery, especially within the first 24 h after surgery. Furthermore, in the on-pump group, there was a significant difference in serum NSE levels of CHD patients between before and after surgery, particularly at 0 h after surgery. In the off-pump group, there was an obvious difference in serum S-100β levels between before and after surgery, especially within 24 h after surgery. Our results also demonstrated that serum S-100β and NSE levels of CHD patients in the on-pump group were significantly higher than those of patients in the off-pump group, especially within 24 h after surgery.

Conclusions: Our findings provide empirical evidence that off-pump and on-pump CABG surgeries may increase serum S-100β and NSE levels in CHD patients, which was most prominent within 24 h after on-pump CABG surgery.

Keywords: S-100β, NSE, Coronary heart disease, Coronary artery bypass grafting, Meta-analysis

Background

As a major public health issue worldwide, coronary heart disease (CHD) is the primary cause of disability and death in the developed countries and is among the leading causes of disease burden in low-and middle-income countries [1, 2]. Evidence has revealed that the prevalence of CHD in persons aged 20 years or older was estimated to be 6.4 % (15.4 million) in the US in 2010, and 386,324 cases of CHD-related deaths were reported in 2009 [3]. Nowadays, three therapeutic options are generally used for patients with CHD, including medical treatment with drugs, coronary interventions such as angioplasty and coronary stent implantation, and coronary artery bypass grafting (CABG) surgery [4, 5].

CABG surgery is a surgical procedure most commonly performed to relieve angina and reduce the risk of death from CHD [6]. The CABG surgery has significantly changed over the years, from traditional surgical operations using cardiopulmonary bypass (on-pump CABG) to a newer approach in cardiovascular surgery (off-pump CABG), both of which are primarily designed to improve the outcomes in CHD patients [7, 8]. Although the operative mortality in CABG surgeries has decreased dramatically, the rate of neurologic complications remains unacceptably high; for example, neurological injury is a major perioperative risk in these patients [9, 10]. Unfortunately, the postoperative brain damage is difficult to

* Correspondence: fanqinming0107@126.com
Department of Cardiovascular Surgery, Yantai Yuhuangding Hospital, No.20 Yuhuangding East Road, Yantai 264000, P.R. China

diagnose early and mainly based on the observation of specific brain injury markers [11]. Recently, it has been reported that the cerebral biomarkers such as S-100 beta (S-100β) and neuron specific enolase (NSE) may serve as biomarkers to reflect brain damages in cardiac surgery [12]. S-100β protein, a specific protein originating from the brain, has been found in the cytosol of both glial and Schwann cells, chondrocytes and adipocytes, having both intracellular and extracellular neurotropic and also neurotoxic functions [13, 14]. Low physiological concentrations of S-100β could protect neurons against apoptosis, stimulate neurite outgrowth and astrocyte proliferation, whereas S-100β at high concentrations may result in neuronal death and exhibit properties of a damage-associated molecular pattern protein [15, 16]. In addition, elevated levels of S-100β might accurately reflect the existence of neuropathological conditions, including neurodegenerative diseases and neuronal injury [17, 18]. NSE has also been suggested to act as a specific serum marker for neuronal damage, which is mainly found in neuronal cells, especially in mature neurons of the central nervous system, and is not secreted; and thus, increased NSE in cerebrospinal fluid or blood may reflect postoperative cognitive dysfunction or structural damage to neuronal cells [19, 20]. Therefore, serum S-100β and NSE levels measured before and after on-pump and off-pump CABG could potentially be diagnostic of ongoing cerebral damage associated with these surgical procedures [21]. To date, evidence supports that both on-pump and off-pump CABG are associated with increased serum levels of NSE and S-100β, but the off-pump CABG exhibits relatively lower serum S-100β protein and NSE levels, suggesting that the off-pump CABG has less influence or impairment on neurocognitive functions in comparison to the on-pump CABG [22, 23]. However, contradictory results have also been reported in the literature. Therefore, we performed this meta-analysis aiming to evaluate serum S-100β and NSE levels in CHD patients after off-pump versus on-pump CABG surgery.

Methods
Literature search and selection criteria
The PubMed (~2013) and the Chinese Biomedical Database (CBM) (from 1982 to 2013) were searched without language restrictions. The keywords and MeSH terms applied in combination with a highly sensitive search strategy were: ("S100 calcium binding protein beta subunit" or "nerve tissue protein S100b" or "neurotrophic protein S100beta" or "S-100β" or "S100beta protein" or "S100beta") and ("phosphopyruvate hydratase" or "2-phospho-D-glycerate hydrolase" or "NSE" or "neuron-specific enolase" or "nervous system specific enolase" or "muscle specific enolase") and ("coronary artery bypass" or "coronary artery bypass grafting"

or "CABG" or "on-pump coronary artery bypass" or "off-pump coronary artery bypass" or "on- and off- coronary artery bypass"). Moreover, a manual search based on the references lists of the searched articles was also carried out to identify other potential articles.

The eligibility criteria for the inclusion of studies in this meta-analysis were as follows: (1) the study must report serum S-100β and NSE levels in CHD patients after off-pump versus on-pump CABG surgery; (2) all patients must have confirmed the diagnostic criteria for CHD; (3) the study must supply sufficient information on serum levels of S-100β and NSE. Studies that did not meet the inclusion criteria were excluded. In case those authors published the same subjects in several studies, the most recent study or the study with largest sample size was selected.

Data extraction and methodological assessment
Using a standardized data extraction form, two authors independently extracted the following information from the studies included: publication year of article, geographical location, language of publication, surname of the first author, sample size, the source of the subjects, design of study, follow-up time, detection method, serum levels of S-100β and NSE, etc. Methodological quality assessment was carried out respectively by two authors through the Newcastle-Ottawa Scale (NOS) criteria [24]. Three aspects were included in the NOS criteria: (1) subject selection: 0 ~ 4; (2) comparability of subject: 0 ~ 2; (3) clinical outcome: 0 ~ 3. The range of NOS scores is from 0 to 9; and a score of ≥ 7 represents a high quality.

Statistical analysis
The STATA statistical software (Version 12.0, Stata Corporation, College Station, TX, USA) was applied for our meta-analysis. Standardized mean difference (SMD) with the corresponding 95 % confidence intervals (95 % CI) was calculated. In addition, the Z test was conducted for estimation of the statistical significance of pooled SMDs. Heterogeneity among studies was estimated by the Cochran's Q-statistic and I^2 tests [25]. If the Q-test showed a $P < 0.05$ or the I^2 test showed > 50 %, which indicate significant heterogeneity and the random-effect model was implemented, otherwise the fixed-effects model was performed [26]. Using sensitivity analysis of variables, the impact on the overall results by removing one single study was evaluated. Moreover, funnel plots and Egger's linear regression test were applied for the investigation of publication bias [27]. Possible sources of heterogeneity were examined through univariate and multivariate meta-regression analyses and verified by Monte Carlo Simulation [28, 29].

Results

Characteristics of included studies

Our search strategy initially identified 138 articles. By reviewing the titles and abstracts, 67 articles were excluded. After systematically reviewing the remaining full texts, we excluded another 55 articles. In addition, 5 studies were excluded for lack of data integrity. Finally, 11 clinical cohort studies containing a total of 411 patients with CHD met the inclusion criteria used for qualitative data analysis [30, 22, 23, 31–38]. The publication years of eligible studies were between 2002 and 2013. Overall, 9 studies were based on Asians, and the other 2 studies on Caucasians. The NOS score of each included studies was ≥ 5 (moderate-high quality). The characteristics of eligible studies are summarized in Table 1.

Quantitative data synthesis

Our meta-analysis showed no significant difference in serum S-100β and NSE levels between the on-pump group and the off-pump group before surgery (S-100β: SMD = 0.14, 95 % CI = −0.07 ~ 0.35, $P = 0.191$; NSE: SMD = −0.12, 95 % CI = −0.42 ~ 0.17, $P = 0.408$; respectively) (Fig. 1).

In the on-pump group, there was a significant difference in serum S-100β levels of CHD patients between before and after surgery (SMD = 2.05, 95 % CI = 1.55 ~ 2.55, $P < 0.001$), especially within 24 h after surgery (0 h: SMD = 4.81, 95 % CI = 3.20 ~ 6.41, $P < 0.001$; 6 h: SMD = 2.41, 95 % CI = 1.26 ~ 3.55, $P < 0.001$; 24 h: SMD = 1.14, 95 % CI = 0.66 ~ 1.62, $P < 0.001$), while no such difference was found after 24 h post-surgery (48 h: SMD = 0.79, 95 % CI = −0.18 ~ 1.75, $P = 0.109$; 72 h: SMD = 0.25, 95 % CI = −0.31 ~ 0.82, $P = 0.380$) (Fig. 2a). In the off-pump group, there was a significant difference in serum S-100β levels between before and after surgery (SMD = 1.29, 95 % CI = 0.86 ~ 1.72, $P < 0.001$), especially within 24 h after surgery (0 h: SMD = 3.15, 95 % CI = 1.74 ~ 4.56, $P < 0.001$; 6 h: SMD = 1.48, 95 % CI = 0.53 ~ 2.44, $P = 0.002$; 24 h: SMD = 0.82, 95 % CI = 0.32 ~ 1.33, $P = 0.001$); however, there was no significant difference observed after 24 h (48 h: SMD = 0.06, 95 % CI = −0.37 ~ 0.49, $P = 0.780$; 72 h: SMD = 0.13, 95 % CI = −0.45 ~ 0.71, $P = 0.669$) (Fig. 3a). Also, our results demonstrated that the serum S-100β of CHD patients in the on-pump group were significantly higher than those of patients in the off-pump group (SMD = 1.08, 95 % CI = 0.67 ~ 1.48, $P < 0.001$), especially within 24 h after surgery (0 h: SMD = 2.91, 95 % CI = 1.64 ~ 4.19, $P < 0.001$; 6 h: SMD = 1.19, 95 % CI = 0.56 ~ 1.83, $P = 0.017$; 24 h: SMD = 0.51, 95 % CI = 0.09 ~ 0.92, $P = 0.001$); after 24 h, the results revealed no such statistical significance (48 h: SMD = 0.29, 95 % CI = −1.03 ~ 1.61, $P = 0.670$; 72 h: SMD = 0.02, 95 % CI = −0.55 ~ 0.59, $P = 0.952$) (Fig. 4a). The difference of the serum S-100β levels between on-pump and off-pump groups was the most significant 0 h after surgery, after which the difference was decreased with time (Fig. 5). According to univariate meta-regression analyses, time may be a source of heterogeneity ($P = 0.016$), while publication year, ethnicity and sample size did not cause heterogeneity (all $P > 0.05$), which was also verified by the multivariate analyses (Table 2).

Furthermore, in the on-pump group, there was a significant difference in serum NSE levels of CHD patients between before and after surgery (SMD = 1.28, 95 % CI = 0.31 ~ 2.25, $P = 0.010$), particularly at 0 h after surgery (SMD = 2.90, 95 % CI = 0.39 ~ 5.42, $P = 0.024$), while it was not significant at other time points (6 h: SMD = 0.17, 95 % CI = −2.69 ~ 3.04, $P = 0.906$; 24 h: SMD = 1.34, 95 % CI = −0.28 ~ 2.95, $P = 0.105$; 48 h: SMD = 1.75, 95 %

Table 1 Main characteristics of included studies

First author	Year	Ethnicity	Case number		Gender (M/F)		Age (years)		Study design
			On-pump	Off-pump	On-pump	Off-pump	On-pump	Off-pump	
van Boven WJ [30]	2013	Caucasians	10	10	9/1	8/2	73.3 ± 1.4	73.1 ± 2.2	RCT
Bayram H [22]	2013	Asians	40	24	31/9	18/6	61.9 ± 9.4	60.4 ± 11.3	NON-RCT
Tian LQ [29]	2012	Asians	25	25	-	-	-	-	RCT
Zhai YJ [31]	2008	Asians	10	8	7/3	6/2	60.2 ± 8.5	57.3 ± 6.6	NON-RCT
Hong T [35]	2008	Asians	15	15	11/4	12/3	72.4 ± 4.3	71.8 ± 5.0	NON-RCT
Liu JT [34]	2007	Asians	25	35	-	-	64.3 ± 9.1	65.1 ± 10.3	NON-RCT
Hong F [36]	2007	Asians	15	15	11/4	9/6	58.2 ± 7.2	57.9 ± 6.8	NON-RCT
Bonacchi M [23]	2006	Caucasians	24	18	17/7	12/6	63.5 ± 7.8	63.7 ± 5.4	RCT
Guo XY [37]	2005	Asians	20	20	20/0	20/0	56.8 ± 5.8	58.2 ± 6.5	NON-RCT
Gao CQ [38]	2003	Asians	20	20	17/3	16/4	64.0 ± 8.7	59.0 ± 10.0	RCT
Yan XZ [32]	2002	Asians	9	8	9/0	8/0	63.5 ± 12.1	62.4 ± 10.2	RCT

M Male, *F* Female, *RCT* Randomized controlled trial

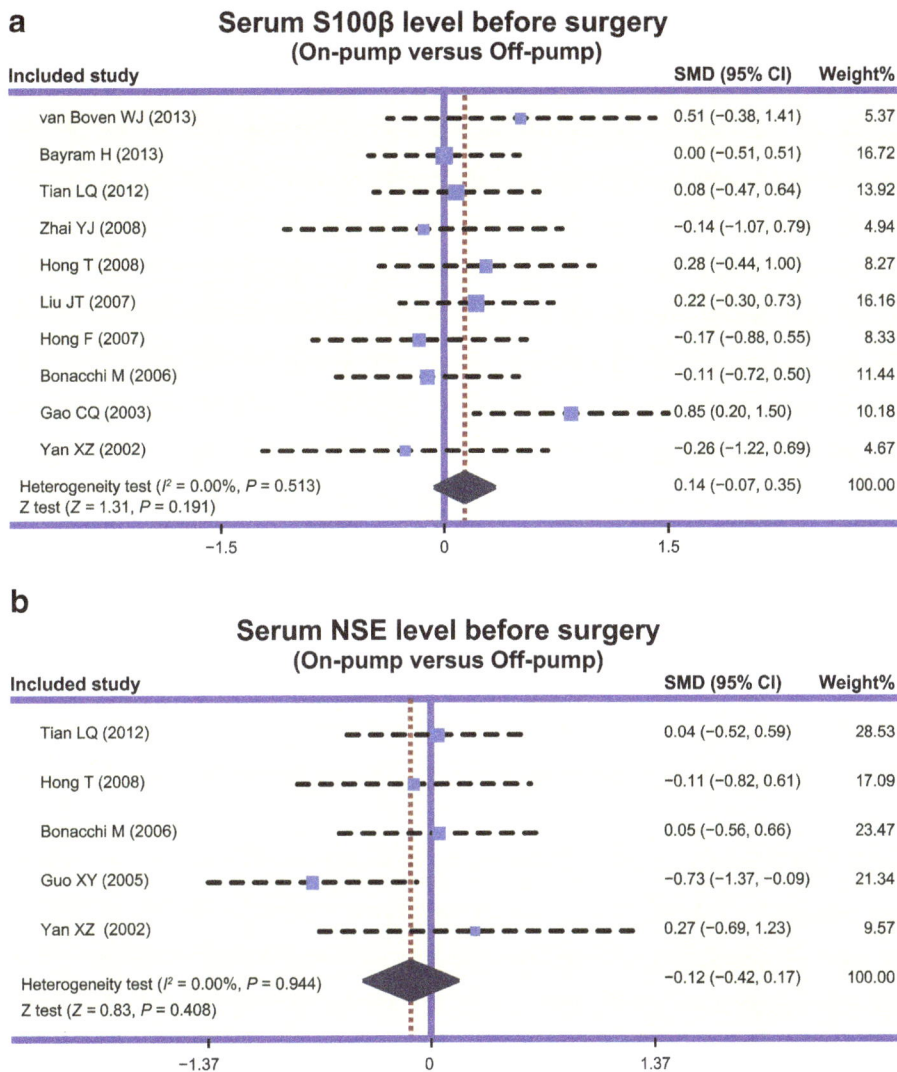

Fig. 1 Forest plots for the differences in serum S-100 beta (S-100β) and neuron specific enolase (NSE) levels between on-pump and off-pump groups before surgery (**a**: S-100β; **b**: NSE; SMD: standardized mean difference; CI: confidence interval)

CI = −1.10 ~ 4.59, $P = 0.229$; 72 h: SMD = 0.52, 95 % CI = −0.05 ~ 1.10, $P = 0.076$) (Fig. 2b). Nevertheless, we found no difference in serum NSE levels before and after off-pump CABG surgery (SMD = 0.42, 95 % CI = −0.24 ~ 1.08, $P = 0.209$) (Fig. 3b). Also, our results demonstrated that the NSE levels of CHD patients in the on-pump group were significantly higher than those of patients in the off-pump group (SMD = 1.19, 95 % CI = 0.66 ~ 1.73, $P < 0.001$), especially within 24 h after surgery (0 h: SMD = 1.56, 95 % CI = 0.72 ~ 2.40, $P < 0.001$; 6 h: SMD = 1.20, 95 % CI = 0.31 ~ 2.09, $P = 0.008$; 24 h: SMD = 1.24, 95 % CI = 0.01 ~ 2.48, $P = 0.048$), but no such difference was found after 24 h (48 h: SMD = 1.48, 95 % CI = −1.61 ~ 4.58, $P = 0.348$; 72 h: SMD = 0.24, 95 % CI = −1.41 ~ 1.89, $P = 0.777$) (Fig. 4b). Based on univariate

meta-regression analyses, time, publication year, ethnicity and sample size were all not sources of heterogeneity (all $P > 0.05$), which was further verified by the multivariate analyses (Table 2).

Sensitivity analysis and publication bias

Results of sensitivity analyses indicated that all the included publications had no significant influence on SMD (Fig. 6). Funnel plots revealed no obvious asymmetry (Fig. 7). Also, Egger's test didn't illustrate strong statistical evidence of publication bias (all $P > 0.05$).

Discussion

The present meta-analysis was identified the influence of off-pump and on-pump CABG surgeries on serum levels

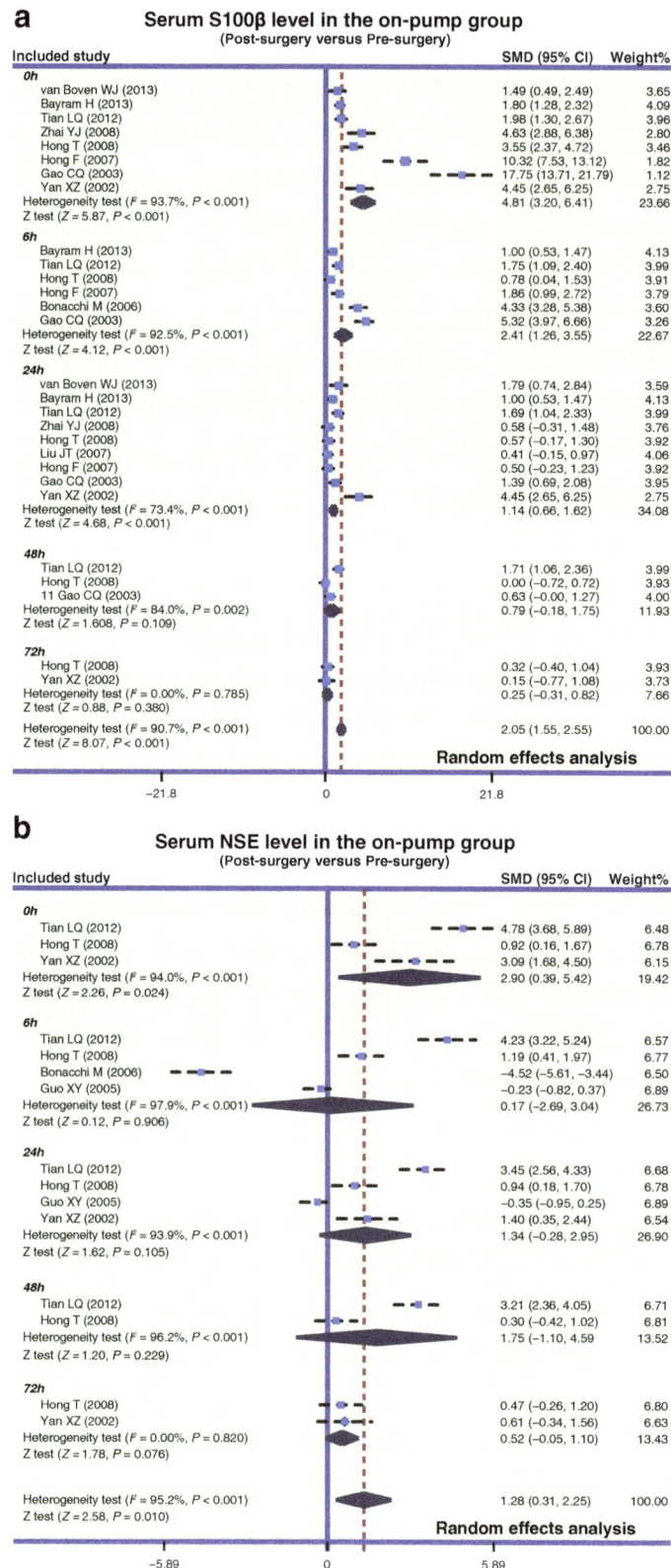

Fig. 2 Forest plots for the differences in serum S-100 beta (S-100β) and neuron specific enolase (NSE) levels between before and after surgery in the on-pump and off-pump groups (**a**: S-100β; **b**: NSE; SMD: standardized mean difference; CI: confidence interval)

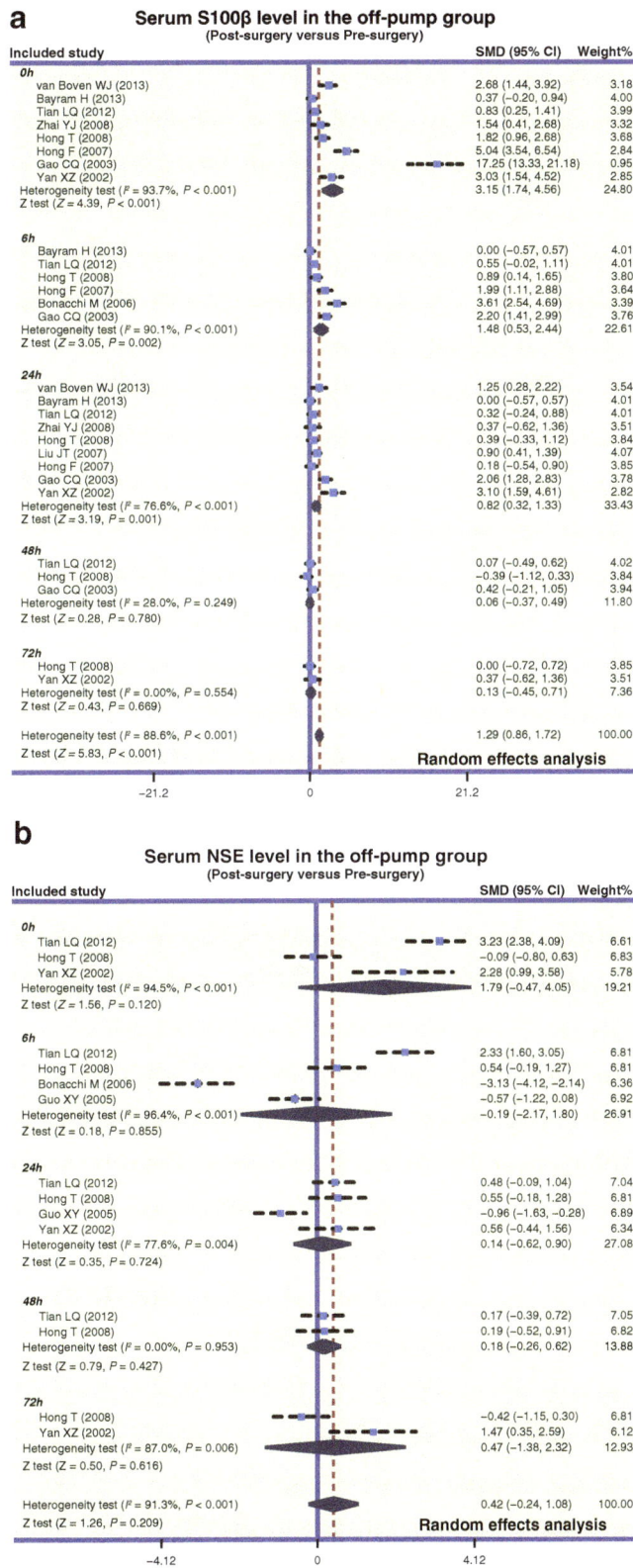

Fig. 3 Forest plots for the differences in serum S-100 beta (S-100β) and neuron specific enolase (NSE) levels between before and after surgery in the off-pump groups (**a**: S-100β; **b**: NSE; SMD: standardized mean difference; CI: confidence interval)

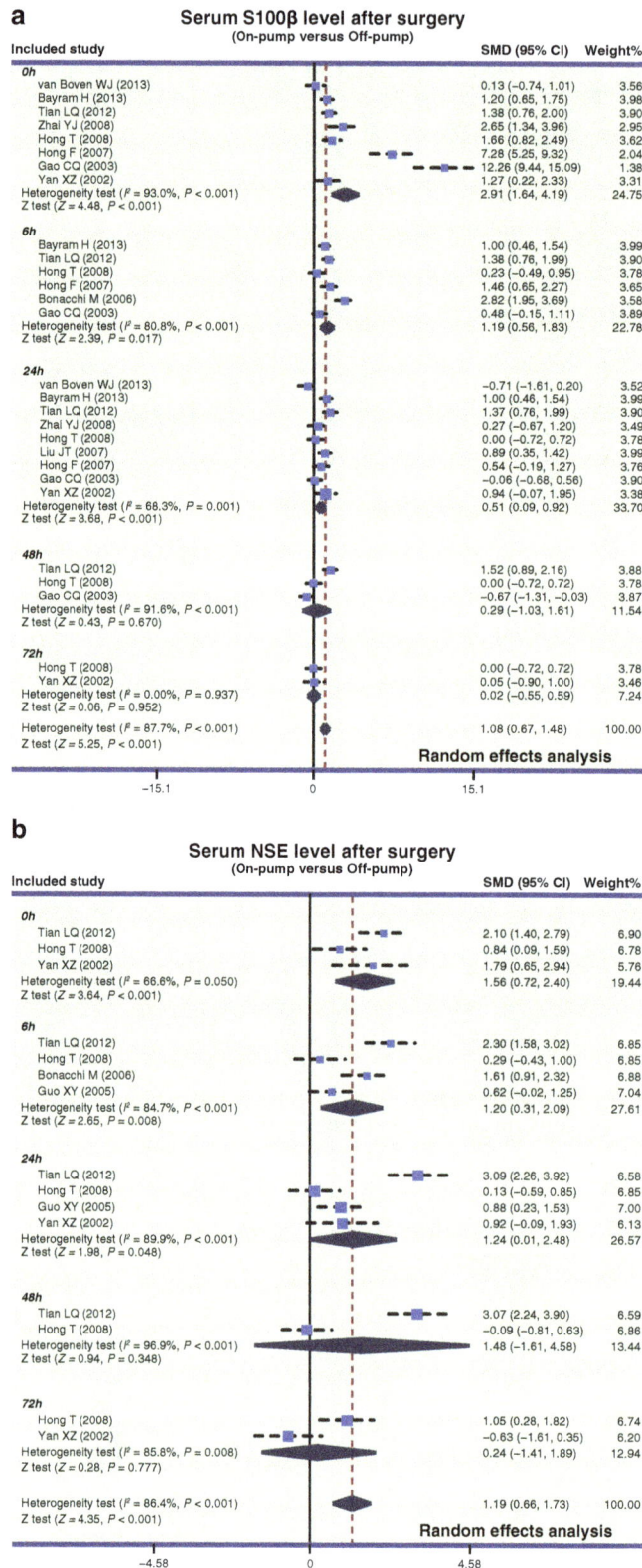

Fig. 4 Forest plots for the differences in serum S-100 beta (S-100β) and neuron specific enolase (NSE) levels between on-pump and off-pump groups after surgery (**a**: S-100β; **b**: NSE; SMD: standardized mean difference; CI: confidence interval)

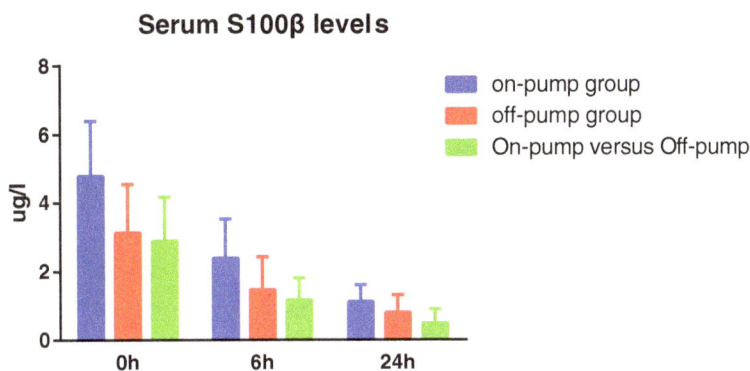

Fig. 5 Box-whiskers plots for the differences in serum S-100 beta (S-100β) levels within 24 hours aftersurgery

of S-100β and NSE in patients with CHD. The findings revealed no significant difference in preoperative serum S-100β and NSE levels between off-pump and on-pump CABG groups. The S-100β and NSE proteins cannot be detected in the serum under normal circumstances; however, they can be detected in serum following traumatic cerebral injury, stroke and cardiopulmonary bypass surgery due to impairment of blood–brain barrier (BBB) [39]. We presume that the lack of significant difference in serum S-100β and NSE protein levels before surgery indicates an intact BBB in the patients. Previous evidence showed a positive correlation between serum levels of S-100β and NSE and the neurocognitive dysfunction, because increased S-100β and NSE proteins could leak out from structurally damaged nerve cells into cerebrospinal fluid and secondarily across the BBB [40]. Interestingly, in previous studies the time of cardiopulmonary

bypass has been proved strongly correlated with the peak release of S-100β and NSE, and the restrictive fluid management may reduce perioperative cerebral injury [23, 30].

The results also showed that the postoperative serum S-100β and NSE levels were markedly elevated in the on-pump group, especially within 24 h after surgery. Cerebral damage remains one of the major problems associated with open-heart surgery and the contribution of on-pump CABG to cerebral damage is still only partially understood. We hypothesized that during extracorporeal circulation in on-pump CABG, blood and its constituents are likely in contact with foreign surfaces, which may activate inflammation, potentially leading to respiratory insufficiency and damage to lung and brain [22]. Furthermore, brain damage may cause disruption of BBB, which may induce dilatation of small capillaries and arterioles in the

Table 2 Univariate and multivariate meta-regression analyses of potential source of heterogeneity

Heterogeneity factors	Serum S100β levels						Serum NSE levels					
	Coefficient	SE	t	P	95 % CI		Coefficient	SE	t	P	95 % CI	
					LL	UL					LL	UL
Publication year												
Univariate	−0.078	0.114	−0.68	0.501	−0.313	0.157	0.189	0.068	2.78	0.016	0.042	0.335
Multivariate	−0.126	0.108	−1.17	0.529	−0.349	0.097	0.125	0.074	1.68	0.336	−0.040	0.290
Ethnicity												
Univariate	−0.583	1.407	−0.41	0.682	−3.474	2.308	0.451	1.165	0.39	0.705	−2.067	2.968
Multivariate	−0.574	1.294	−0.44	0.983	−3.252	2.103	0.050	0.936	0.05	1.000	−2.035	2.136
Time												
Univariate	−0.801	0.311	−2.58	0.016	−1.439	−0.163	−0.219	0.223	−0.98	0.344	−0.702	0.263
Multivariate	−0.896	0.327	−2.74	0.016	−1.571	−0.220	−0.086	0.178	−0.48	0.964	−0.483	0.312
Sample size												
Univariate	0.647	0.866	0.75	0.462	−1.133	2.427	1.408	0.442	3.18	0.007	−0.452	2.364
Multivariate	0.649	0.792	0.82	0.807	−0.990	2.287	0.970	0.534	1.82	0.265	−0.220	2.161

SE Standard error. 95 % CI: 95 % confidence interval. *NSE* Neuron specific enolase. *UL* Upper limit. *LL* Lower limit

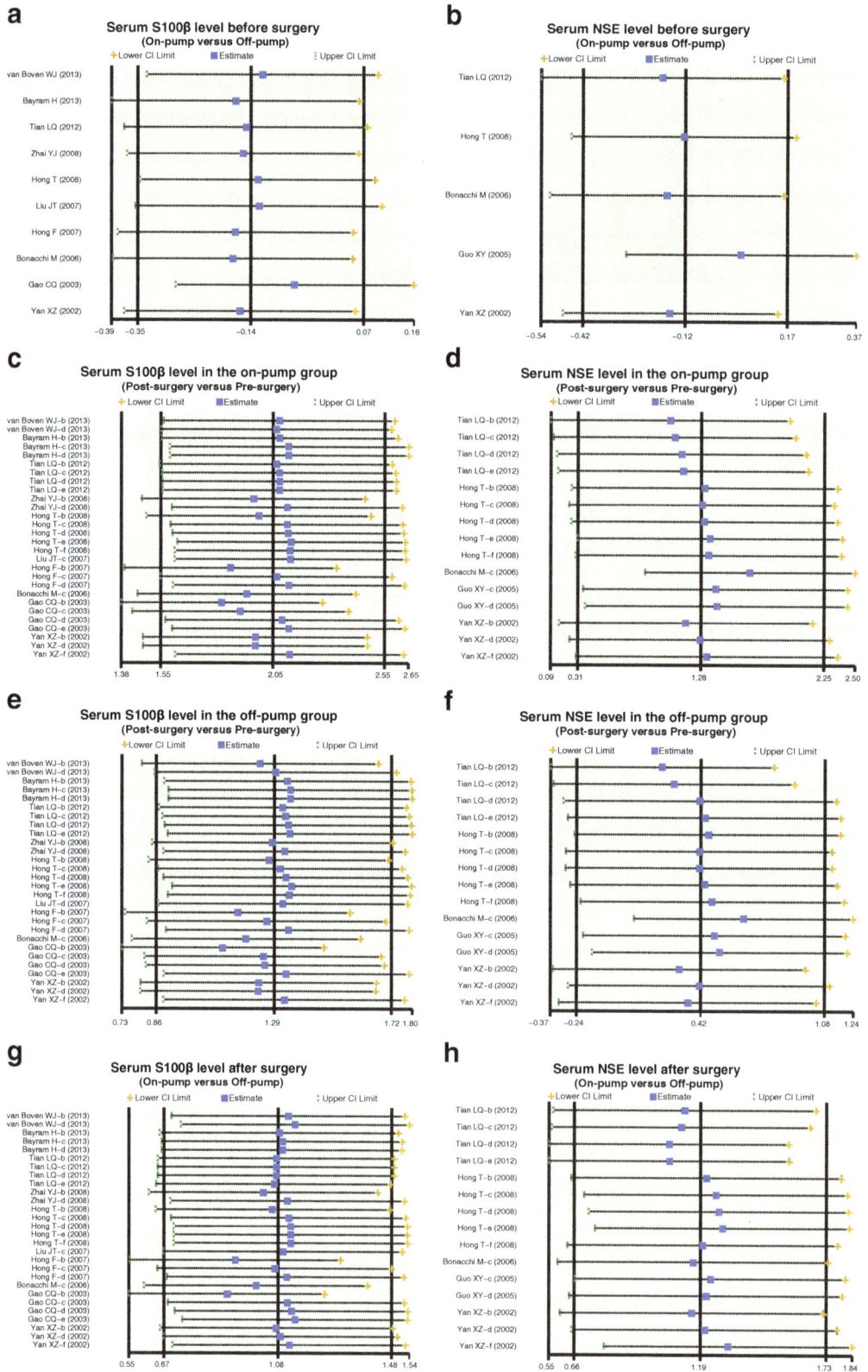

Fig. 6 (See legend on next page.)

(See figure on previous page.)
Fig. 6 Sensitivity analyses to evaluate the impact of removing one single study on the overall results. **a**: Serum S100ß level before surgery (On-pump versus Off-pump); **b**: Serum NSE level before surgery (On-pump versus Off-pump); **c**: Serum S100ß level in the on-pump group (Post-surgery versus Pre-surgery); **d**: Serum NSE level in the on-pump group (Post-surgery versus Pre-surgery); **e**: Serum S100ß level in the off-pump group (Post-surgery versus Pre-surgery); **f**: Serum NSE level in the off-pump group (Post-surgery versus Pre-surgery); **g**: Serum S100ß level after surgery (On-pump versus Off-pump); **h**: Serum NSE level after surgery (On-pump versus Off-pump)

brain and then both S-100β and NSE protein may be allowed to release from cerebrospinal fluid to blood fluid in the patients [41]. Thereby, serum levels of S-100β and NSE may increase markedly after on-pump CABG surgery, confirmed by our results, further suggesting that perioperative care should be modified accordingly to control such adverse effects. Additionally, another mechanism of neurocognitive dysfunction in patients undergoing on-pump CABG is cerebral microembolization, which mostly generates from pump circuits and is partially related to the manipulation and instrumentation of the heart using surgical instrumentation, especially the aorta [42]. These embolic events can also result in increased serum S-100β and NSE levels postoperatively in patients [43].

We found a significant difference in the serum S-100β levels before and after off-pump CABG surgery, while no significant difference in serum NSE levels were observed in the off-pump group before and after surgery. In a previous study, the peak release of S-100β occurs at 6 h postoperatively and signifies perioperative brain damage, while the NSE peak serum levels occurred beyond 24 h after the surgery in patients undergoing off-pump CABG [44, 45]. Therefore, the different peak times of the peak serum S-100β and NSE levels may be a the reason that significant changes are observed in S-100β levels and not in NSE levels before and after off-pump CABG. Bonacchi et al. also found that in the off-pump group, serum levels of S-100β and NSE were almost within the normal range preoperatively; but only the S-100β serum levels increased significantly postoperatively [23].

Another principal finding in our meta-analysis is that postoperative serum S-100β and NSE protein levels were significantly higher in the on-pump group than those in the off-pump group, especially within 24 h after surgery, implying that off-pump CABG may be associated with lower risk of neurocognitive dysfunction than on-pump CABG. Although the precise mechanism through which off-pump CABG reduces systemic inflammation in brain damage and postoperative mortality is still not fully understood, it may be reasonable to postulate that off-pump CABG and decrease the frequency of cerebral embolism [46]. Huseyin Bayram et al. has showed that the postoperative serum S-100β levels in the off-pump group were significantly lower than that in the on-pump CABG group [22]. Similarly, Lee et al. have observed that off-pump CABG surgery may decrease neurological

and clinical morbidity in comparison to on-pump CABG in a randomized group of 60 patients undergoing on-pump and off-pump procedures and complemented by neurocognitive testing before surgery and 2 week/1 year after surgery [47]. By contrast, Edwards compared on-pump and off-pump CABG with a year of follow-up study, reporting that on-pump CABG is superior to off-pump CABG, although off-pump CABG had advantages of time on mechanical ventilation, bleeding and need for reoperation etc. [48]. Despite these contradictory results on whether off-pump CABG is superior to the on-pump CABG [49], our results are in accordance with several studies that demonstrated that the preoperative brain injury evaluated by the release of NSE and S-100β protein is significantly higher in patients undergoing off-pump CABG than patients receiving on-pump CABG. Our study has limitations which should be interpreted. First, through searching the databases, only 5 randomized controlled trials relevant to the topic were identified (the other 6 studies were non-randomized controlled trials), which may cause bias due to the small sample size. Second, because all the included randomized controlled trials could not demonstrated any significant impairment of cognitive function after both on-pump and off-pump surgeries, these studies are more likely to provide "academic" rather than clinical evidence, therefore future clinical evidence are needed. Third, the meta-analysis could not acquire the original data and information on the techniques used in the surgeries was limitedly provided in the studies included, which may restrict further evaluation of the plausible effect of off-pump and on-pump CABG on serum S-100β and NSE levels. Moreover, Due to the lack of data on neurological complications in the enrolled studies, we failed to identify a relationship between higher marker levels and neurological events. Even though there are several limitations, our study is the first meta-analysis on the comparison of serum levels of S-100β and NSE between patients treated with on-pump and off-pump CABG. More importantly, a literature search strategy with high sensitivity was implemented for electronic databases. In order to identify other potential articles, we also manually searched the reference lists of relevant articles, and the eligible articles were selected on the basis of strict inclusion and exclusion criteria. Besides, pooling of information from each study is founded on rigorous statistical analysis.

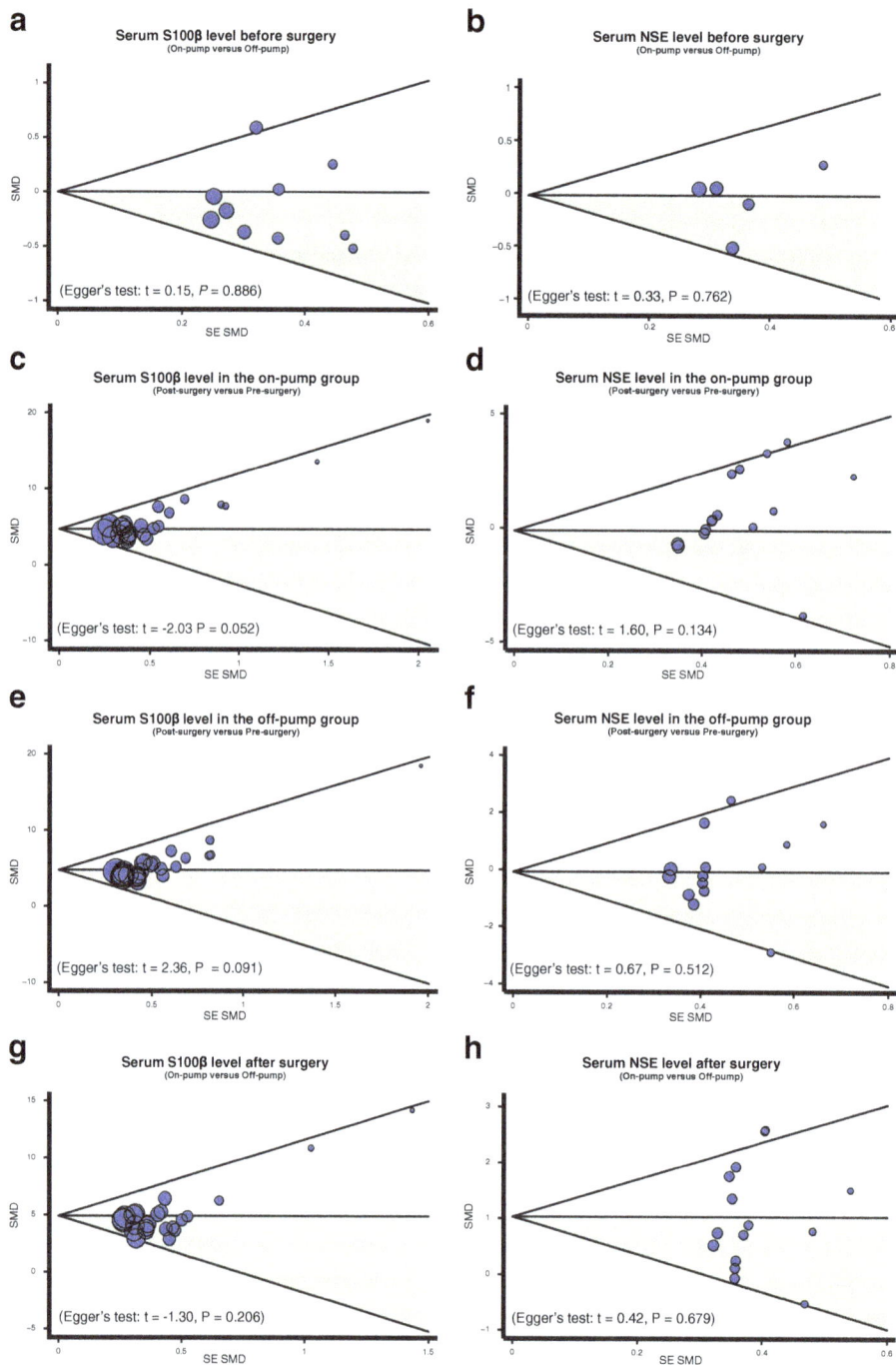

Fig. 7 Funnel plots for the differences in serum S-100 beta (S-100ß) and neuron specific enolase (NSE) levels before and after on-pump versus off-pump coronary artery bypass graft surgeries. **a**: Serum S100ß level before surgery (On-pump versus Off-pump); **b**: Serum NSE level before surgery (On-pump versus Off-pump); **c**: Serum S100ß level in the on-pump group (Post-surgery versus Pre-surgery); **d**: Serum NSE level in the on-pump group (Post-surgery versus Pre-surgery); **e**: Serum S100ß level in the off-pump group (Post-surgery versus Pre-surgery); **f**: Serum NSE level in the off-pump group (Post-surgery versus Pre-surgery); **g**: Serum S100ß level after surgery (On-pump versus Off-pump); **h**: Serum NSE level after surgery (On-pump versus Off-pump)

Conclusions

Our findings revealed that off-pump and on-pump CABG surgeries may increase serum S-100ß and NSE levels in CHD patients, especially within 24 h of on-pump CABG surgery. However, more researches with more detailed data and large sample size are necessary to confirm our findings and validate the clinical use of S-100ß and NSE as reliable biomarkers to predict outcomes.

Abbreviations
CABG: Coronary artery bypass graft; CHD: Coronary heart disease; NSE: Neuron specific enolase; CBM: Chinese Biomedical Database; NOS: The Newcastle-Ottawa Scale; SMD: Standardized mean difference; CI: Confidence intervals; BBB: Blood–brain barrier.

Competing interests
The authors declare that they have no competing interests.

Authors' contributions
LZ, Q-M F designed, conceived and supervised the study. LZ and Z-Y W selected the studies. Z-Y W performed the statistical analysis and interpreted the results. All authors drafted and revised the paper. All authors read and approved the final paper.

Acknowledgments
We would like to acknowledge the reviewers for their helpful comments on this paper.

References
1. Gaziano TA, Bitton A, Anand S, Abrahams-Gessel S, Murphy A. Growing epidemic of coronary heart disease in low- and middle-income countries. Curr Probl Cardiol. 2010;35(2):72–115.
2. Odegaard AO. Coronary heart disease: what hope for the developing world? Heart. 2013;99(17):1227–9.
3. Go AS, Mozaffarian D, Roger VL, Benjamin EJ, Berry JD, Borden WB, et al. Heart disease and stroke statistics–2013 update: a report from the American Heart Association. Circulation. 2013;127(1):e6–e245.
4. Serruys PW, Morice MC, Kappetein AP, Colombo A, Holmes DR, Mack MJ, et al. Percutaneous coronary intervention versus coronary-artery bypass grafting for severe coronary artery disease. N Engl J Med. 2009;360(10):961–72.
5. Ho PM, Bryson CL, Rumsfeld JS. Medication adherence: its importance in cardiovascular outcomes. Circulation. 2009;119(23):3028–35.
6. ElBardissi AW, Aranki SF, Sheng S, O'Brien SM, Greenberg CC, Gammie JS. Trends in isolated coronary artery bypass grafting: an analysis of the Society of Thoracic Surgeons adult cardiac surgery database. J Thorac Cardiovasc Surg. 2012;143(2):273–81.
7. Lamy A, Devereaux PJ, Prabhakaran D, Taggart DP, Hu S, Paolasso E, et al. Off-pump or on-pump coronary-artery bypass grafting at 30 days. N Engl J Med. 2012;366(16):1489–97.
8. Palmerini T, Biondi-Zoccai G, Riva DD, Mariani A, Savini C, Di Eusanio M, et al. Risk of stroke with percutaneous coronary intervention compared with on-pump and off-pump coronary artery bypass graft surgery: Evidence from a comprehensive network meta-analysis. Am Heart J. 2013;165(6):910–7. e914.
9. Selnes OA, Gottesman RF, Grega MA, Baumgartner WA, Zeger SL, McKhann GM. Cognitive and neurologic outcomes after coronary-artery bypass surgery. N Engl J Med. 2012;366(3):250–7.
10. Kennedy ED, Choy KC, Alston RP, Chen S, Farhan-Alanie MM, Anderson J, et al. Cognitive outcome after on- and off-pump coronary artery bypass grafting surgery: a systematic review and meta-analysis. J Cardiothorac Vasc Anesth. 2013;27(2):253–65.
11. Dabrowski W, Rzecki Z, Czajkowski M, Pilat J, Wacinski P, Kotlinska E, et al. Volatile anesthetics reduce biochemical markers of brain injury and brain magnesium disorders in patients undergoing coronary artery bypass graft surgery. J Cardiothorac Vasc Anesth. 2012;26(3):395–402.
12. Yuan SM. Biomarkers of cerebral injury in cardiac surgery. Anadolu Kardiyol Derg. 2014;14(7):638–45.
13. Astrand R, Unden J, Romner B. Clinical use of the calcium-binding S100B protein. Methods Mol Biol. 2013;963:373–84.
14. Seco M, Edelman JJ, Wilson MK, Bannon PG, Vallely MP. Serum biomarkers of neurologic injury in cardiac operations. Ann Thorac Surg. 2012;94(3):1026–33.
15. Sorci G, Bianchi R, Riuzzi F, Tubaro C, Arcuri C, Giambanco I, Donato R: S100B Protein, A Damage-Associated Molecular Pattern Protein in the Brain and Heart, and Beyond. Cardiovasc Psychiatry Neurol 2010, 2010; PMID: 20827421.
16. Donato R, Cannon BR, Sorci G, Riuzzi F, Hsu K, Weber DJ, et al. Functions of S100 proteins. Curr Mol Med. 2013;13(1):24–57.
17. Beharier O, Kahn J, Shusterman E, Sheiner E. S100B - a potential biomarker for early detection of neonatal brain damage following asphyxia. J Matern Fetal Neonatal Med. 2012;25(9):1523–8.
18. Michetti F, Corvino V, Geloso MC, Lattanzi W, Bernardini C, Serpero L, et al. The S100B protein in biological fluids: more than a lifelong biomarker of brain distress. J Neurochem. 2012;120(5):644–59.
19. Yee KM, Ross-Cisneros FN, Lee JG, Da Rosa AB, Salomao SR, Berezovsky A, et al. Neuron-specific enolase is elevated in asymptomatic carriers of Leber's hereditary optic neuropathy. Invest Ophthalmol Vis Sci. 2012;53(10):6389–92.
20. Streitburger DP, Arelin K, Kratzsch J, Thiery J, Steiner J, Villringer A, et al. Validating serum S100B and neuron-specific enolase as biomarkers for the human brain - a combined serum, gene expression and MRI study. PLoS One. 2012;7(8), e43284.
21. Kobayashi J, Tashiro T, Ochi M, Yaku H, Watanabe G, Satoh T, et al. Early outcome of a randomized comparison of off-pump and on-pump multiple arterial coronary revascularization. Circulation. 2005;112(9 Suppl):I338–43.
22. Bayram H, Hidiroglu M, Cetin L, Kucuker A, Iriz E, Uguz E, et al. Comparing S-100 beta protein levels and neurocognitive functions between patients undergoing on-pump and off-pump coronary artery bypass grafting. J Surg Res. 2013;182(2):198–202.
23. Bonacchi M, Prifti E, Maiani M, Bartolozzi F, Di Eusanio M, Leacche M. Does off-pump coronary revascularization reduce the release of the cerebral markers, S-100beta and NSE? Heart Lung Circ. 2006;15(5):314–9.
24. Stang A. Critical evaluation of the Newcastle-Ottawa scale for the assessment of the quality of nonrandomized studies in meta-analyses. Eur J Epidemiol. 2010;25(9):603–5.
25. Zintzaras E, Ioannidis JP. HEGESMA: genome search meta-analysis and heterogeneity testing. Bioinformatics. 2005;21(18):3672–3.
26. Zintzaras E, Ioannidis JP. Heterogeneity testing in meta-analysis of genome searches. Genet Epidemiol. 2005;28(2):123–37.
27. Peters JL, Sutton AJ, Jones DR, Abrams KR, Rushton L. Comparison of two methods to detect publication bias in meta-analysis. JAMA. 2006;295(6):676–80.
28. Huizenga HM, Visser I, Dolan CV. Testing overall and moderator effects in random effects meta-regression. Br J Math Stat Psychol. 2011;64(Pt 1):1–19.
29. Jackson D, White IR, Riley RD. Quantifying the impact of between-study heterogeneity in multivariate meta-analyses. Stat Med. 2012;31(29):3805–20.
30. van Boven WJ, Morariu A, Salzberg SP, Gerritsen WB, Waanders FG, Korse TC, et al. Impact of different surgical strategies on perioperative protein S100beta release in elderly patients undergoing coronary artery bypass grafting. Innovations (Phila). 2013;8(3):230–6.
31. Zhai YJ, Wang XL, Ji SY, Liu YR. Brain injuries in patients during cornonary artery bypass graft with or without cardiopulmonary bypass. Academic J Guangzhou Med Col. 2008;36(5):13–5.
32. Yan XZ, Yang SY, Sun ZL, Huang FJ, Zhang DG, Xiang DK, et al. Off-pump coronary artery bypass grafting and neuronal injury. Guizhou Med J. 2002;26(6):483–5.
33. Tian LQ, Cheng ZY, Li XH, Liu C. Effects of on-pump and off-pump coronary artery bypass grafting on plasma neuron specific enolase and S100 protein levels. Chin J Practical Nerv Dis. 2012;15(1):17–9.
34. Liu JT, Li HY, He GX, Wang SB, Pu RF, Zhou F. The change and meaning of serum s100β protein during CABG with or without extracorporeal circulation. Chin J Extracorporeal Circulation. 2007;5(2):81–3. 120.
35. Hong T, Wen DX, Hang YN. Effects of off-pump and on-pump on cerebral neurologic injuries in elder patients undergoing coronary artery bypass grafting. Jiangsu Med J. 2008;34(2):117–9.
36. Hong F, Peng JM, Zhang RX, Chen JP. Serum concentration of S100 -B protein in patients during CABG with or without cardiopulmonary bypass. Chin J Pathophysiol. 2007;23(7):1293–5.
37. Guo XY, Luo AL, Yin YQ, Ren HZ, Ye TH, Huang YG, et al. Perioperative plasma concentrations of neuron-specific enolase and postoperative cognitive function in patients undergoing coronary artery bypass grafting surgery. Basic & Clin Med. 2005;25(10):934–7.
38. Gao CQ, He T, Li BJ, Wang G, Li JC, Mu YL. Comparison of cerebral Injury in patients during coronary artery bypass graft without versus with cardiopulmonary bypass. Chin Circulation J. 2003;18(6):449–52.
39. Iriz E, Kolbakir F, Akar H, Adam B, Keceligil HT. Comparison of hydroxyethyl starch and ringer lactate as a prime solution regarding S-100beta protein levels and informative cognitive tests in cerebral injury. Ann Thorac Surg. 2005;79(2):666–71.

40. Berger RP, Pierce MC, Wisniewski SR, Adelson PD, Clark RS, Ruppel RA, et al. Neuron-specific enolase and S100B in cerebrospinal fluid after severe traumatic brain injury in infants and children. Pediatrics. 2002;109(2), E31.

41. Kapural M, Krizanac-Bengez L, Barnett G, Perl J, Masaryk T, Apollo D, et al. Serum S-100beta as a possible marker of blood–brain barrier disruption. Brain Res. 2002;940(1–2):102–4.

42. Mackensen GB, Ti LK, Phillips-Bute BG, Mathew JP, Newman MF, Grocott HP. Cerebral embolization during cardiac surgery: impact of aortic atheroma burden. Br J Anaesth. 2003;91(5):656–61.

43. Schoenburg M, Kraus B, Muehling A, Taborski U, Hofmann H, Erhardt G, et al. The dynamic air bubble trap reduces cerebral microembolism during cardiopulmonary bypass. J Thorac Cardiovasc Surg. 2003;126(5):1455–60.

44. Grocott HP, Arrowsmith JE. Serum S100 protein as a marker of cerebral damage during cardiac surgery. Br J Anaesth. 2001;86(2):289–90.

45. Woertgen C, Rothoerl RD, Brawanski A. Neuron-specific enolase serum levels after controlled cortical impact injury in the rat. J Neurotrauma. 2001;18(5):569–73.

46. Bowles BJ, Lee JD, Dang CR, Taoka SN, Johnson EW, Lau EM, et al. Coronary artery bypass performed without the use of cardiopulmonary bypass is associated with reduced cerebral microemboli and improved clinical results. Chest. 2001;119(1):25–30.

47. Lee JD, Lee SJ, Tsushima WT, Yamauchi H, Lau WT, Popper J, et al. Benefits of off-pump bypass on neurologic and clinical morbidity: a prospective randomized trial. Ann Thorac Surg. 2003;76(1):18–25. discussion 25–16.

48. Edwards JH, Huang DT. Using pump for bypass surgery–on-off-on again? Crit Care. 2010;14(5):319.

49. Velissaris T, Jonas MM, Ohri SK. Hemodynamic advantages of right heart decompression during off-pump surgery. Asian Cardiovasc Thorac Ann. 2010;18(1):17–21.

17

Comprehensive geriatric assessment in patients undergoing transcatheter aortic valve implantation – results from the CGA-TAVI multicentre registry

Andrea Ungar[1][*], Giulio Mannarino[1], Nathalie van der Velde[2], Jan Baan[3], Marie-Pierre Thibodeau[4], Jean-Bernard Masson[4], Gennaro Santoro[1], Martijn van Mourik[3], Sofie Jansen[2], Cornelia Deutsch[5], Peter Bramlage[5] [iD], Jana Kurucova[6], Martin Thoenes[6], Stefania Maggi[7] and Andreas W. Schoenenberger[8]

Abstract

Background: In older patients with aortic stenosis (AS) undergoing TAVI, the potential role of prior CGA is not well established. To explore the value of comprehensive geriatric assessment (CGA) for predicting mortality and/or hospitalisation within the first 3 months after transcatheter aortic valve implantation (TAVI).

Methods: An international, multi-centre, prospective registry (CGA-TAVI) was established to gather data on CGA results and medium-term outcomes in geriatric patients undergoing TAVI. Logistic regression was used to evaluate the predictive value of a multidimensional prognostic index (MPI); a short physical performance battery (SPPB); and the Silver Code, which was based on administrative data, for predicting death and/or hospitalisation in the first 3 months after TAVI (primary endpoint).

Results: A total of 71 TAVI patients (mean age 85.4 years; mean log EuroSCORE I 22.5%) were enrolled. Device success according to VARC criteria was 100%. After adjustment for selected baseline characteristics, a higher (poorer) MPI score (OR: 3.34; 95% CI: 1.39–8.02; $p = 0.0068$) and a lower (poorer) SPPB score (OR: 1.15; 95% CI: 1.01–1.54; $p = 0.0380$) were found to be associated with an increased likelihood of the primary endpoint. The Silver Code did not show any predictive ability in this population.

Conclusions: Several aspects of the CGA have shown promise for being of use to physicians when predicting TAVI outcomes. While the MPI may be useful in clinical practice, the SPPB may be of particular value, being simple and quick to perform. Validation of these findings in a larger sample is warranted.

Keywords: Transcatheter aortic valve implantation (TAVI), Comprehensive geriatric assessment (CGA), Multidimensional prognostic index (MPI), Short physical performance battery (SPPB), Silver code

* Correspondence: aungar@unifi.it
[1]Geriatric Intensive Care Unit, Department of Geriatrics and Medicine, Careggi Hospital and University of Florence, Florence, Italy
Full list of author information is available at the end of the article

Background

Severe symptomatic stenosis of the aortic valve (aortic stenosis; AS) is associated with mortality of up to 50% at 1 year if left untreated [1, 2]. The outcome of surgical aortic valve replacement (SAVR) is generally predicted with the aid of quantitative scales such as the EuroSCORE or the Society of Thoracic Surgeons (STS) risk score. However, the accuracy of such algorithms for assessing older-age, multi-morbid patients undergoing transcatheter aortic valve implantation (TAVI) is low [3–5]. This is mainly due to the absence of variables related to ageing, such as frailty, mental status, social support, and overall health. There is evidence that additionally evaluating these factors can help provide a more precise estimation of an older person's response to treatment [3, 6, 7]. Indeed, a recent report from the American College of Cardiology (ACC) advocates assessment of frailty and cognitive function prior to determining a patient's suitability for TAVI [8]. The inclusion of a geriatrician in the Heart Team responsible for assessing patients prior to TAVI may therefore be warranted [9].

A comprehensive geriatric assessment (CGA) is a multidimensional diagnostic process for evaluating an individual's clinical, psychosocial, and functional characteristics [10, 11]. It usually consists of functional tests complementing usual clinical evaluation. For example, CGA may include the calculation of a multidimensional prognostic index (MPI) based on mental and nutritional status, number of co-morbid conditions and medications, living arrangements, and the ability to cope with activities of daily living [12, 13]. Pilotto et al. showed that the MPI had high predictive power for assessing mortality after hospitalisation of older patients [13]. For TAVI specifically, few studies have evaluated CGA and its components for outcome prediction [3, 14–16]. For example, Stortecky et al. evaluated a geriatric assessment that contained many of the same components as the MPI, and found that many of the included items were predictive of mortality and the occurrence of a major adverse cardiac or cerebrovascular event (MACCE) at 30 days and 1 year after the procedure [14]. All previous studies originated from single-centre experiences.

We aimed to determine the power of CGA for predicting the combined endpoint of mortality and stroke within the 3 months subsequent to TAVI based on data from a multi-centre, prospective cohort. We further characterised changes in CGA over time, and provide additional evidence for the utility of TAVI in a geriatric, comorbid population.

Methods

Patients and registry design

The CGA-TAVI registry is a prospective, international, multi-centre, observational registry [17].

Patients were enrolled at three centres in Italy (Careggi Hospital, Florence), the Netherlands (Academic Medical Center, Amsterdam) and Canada (Centre Hospitalier de l'Université de Montréal) between August 2013 and December 2015. Individuals were eligible if they were aged >80 years, had symptomatic severe calcific aortic valve (AV) stenosis, and were assigned to undergo transaortic, transapical or transfemoral TAVI. Patients were excluded if TAVI was being performed as an emergency procedure or if patients were unable to participate in the follow-up. Overall, 603 patients underwent TAVI at one of the three study centres during the study period (Italy: 68, Canada: 95; the Netherlands: 440. Of these, 71 patients were enrolled in the CGA-TAVI registry: 41, 15 and 15 from the sites in Italy, Canada and the Netherlands, respectively.

Baseline assessment

A detailed description of the information documented has been previously published [17]. Briefly, data regarding demographics, comorbidities, and prior cardiovascular interventions were collected at hospital admission. A CGA was performed by a geriatrician for each patient. This included calculation of the MPI [12, 13], which consisted of the following components: Activities of Daily Living (ADL; 6 items) [18, 19]; Instrumental Activities of Daily Living (IADL; 8 items) [20]; Short Portable Mental Status Questionnaire (SPMSQ; 10 items) [21]; Cumulative Illness Rating Scale (CIRS; 14 items) [22, 23]; Mini Nutritional Assessment (MNA; 18 items) [24]; Exton-Smith Scale (ESS; 5 items) [25]; number of drugs used (1 item); and cohabitation status (1 item). In each case, a tripartite hierarchy was used for scoring (no problems: 0 points; minor problems: 0.5 points; severe problems: 1 point). The boundaries for these scores were based on the cut-off points derived from the associated literature [12]. A Silver Code value was also calculated from administrative data for further prognostic stratification [26] and a Short Physical Performance Battery (SPPB) was performed, which involved repeated chair stands, balance testing, and an 8-ft (2.44 m) walk [27]. Detailed breakdowns of the three assessment scores can be found in Appendices 1, 2 (MPI), 3 (Silver Code) and 4 (SPPB). Procedural characteristics were also documented.

Follow-up assessment and outcomes

Patients were scheduled for follow-up at discharge, 30 days and 3 months post-procedure. These visits were conducted at the patient's enrolling centre and involved repetition of the CGA performed at the baseline assessment. Death, all-cause hospitalisation, TAVI-related hospitalisation, stroke, transient ischaemic attack (TIA), myocardial infarction (MI), life-threatening bleeding, acute kidney injury, coronary artery obstruction requiring intervention, major vascular complications, valve dysfunction requiring repeat procedure, or worsening congestive heart failure (CHF) were recorded, as defined in the Valve Academic Research Consortium-2 (VARC-2) consensus document [28].

Endpoints

The primary endpoint was death and/or hospitalisation within the first 3 months after TAVI. The secondary endpoint was death and/or non-fatal stroke within the same period. Changes in the scores of the components of the CGA from baseline to 3 months were also evaluated.

Data management and statistics

Data were entered into an online database via the completion of an electronic case report form (eCRF; s4trials, Berlin, Germany). Details were automatically checked for plausibility and completeness.

Data were analysed using descriptive statistics, with categorical variables presented as absolute values and percentages and continuous variables as means with standard deviations (SD). A logistic regression was used to evaluate the predictive value of CGA components (MPI, SPBB and Silver Code) for the primary/secondary endpoints. Age, gender, New York Heart Association (NYHA) class and surgical risk (EuroSCORE/STS) were used as co-variables. Logistic regression results are presented as odds ratios (OR) with 95% Wald confidence limits (95% CI) and p-values. CGA changes from baseline to 3-month follow-up were tested for significance using a t-test. P-values of <0.05 were considered significant.

Data were analysed using IBM SPSS statistics version 24 (IBM corporation, Amonk, New York, USA).

Results

Baseline patient characteristics

Overall, 44 patients (62%) were female. Means for age and body mass index (BMI) were 85.4 ± 2.9 years and 24.7 ± 3.7 kg/m^2, respectively (Table 1). The most prevalent comorbidity was hypertension (83.1%), followed by coronary artery disease (53.5%), peripheral artery disease (28.2%), diabetes mellitus (26.8%), prior MI (23.9%), and pulmonary disease (15.5%). In terms of surgical risk, the mean log EuroSCORE and STS scores were $22.5 \pm 13.2\%$ and $5.8 \pm 3.9\%$, respectively.

Table 1 Patient characteristics

	Mean ± SD (n) / n/N (%)
Age [years]	85.4 ± 2.9 ($n = 71$)
Gender [female]	44/71 (62.0)
BMI [kg/m²]	24.7 ± 3.7 ($n = 71$)
Comorbidities	
Hypertension	59/71 (83.1)
Diabetes mellitus	19/71 (26.8)
PAD	20/71 (28.2)
Prior stroke/TIA	6/71 (8.5)
CAD	38/71 (53.5)
Prior MI	17/71 (23.9)
Pulmonary disease[a]	11/71 (15.5)
Pulmonary hypertension	35/71 (49.3)
Creatinine ≥2.0 mg/dl[b]	5/71 (7.0)
Dialysis	2/71 (2.8)
Prior cardiovascular intervention	
PCI	16/71 (22.5)
CABG	13/71 (18.3)
Mitral valve replacement	2/71 (2.8)
Tricuspid valve replacement	0/71 (0)
Balloon aortic valvuloplasty	6/71 (8.5)
PPI	5/71 (7.0)
Surgical risk	
Log EuroSCORE I	22.5 ± 13.2 ($n = 71$)
STS risk score	5.8 ± 3.9 ($n = 71$)
AS-related symptoms (%)	
Syncope	5/71 (7.0)
Dizziness with exertion	5/71 (7.0)
CCS angina grade	
Class III	7/70 (10.0)
Class IV	0/70 (0)
NYHA classification	
Class III	50/71 (70.4)
Class IV	7/71 (9.9)
AS echocardiographic parameters	
AV peak gradient (mmHg)	78.5 ± 17.8 ($n = 59$)
AV mean gradient (mmHg)	50.5 ± 14.1 ($n = 61$)
V$_{max}$ (m/s)	4.2 ± 0.9 ($n = 24$)
Effective orifice area (cm²)	0.9 ± 0.6 ($n = 37$)
LVEF (%)	50.9 ± 12.0 ($n = 62$)

Legend: *BMI* body mass index, *PAD* peripheral artery disease, *TIA* transient ischaemic attack, *CAD* coronary artery disease, *MI* myocardial infarction, *PCI* percutaneous coronary intervention, *CABG* coronary artery bypass grafting, *PPI* permanent pacemaker implantation, *log Euro SCORE* logistic European System for Cardiac Operative Risk Evaluation, *STS* Society of Thoracic Surgeons, *AS* aortic stenosis, *LVEF* left ventricular ejection fraction, *AV* aortic valve, *CCS* Canadian Cardiovascular Society, *NYHA* New York Heart Association, *V$_{max}$* maximum velocity
[a]Defined as chronic obstructive pulmonary disease, asthma, a forced expiratory volume-1 of < 1.0, or oxygen dependency
[b]Excluding patients with dialysis

The majority of patients were at NYHA class III (70.4%) or IV (9.9%). Further AS-related symptoms were class III angina (10.0%), dizziness with exertion (7.0%), and syncope (7.0%). Regarding echocardiography, peak and mean AV gradients were 78.5 ± 17.8 and 50.5 ± 14.1 mmHg, respectively, with a left ventricular ejection fraction (LVEF) of $50.9 \pm 12.0\%$, a mean V_{max} of 4.2 ± 0.9 m/s, and an effective orifice area of 0.9 ± 0.6 cm^2.

Procedural characteristics and periprocedural outcomes

Details about procedural aspects are provided in the supplementary data (Appendix 5). Devices were placed successfully (as defined by VARC-2 [28]) in all patients (Appendix 6). The rate of intraoperative complications was 17.1%, which were vascular complications requiring treatment in 10.0% of patients and access-related in 5.6%. No conversion to open surgery was necessary. Paravalvular regurgitation was moderate in 2.9%, with no severe regurgitation. Post-procedural AV peak and mean gradients were 20.0 ± 12.4 and 11.3 ± 7.2 mmHg, respectively.

Outcomes at 3-months

In total, 6 patients died (8.5%) and 9 were hospitalised (13.8%) by the 3-month follow-up. The primary endpoint (death and/or hospitalisation in the first 3 months) was observed in 13/71 patients (18.3%) (Table 2). After adjustment for baseline characteristics, a higher (poorer) MPI score (OR: 3.34; 95% CI: 1.39–8.02; p = 0.0068) and a lower (poorer) SPPB

Table 2 Short- and medium-term outcomes

	≤30 days[a] n/N (%)	≤3 months n/N (%)
Primary endpoint (Death and/or hospitalisation)	5/70 (7.1)	13/71 (18.3)
Secondary endpoint (Death and/or non-fatal stroke)	2/71 (2.8)	6/71 (8.5)
All-cause mortality	2/71 (2.8)	6/71 (8.5)
Non-fatal complications	(n = 69)	(n = 65)
All-cause hospitalisation	5/69 (7.2)	9/65 (13.8)
Valve-related hospitalisation	3/69 (4.3)	2/65 (6.2)
Non-fatal stroke	0/69 (0.0)	0/62 (0.0)
Acute kidney injury (stage 2 or 3)	3/69 (4.3)	5/64 (7.8)
Major vascular complication	1/69 (1.4)	0/64 (3.1)
Repeat procedure for valve dysfunction	0/69 (0)	1/62 (1.6)
Myocardial infarction	0/69 (0)	0/62 (0)
PPI	9/69 (13.0)	9/65 (13.8)

Legend: *CHF* congestive heart failure, *MI* myocardial infarction, *NYHA* New York Heart Association, *CCS* Canadian Cardiovascular Society, *PPI* permanent pacemaker implantation
[a] ≤ 30 days includes all complications which occurred periprocedurally, during the phase of hospitalisation for TAVI and after discharge within 30 days

score (OR: 1.15; 95% CI: 1.01–1.54; p = 0.0380) were found to be associated with an increased odds of primary endpoint achievement (Table 3).

The secondary endpoint (death and/or non-fatal stroke in the first 3 months) was observed in 6 patients (8.5%) (Table 2). After multivariate adjustment, a higher (poorer) MPI score (OR: 4.75; 95% CI: 1.40–16.08; p = 0.0123) and a lower (poorer) SPPB score (OR: 1.62; 95% CI: 1.08–2.43; p = 0.0188) were associated with a greater odds of secondary endpoint achievement (Table 3).

CGA change from baseline to 3 months

Between baseline and 3 months, the total MPI score decreased only slightly, from a mean of 0.34 ± 0.11 to 0.30 ± 0.13 (mean intra-individual change: -0.02 ± 0.12; p = 0.25) (Appendix 7). However, the CIRS and ESS components changed by a statistically significant amount (-0.12 ± 0.25; p < 0.001 and -0.04 ± 0.13; p = 0.04, respectively). While the change in Silver Code was small, the SPPB score increased significantly (+1.86 ± 2.76; p < 0.001).

Discussion

Of the multiple components of the CGA that were evaluated, the MPI and the SPPB both had value for predicting the likelihood of death and/or hospitalisation in the first 3 months following TAVI. In terms of time-efficiency, the SPPB appears to be the favourable approach, with the MPI perhaps not adding sufficient additional predictive value to warrant such a time-consuming assessment.

Outcomes

In our patients, the rate of all-cause mortality at 30 days (2.8%) was within the range (1.1%–5.9%) reported by large-scale studies in patients with a similar level of surgical risk and mean ages above 80 years, such as the PARTNER II trial and SOURCE 3, WIN-TAVI, Swiss TAVI, and PRAGMATIC registries [29–33]. Though a less commonly reported outcome, the same was true of the rate of rehospitalisation (7.2% vs. 4.6% in the PARTNER II SAPIEN 3 trial and 6.5% in the overall PARTNER II trial) [29, 34]. Variations in rates between studies are likely due to differing patient characteristics, access routes, and the valves/delivery devices available during study periods. Our findings regarding three-month outcomes could not be easily compared to previous studies, as this time-point is not largely reported upon in the literature.

Table 3 Logistic regression for the prediction of events at 3 months by CGA at baseline

	Univariable OR (95% CI)	p-value	Multivariable OR (95% CI)	p-value
Death and/or hospitalisation				
Increasing MPI score (high vs. low)	0.66 (0.54–0.81)	< 0.0001	3.34 (1.39–8.02)[a]	0.0068
Decreasing SPPB (low vs. high)	1.35 (1.19–1.53)	< 0.0001	1.15 (1.01–1.54)	0.0380
Increasing Silver Code (high vs. low)	0.94 (0.92–0.97)	< 0.0001	1.03 (0.91–1.15)	0.6576
Death and/or non-fatal stroke				
Increasing MPI score (high vs. low)	0.49 (0.36–0.63)	< 0.0001	4.75 (1.40–16.08)	0.0123
Decreasing SPPB (low vs. high)	1.89 (1.36–2.64)	0.0002	1.62 (1.08–2.43)	0.0188
Increasing Silver Code (high vs. low)	0.90 (0.87–0.94)	< 0.0001	1.04 (0.87–1.23)	0.6938

Legend: *MPI* multidimensional prognostic index, *SPPB* short physical performance battery. All values adjusted for age, gender, NYHA class and surgical risk (EuroSCORE)
[a]The direction of the OR changed with the introduction of age into the model

Surgical risk scores
EuroSCORE and STS algorithms are conventional tools for assessing cardiac operative risk. It has been suggested that the latter is slightly more accurate in TAVI patients [4, 5], though neither are ideal. Patients in the present study had expected mortality rates of 22.5% (EuroSCORE I) and 5.8% (STS), and though the latter was closer to the observed rate, both were excessively elevated. Even the more up-to-date EuroSCORE II has been shown to have suboptimal discriminatory power, suggesting the need for alternative or additional assessment tools [35, 36].

Multidimensional prognostic index
Use of a CGA during clinical assessment of operative risk in AS patients has been suggested as a way to address the shortcomings of the EuroSCORE and STS score, and better predict outcomes [17, 36]. In the present study, both MPI and SPPB were found to have predictive value for determining the likelihood of short-term mortality/hospitalisation or stroke after TAVI. Interestingly, while high MPI was a "negative predictor" in the univariate analysis, it became a "positive predictor" after adjusting for age, gender, NYHA class and surgical risk. This change of direction can be explained by the clinical setting; younger patients with a low MPI are typically treated with SAVR, while elderly patients with a high MPI are unlikely to be treated at all. Consequently, our TAVI population was likely composed of patients with a lower age and high MPI or a higher age and low MPI, resulting in a switch of the direction of the odds ratio at multivariate analysis. This reflection of the clinical context is supportive of the "real" association between MPI score and outcomes.

Though no other studies appear to have specifically reported on the predictive value of MPI in TAVI, several have shown higher MPI scores to be significantly associated with greater rates of mortality in older patients with a variety of acute illnesses, including heart failure and TIA [12, 13, 37–40]. Other studies have evaluated other multi-component models for predicting mortality and morbidity after cardiac surgery [41]. For TAVI specifically, Green et al. found that patients with a high frailty score, as determined by gait speed, grip strength, serum albumin and ADL, were at greater risk of one-year mortality [15]. The five-component frailty score proposed by Kamga et al. was found to predict one-year mortality after transfemoral TAVI [16]. Stortecky et al. identified numerous parameters in their Multidimensional Geriatric Assessment that were predictive of 30-day and one-year mortality and MACCE after TAVI [14]. Data from the PARTNER trial were used to construct models for predicting a poor outcome, defined as death or a low/significantly decreased quality of life, after TAVI [42]. These models were subsequently validated in a large multi-centre cohort of TAVI patients, with an incremental increase in discriminative ability identified on the addition of markers of frailty and disability [43]. In agreement with the data from our CGA registry, these studies demonstrate the potential value of such multi-component analyses for predicting outcome after TAVI.

Short physical performance battery
A significant drawback of these multidimensional evaluation tools, however, is that they are extremely time-consuming. In the present work, we found that use of the SPPB alone was equally as effective as the MPI for predicting death and/or hospitalisation, and death and/or non-fatal stroke, in the first 3 months after TAVI. This short series of tests is

recommended by the European Union Geriatric Medicine Society (EUGMS) as part of a CGA in older AS patients [17], although it appears that there is little published evidence in support of using it for assessing TAVI candidates specifically. The concept of tests of physical ability to predict outcome after cardiac surgery has been evaluated in other studies. Afilalo et al. demonstrated that a slow 5-m gait speed was associated with a greater risk of operative mortality and in-hospital mortality and major morbidity in older patients undergoing cardiac surgery [7, 44]. They further determined that use of this parameter alone was superior to a variety of other frailty scales [6]. In patients undergoing TAVI specifically, 5-m gait speed has been shown to be independently associated with 30-day mortality after adjustment for STS score and other relevant baseline characteristics [45]. Stortecky et al. reported that the "timed get-up and go" (TUG) test had the greatest predictive ability of all of the individual geriatric assessment tools that they investigated [14]. In combination with either the STS or EuroSCORE, the TUG was superior to the other components evaluated for predicting all-cause mortality and MACCE during the first year after TAVI. A recent report by the ACC recommends that a 5-m gait speed test and a 6 min walk test be used to assess frailty and physical functioning, respectively, when determining a patient's suitability for TAVI [8].

The simplicity of physical tests such as the SPPB is not their only advantage, with the lack of subjectivity on the part of both physician and patient providing a level of accuracy that cannot be obtained using questionnaire-based assessment. This is particularly relevant for the advanced-age TAVI population, where cognitive impairment is a potentially significant confounding factor when evaluating self-reported parameters [6].

Silver code

According to our data, the Silver Code had no value for predicting death/hospitalisation or death/stroke during the first 3 months after TAVI. The calculation of this parameter prior to deciding on the suitability of a patient for TAVI is another recommendation of the EUGMS [17]. Previous studies have demonstrated a relationship between Silver Code and one-year mortality, although this was in the setting of the Emergency Department [26, 46]. As the Silver Code is determined from administrative data, it is particularly suited to planned procedures such as TAVI. Therefore, although it was not found to be an independent predictor of outcome in the present analysis, it should perhaps not be discounted. Further evaluation in a larger population may clarify its utility as part of a CGA prior to TAVI.

Limitations

Firstly, as an observational study, inherent limitations such as a higher potential for missing data are present. However, the observational aspect carried several advantages, such as an evaluation of TAVI patients in a real-world setting, avoiding the confounding issue of the strict inclusion and exclusion criteria used for clinical trials. This is particularly important, as geriatric patients are often those excluded due to high levels of comorbidity. Secondly, our findings are currently only applicable to geriatric patients at higher surgical risk. Considering that there is a current shift in clinical practice towards TAVI in lower-risk patients who are normally eligible for surgical heart valve replacement, re-evaluation of CGA in different populations may become necessary. In addition, we were only able to obtain data for a modest number of patients from three participating sites, limiting statistical power and generalisability. Indeed, the relatively low incidence of mortality and stroke at 3 months in a fairly small sample may have resulted in suboptimal power to detect baseline characteristics that are predictive for this outcome. Future studies in larger samples would be useful for clarification.

Conclusion

Several aspects of the CGA have shown promise for being of use to physicians when predicting the likelihood of death, rehospitalisation and non-fatal stroke following TAVI. The strong association between MPI and such outcomes indicates its potential utility in clinical practice. In addition, the SPPB may have significant value, being simple and quick to perform; however, the modest sample size included herein limit the formation of firm conclusions, and validation of these findings in a larger sample of TAVI patients with a greater range of surgical risk is warranted.

Clinical perspectives

The accuracy of conventional surgical risk scores is known to be suboptimal for predicting the outcomes of TAVI in elderly aortic stenosis patients. This study shows a potential benefit of adding items from a comprehensive geriatric assessment (CGA) to pre-intervention assessments. This now requires further validation in larger cohorts.

Appendix 1
Provides an overview about the Multidimensional Prognostic Index (MPI).

Table 4 Calculation of the Multidimensional Prognostic Index (MPI)

	Problem severity		
	No (= 0 points)	Minor (= 0.5 points)	Severe (= 1 point)
1. Co-habitation status	Living with relatives/nurse	Living in an institution	Living alone
2. Current medication use	0–3 medications	4–6 medications	≥7 medications
3. ADL score	6–5	4–3	2–0
4- IADL score	8–6	5–4	3–0
5. SPMSQ score	0–3	4–7	8–10
6. ESS score	16–20	10–15	5–9
7. CIRS CI	0	1–2	≥3
8. MNA score	≥24	17–23.5	<17
Total MPI score (sum of points/8):			
Low-risk:	≤0.33		
Moderate-risk:	0.34–0.66		
High-risk:	>0.66		

Legend: *ADL* activities of daily living, *IADL* instrumental ADL, *SPMSQ* short portable mental status questionnaire, *ESS* Exton-Smith scale, *CIRS* cumulative illness raiting scale, *CI* comorbidity index, *MNA* mini nutritional assessment, *MPI* multidimensional prognostic index. The numbering on the left-hand side of factors corresponds to the numbering in Appendix 2

Appendix 2
Provides a breakdown of the Multidimensional Prognostic Index (MPI).

Table 5 Breakdown of MPI Scoring

3. Activities of Daily Living (ADL)	Points
Bathing (sponge bath, tub bath, or shower)	
Receives no assistance (gets in and out of the tub by self if tub is usual means of bathing)	1
Receives no assistance in bathing only one part of the body (such as back or leg)	1
Receives assistance in bathing more than one part of the body (or not bathed)	0
Dressing (gets clothes from closets and drawers, including underclothes/outer garments and using fasteners/braces, if worn)	
Gets clothes and gets completely dressed without assistance	1
Gets clothes and gets dressed without assistance except for assistance in tying shoes	1
Receives assistance in getting clothes or in getting dressed, or stays partly or completely undressed	0
Toileting	
Goes to "toilet room" cleans self, and arranges clothes without assistance (may use object for support such as cane, walker, or wheelchair and may manage night bedpan or commode, emptying same in morning)	1
Receives assistance in going to "toilet room" or in cleaning self or in arranging clothes after elimination or in use of night bedpan or commode	0
Doesn't go to room termed "toilet" for the elimination process	0
Transfer	
Moves in and out of bed as well as in and out of chair without assistance (may be using object for support such as cane or walker)	1
Moves in and out of bed or chair with assistance	0
Doesn't get out of bed	0
Continence	

Table 5 Breakdown of MPI Scoring *(Continued)*

Controls urination and bowel movement completely by self	1
Has occasional "accidents"	0
Supervision helps keep urine or bowel control, catheter is used, or is incontinent	0
Feeding	
Feeds self without assistance	1
Feeds self except for getting assistance in cutting meat or buttering bread	1
Receives assistance in feeding or is fed partly or completely by using tubes or intravenous fluids	0
Max ADL score (best performance):	6
4. Instrumental Activities of Daily Living Scale (IADL)	
Ability to use telephone	
Operates telephone on own initiative: looks up and dials numbers, etc.	1
Dials a few well-known numbers	1
Answers telephone but does not dial	1
Does not use telephone at all	0
Shopping	
Takes care of all shopping needs independently	1
Shops independently for small purchases	0
Needs to be accompanied on any shopping trip	0
Completely unable to shop	0
Food preparation	
Plans, prepares and serves adequate meals independently	1
Prepares adequate meals if supplied with ingredients	1
Heats, serves and prepares meals or prepares meals but does not maintain adequate diet	0
Needs to have meals prepared and served	0
Housekeeping	
Maintains house alone or with occasional assistance (e.g. "heavy work domestic help")	1
Performs light daily tasks such as dishwashing, bed-making	1
Performs light daily tasks but cannot maintain acceptable level of cleanliness	1
Needs help with all home maintenance tasks	0
Does not participate in any housekeeping tasks	0
Laundry	
Does personal laundry completely	1
Launders small items; rinses stockings, etc.	1
All laundry must be done by others	0
Mode of transportation	
Travels independently on public transportation or drives own car	1
Arranges own travel via taxi, but does not otherwise use public transportation	1
Travels on public transportation when accompanied by another	1
Travel limited to taxi or automobile with assistance of another	0
Does not travel at all	0
Responsibility for own medications	
Is responsible for taking medication in correct dosages at correct time	1
Takes responsibility if medication is prepared in advance in separate dosage	0
Is not capable of dispensing own medication	0

Table 5 Breakdown of MPI Scoring *(Continued)*

Ability to handle finances	
Manages financial matters independently (budgets, writes checks, pays rent, bills, goes to bank), collects and keeps track of income	1
Manages day-to-day purchases, but needs help with banking, major purchases, etc	1
Incapable if handling money	0
Max IADL score (best performance):	8
5. Short Portable Mental Status Questionnaire (SPMSQ)	
What is the date today? (Correct only when the month, date, and year are all correct)	If incorrect: 1
What day of the week is it?	If incorrect: 1
What is the name of this place? (Correct if any of the description of the location is given)	If incorrect: 1
What is your street address?	If incorrect: 1
How old are you?	If incorrect: 1
When were you born?	If incorrect: 1
Who is the president (or the Pope) now? (Requires only the correct last name)	If incorrect: 1
Who was president (or the Pope) just before him?	If incorrect: 1
What was your mother's maiden name?	If incorrect: 1
Subtract 3 from 20 and keep subtracting 3 from each new number at least for 3 times (the entire series must be performed correctly to be scored as correct)	If incorrect: 1
Max SPMQ score (worst performance):	10
6. Exton-Smith Scale (ESS)	
General Condition	
Bad	1
Poor	2
Fair	3
Good	4
Mental State	
Stuporous	1
Confused	2
Apathetic	3
Alert	4
Activity	
In bed all day	1
Chairfast	2
Walks with help	3
Ambulant	4
Incontinence	
Doubly incontinent	1
Usually of urine	2
Occasional	3
None	4
Mobility in Bed	
Immobile	1
Very limited	2
Slightly limited	3
Full	4

Table 5 Breakdown of MPI Scoring *(Continued)*

Max ESS score (best performance):					20

7. Cumulative Illness Rating Scale

	Point allocation based on disease severity				
	None	Mild	Moderate	Severe	Extremely severe
Cardiac (heart only)	1	2	3	4	5
Hypertension (rating is based on severity)	1	2	3	4	5
Vascular (arteries, veins, lymphatics)	1	2	3	4	5
Respiratory (lungs, bronchi, trachea)	1	2	3	4	5
EENT (eye, ear, nose, throat, larynx)	1	2	3	4	5
Upper GI (esophagus, stomach, duodenum, biliary and pancreatic trees)	1	2	3	4	5
Lower GI (intestines, hernias)	1	2	3	4	5
Hepatic (liver only)	1	2	3	4	5
Renal (kidneys only)	1	2	3	4	5
Other GU (urethers, bladder, urethra, prostate, genitals)	1	2	3	4	5
Musculo-skeletal-integumentary (muscles, bone, skin)	1	2	3	4	5
Neurological (brain, spinal cord, nerves)	1	2	3	4	5
Endocrine-metabolic (including diabetes, hyperlipidemia, infections, toxicity)	1	2	3	4	5
Psychiatric (dementia, depression, anxiety, agitation, psychosis)	1	2	3	4	5

Max comorbidity index (number of items with a score of ≥3; excluding the psychiatric item; most severe):	13

8. Mini Nutritional Assessment (MNA)   Points

Anthropometric Assessment

Body Mass Index

< 19	0
19–20	1
21–22	2
≥ 23	3

Mid-arm circumference (cm)

< 21	0
22	0.5
> 22	1

Calf circumference (cm)

< 31	0
> 31	1

Weight loss (last 3 months)

Loss of >3 kg	0
Do not know	1
Loss between 1 and 3 kg	2
No weight loss	3

General Assessment

Lives independently (not in a nursing home or hospital)

No	0
Yes	1

Takes more than 3 prescription drugs per day

Table 5 Breakdown of MPI Scoring *(Continued)*

Yes	0
No	1
Has suffered psychological stress or acute disease in the past 3 months	
Yes	0
No	1
Mobility	
Bed/chair-bound	0
Able to get out of bed / chair but does not go out	1
Goes out	2
Neuropsychological problems	
Severe dementia/depression	0
Mild dementia	1
Psychological problems	2
Pressure sores or skin ulcers	
Yes	0
No	1
Dietary Assessment	
How many full meals does the patient eat daily?	
1 meal	0
2 meals	1
3 meals	2
Consumes at least 1 serving of dairy products (milk, cheese, yogurt) per day	
No	1
Yes	0
Consumes 2 or more servings of Legumes or eggs per week	
No	0
Yes	0.5
Consumes meat, fish or poultry every day	
No	0
Yes	1
Consumes 2 or more servings of fruits or vegetables per day?	
No	0
Yes	1
Has food intake declined over the past 3 months due to loss of appetite?	
Severe loss of appetite	0
Moderate loss of appetite	1
No loss of appetite	2
How much fluids consumed per day?	
< 5 glasses	0
5–9 glasses	0.5
> 9 glasses	1
Mode of feeding	
With assistance	0
Self-feed with some difficulty	1

Table 5 Breakdown of MPI Scoring *(Continued)*

Self-feed without any problem	2
Self Assessment	
Do they view themselves as having nutritional problems?	
Major malnutrition	0
Does not know	1
No nutritional problems	2
In comparison with other people of same age, how they consider their health status?	
Not as good	0
Does not know	0.5
As good	1
Better	2
Max MNA score (best-nourished)	30

Legend: The numbering on the left-hand side of score titles corresponds to the numbering of factors in Appendix 1

Appendix 3
Illustrates how the Silver Code is calculated.

Table 6 Calculation of the Silver Code

Factor	Points
Age	
75–79	0
80–84	3
85+	9
Gender	
Female	0
Male	2
Marital status	
Married	0
Unmarried/widowed/divorced	1
Previous admission to a day hospital	
No	0
Yes	5
Previous admission to a regular ward and discharge diagnosis	
No admission (0)	0
Respiratory disease (6)	6
Cancer (11)	11
Other (2)	2
Number of drugs in the previous 3 mo	
0–8	0
8+	2

Total score: 0 pts. = best possible performance, 36 pts. = worst possible performance– Corresponds to gradient risk for mortality

Appendix 4

Describes the components of the Short Physical Performance
Battery (SPPB).

Table 7 Short Physical Performance Battery (SPPB)

Instructions	Scoring
1. Repeated Chair Stands	
• Ask patient if they think it is safe for them to try and stand up from a chair five times without using their arms. • If yes, instruct patient to stand up straight and then sit back down again as quickly as they can five times, without stopping in between, keeping their arms folded over their chest. • Demonstrate. • Begin the stopwatch when patient begins to stand up. Count aloud each time patient rises. • Stop the stopwatch when subject has straightened up completely for the fifth time. Also stop if the subject uses arms, if they have not completed rises after 1 min, or if concerned about their safety.	- <5 stands completed in ≤1 min = 0 pts. - 5 stands in >16.7 s and ≤1 min = 1 pt. - 5 stands in 16.6–13.7 s = 2 pts. - 5 stands in 13.6–11.2 s = 3 pts. - 5 stands in <11.1 s = 4 pts
2. Balance Testing	
Semitandem: • Instruct patient to stand with the side of the heel of one foot touching the big toe of the other foot for 10 s (left/right feet as preferred by patient). • Demonstrate • Stand next to patient to help them into a semitandem position, allowing them to hold onto your arms to establish balance. • Begin timing when patient has the feet in position. • If *unable* to hold the semitandem position for 10 s → *side-by-side.* • If *able* to hold the semitandem position for 10 s → *tandem.* → *Side-by-side:* As for semitandem but with feet together. Patients may use their arms, bend their knees, or move their body to maintain balance, but may not move their feet. → *Tandem:* As for semitandem but with the heel of one foot in-front-of and touching the toes of the other foot.	- Side-by-side: <10 s or unable = 0 pts. - Side-by-side: ≥10 s; semitandem: <10 s = 1 pt. - Semitandem: ≥10 s; tandem: 0–2 s = 2 pts. - Semitandem: ≥10 s; tandem: 3–9 s = 3 pts. - Tandem: ≥10 s = 4 pts
3. Eight-foot (2.44 m) walk	
• Instruct patient to walk at their usual pace to the other end of course (a distance of 8 ft) and to continue walking until they pass the end of the tape. If they use a cane or other walking aid outside of their home, they should use it for the test. • Press the start button on the stopwatch as the participant begins walking. Walk with the patient. • Measure the time they take to complete the 8-ft course.	- Unable to complete course = 0 pts. - Completed course in >5.7 s = 1 pt. - Completed course in 4.1–6.5 s = 2 pts. - Completed course in 3.2–4.0 s = 3 pts. - Completed course in <3.1 s = 4 pts

SPPB score: 0 pts. = worst possible performance, 12 pts. = best performance
Score corresponds to gradient risk for mortality, nursing home admission, and disability

Legend: *pt.* point, *SPPB* short physical performance battery

Appendix 5

Details about procedural aspects are provided.

Table 8 Procedural characteristics

	n/N (%)
Access route	
Transfemoral	55/71 (77.5)
Transapical	9/71 (12.7)
Transaortic	7/71 (9.9)
Type of THV	
SAPIEN XT	26/71 (36.6)
SAPIEN 3	40/71 (56.3)
Other	5/71 (7.0)
THV diameter	
23 mm	37/70 (52.9)
26 mm	26/70 (37.1)
29 mm	7/70 (10.0)
Second valve used	2/71 (2.8)
Pre-implantation balloon dilatation	63/71 (88.7)
Post-delivery balloon dilatation	9/71 (12.7)

Legend: *THV* transcatheter heart valve

Appendix 6
Details about periprocedural outcomes are provided.

Table 9 Periprocedural outcomes

	Mean ± SD / n/N (%)
Device success (VARC-2)[a]	
Absence of procedural mortality	70/70 (100.0)
Correct positioning of THV	70/70 (100.0)
Intended performance of THV	70/70 (100.0)
Intraoperative complications[b]	12/70 (17.1)
Vascular complications requiring treatment[c]	7/70 (10.0)
Access-related complications (dissection, rupture)	4/71 (5.6)
Conversion to open surgery (%)	0/70 (0.0)
Paravalvular regurgitation (%)	
None/trace	46/70 (65.7)
Mild	22/70 (31.4)
Moderate	2/70 (2.9)
Severe	0/70 (0.0)
Transvalvular leakage (%)	
None/trace	62/70 (88.6)
Mild	8/70 (11.4)
Moderate/severe	0/70 (0.0)
AV peak gradient (mmHg)	20.0 ± 12.4 ($n = 31$)
AV mean gradient (mmHg)	11.3 ± 7.2 ($n = 32$)

Legend: *THV* transcatheter heart valve, *AV* aortic valve
[a]Valve Academic Research Consortium criteria: absence of procedural mortality, correct positioning of a single prosthetic heart valve into proper anatomical position, and intended performance of the prosthetic heart valve (no prosthesis–patient mismatch) and mean aortic valve gradient
[b]Includes access-related complications (8 pts), asystole/arrhythmia (2 pts), haemorrhagic stroke (1 pt) [one patient no further information available]
[c]Includes aneurysm, haematoma, pericardial haematoma/effusion (2 pts), apical bleeding (1 pt)

Appendix 7
Changes of the CGA over 3 month.

Table 10 CGA baseline vs 3 months

	Baseline		3 months		Intra-individual change			
	N	Mean ± SD	N	Mean ± SD	N	Mean ± SD	95% CI	p-value
MPI total score	71	0.34 ± 0.11	56	0.30 ± 0.13	56	−0.02 ± 0.12	−0.05, 0.01	0.25
ADL	71	0.05 ± 0.15	60	0.07 ± 0.22	60	0.04 ± 0.25	−0.02, 0.11	0.20
IADL	71	0.16 ± 0.29	60	0.21 ± 0.32	60	0.06 ± 0.32	−0.02, 0.14	0.16
SPMSQ	71	0.01 ± 0.06	57	0.02 ± 0.09	57	0.01 ± 0.12	−0.02, 0.04	0.57
CIRS	71	0.82 ± 0.27	56	0.71 ± 0.38	56	−0.12 ± 0.25	−0.18, −0.05	< 0.001
MNA	71	0.30 ± 0.33	56	0.21 ± 0.28	56	−0.07 ± 0.37	−0.17, 0.03	0.16
ESS	71	0.08 ± 0.22	56	0.02 ± 0.09	56	−0.04 ± 0.13	−0.07, 0.0	0.04
Medication use	71	0.86 ± 0.24	60	0.88 ± 0.21	60	0.04 ± 0.27	−0.03, 0.11	0.23
Co-habitation status	71	0.42 ± 0.50	60	0.31 ± 0.46	60	−0.08 ± 0.39	−0.18, 0.03	0.14
Silver code	71	22.53 ± 6.44	57	22.8 ± 6.33	57	−0.31 ± 3.55	−0.64, 1.25	0.52
SPPB	71	5.69 ± 3.33	56	7.82 ± 2.84	56	1.86 ± 2.76	1.12, 2.60	< 0.001

Legend: *MPI* Multidimensional Prognostic Index, *ADL* Activities of Daily Living, Instrumental Activities of Daily Living, *SPMSQ* Short Portable Mental Status Questionnaire, *CIRS* Cumulative Illness Rating Scale, *MNA* Mini Nutritional Assessment, *ESS* Exton-Smith Scale, *SPPB* short physical performance battery

Abbreviations
ACC: American College of Cardiology; AS: Aortic stenosis; AV: Aortic valve; BMI: Body mass index; CGA: Comprehensive geriatric assessment; CHF: Congestive heart failure; CI: Confidence interval; CIRS: Cumulative illness rating scale; eCRF: Electronic case report form; ESS: Exton-Smith Scale; EUGMS: European union geriatric medicine society; IADL: Instrumental Activities of Daily Living; LVEF: Left ventricular ejection fraction; MACCCE: Major adverse cardiac or cerebrovascular event; MI: Myocardial infarction; MNA: Mini nutritional assessment; MPI: Multidimensional prognostic index; NYHA: New York Heart Association; OR: Odds ratio; SAVR: Surgical aortic valve replacement; SPMSQ: Short portable mental status questionnaire; SPPB: Short physical performance battery; STS: Society of thoracic surgeons; TAVI: Transcatheter aortic valve implantation; TIA: Transient ischaemic attack; TUG: Timed get-up and go; VARC: Valve Academic Research Consortium

Acknowledgements
Data were captured using the s4trials Software provided by Software for Trials Europe GmbH, Berlin, Germany. Helen Sims and Katherine Smith (Institute for Pharmacology and Preventive Medicine; IPPMed) provided editorial support during the preparation of this manuscript.

Funding
This work was supported by a research grant that was provided by Edwards Lifesciences (Nyon, Switzerland) to the Sponsor, IPPMed (Cloppenburg, Germany). JK and MT are representatives of the funder. They discussed the study design with the principal investigators and the sponsor, had no role in data collection, had no role in the analysis, but revised the manuscript along with the other authors for important intellectual content.

Authors' contributions
The authors take responsibility for all aspects of the reliability and freedom from bias of the data presented and their discussed interpretation. The specific contributions of the respective authors are as follows: AU, PB, JK, MT, SM and AWS were involved in the conception and design of the study; GM, NvV, MT, JB, MPT, JBM, GS, MvM, and SJ collected the data, which were analyzed by AU, GM, CD, and PB and interpreted by the author group; PB drafted the manuscript and all other authors revised the article for important intellectual content. All authors have given final approval for the version to be submitted.

Competing interests

Jan Baan and Peter Bramlage received research funding from Edwards Lifesciences, as did Andrea Ungar. Jean-Bernard Masson is a consultant for Edwards Lifesciences. Jana Kurucova is an employee of Edwards Lifesciences. The other authors declare no conflict of interest in relation to this manuscript.

Author details

[1]Geriatric Intensive Care Unit, Department of Geriatrics and Medicine, Careggi Hospital and University of Florence, Florence, Italy. [2]Internal Medicine, Section of Geriatric Medicine, Academic Medical Center, Amsterdam, Netherlands. [3]Cardiology, Academic Medical Center, Amsterdam, Netherlands. [4]Centre Hospitalier de l'Université de Montréal, Montréal, Canada. [5]Institute for Pharmacology und Preventive Medicine, Cloppenburg, Germany. [6]Edwards Lifesciences, Nyon, Switzerland. [7]CNR–Institute of Neuroscience, Aging Branch, Padua, Italy. [8]Department of Geriatrics, Inselspital, Bern University Hospital, University of Bern, Bern, Switzerland.

References

1. Bonow RO, Leon MB, Doshi D, Moat N. Management strategies and future challenges for aortic valve disease. Lancet (London, England). 2016; 387(10025):1312–23.
2. Leon MB, Smith CR, Mack M, Miller DC, Moses JW, Svensson LG, Tuzcu EM, Webb JG, Fontana GP, Makkar RR, et al. Transcatheter aortic-valve implantation for aortic stenosis in patients who cannot undergo surgery. N Engl J Med. 2010;363(17):1597–607.
3. Schoenenberger AW, Stortecky S, Neumann S, Moser A, Juni P, Carrel T, Huber C, Gandon M, Bischoff S, Schoenenberger CM, et al. Predictors of functional decline in elderly patients undergoing transcatheter aortic valve implantation (TAVI). Eur Heart J. 2013;34(9):684–92.
4. Piazza N, Wenaweser P, van Gameren M, Pilgrim T, Tzikas A, Otten A, Nuis R, Onuma Y, Cheng JM, Kappetein AP, et al. Relationship between the logistic EuroSCORE and the society of thoracic surgeons predicted risk of mortality score in patients implanted with the CoreValve ReValving system–a Bern-Rotterdam study. Am Heart J. 2010;159(2):323–9.
5. Ben-Dor I, Gaglia MA Jr, Barbash IM, Maluenda G, Hauville C, Gonzalez MA, Sardi G, Laynez-Carnicero A, Torguson R, Okubagzi P, et al. Comparison between Society of Thoracic Surgeons score and logistic EuroSCORE for predicting mortality in patients referred for transcatheter aortic valve implantation. Cardiovasc Revasc Med. 2011;12(6):345–9.
6. Afilalo J, Mottillo S, Eisenberg MJ, Alexander KP, Noiseux N, Perrault LP, Morin JF, Langlois Y, Ohayon SM, Monette J, et al. Addition of frailty and disability to cardiac surgery risk scores identifies elderly patients at high risk of mortality or major morbidity. Circ Cardiovasc Qual Outcomes. 2012;5(2):222–8.
7. Afilalo J, Eisenberg MJ, Morin JF, Bergman H, Monette J, Noiseux N, Perrault LP, Alexander KP, Langlois Y, Dendukuri N, et al. Gait speed as an incremental predictor of mortality and major morbidity in elderly patients undergoing cardiac surgery. J Am Coll Cardiol. 2010;56(20):1668–76.
8. Otto CM, Kumbhani DJ, Alexander KP, Calhoon JH, Desai MY, Kaul S, Lee JC, Ruiz CE, Vassileva CM. 2017 ACC expert consensus decision pathway for transcatheter aortic valve replacement in the management of adults with aortic stenosis: a report of the American College of Cardiology Task Force on clinical expert consensus documents. J Am Coll Cardiol. 2017;69(10):1313–46.
9. Ungar A, Bramlage P, Thoenes M, Zannoni S, Michel JP. A call to action - geriatricians' experience in treatment of aortic stenosis and involvement in transcatheter aortic valve implantation. Eur Geriatr Med. 2013;4(3):176–82.
10. Ellis G, Langhorne P. Comprehensive geriatric assessment for older hospital patients. Br Med Bull. 2004;71:45–59.
11. Lilamand M, Dumonteil N, Nourhashemi F, Hanon O, Marcheix B, Toulza O, Elmalem S, van Kan GA, Raynaud-Simon A, Vellas B, et al. Gait speed and comprehensive geriatric assessment: two keys to improve the management of older persons with aortic stenosis. Int J Cardiol. 2014;173(3):580–2.
12. Pilotto A, Ferrucci L, Franceschi M, D'Ambrosio LP, Scarcelli C, Cascavilla L, Paris F, Placentino G, Seripa D, Dallapiccola B, et al. Development and validation of a multidimensional prognostic index for one-year mortality from comprehensive geriatric assessment in hospitalized older patients. Rejuvenation Res. 2008;11(1):151–61.
13. Pilotto A, Rengo F, Marchionni N, Sancarlo D, Fontana A, Panza F, Ferrucci L. Comparing the prognostic accuracy for all-cause mortality of frailty instruments: a multicentre 1-year follow-up in hospitalized older patients. PLoS One. 2012;7(1):e29090.
14. Stortecky S, Schoenenberger AW, Moser A, Kalesan B, Juni P, Carrel T, Bischoff S, Schoenenberger CM, Stuck AE, Windecker S, et al. Evaluation of multidimensional geriatric assessment as a predictor of mortality and cardiovascular events after transcatheter aortic valve implantation. JACC Cardiovasc Interv. 2012;5(5):489–96.
15. Green P, Woglom AE, Genereux P, Daneault B, Paradis JM, Schnell S, Hawkey M, Maurer MS, Kirtane AJ, Kodali S, et al. The impact of frailty status on survival after transcatheter aortic valve replacement in older adults with severe aortic stenosis: a single-center experience. JACC Cardiovasc Interv. 2012;5(9):974–81.
16. Kamga M, Boland B, Cornette P, Beeckmans M, De Meester C, Chenu P, Gurne O, Renkin J, Kefer J. Impact of frailty scores on outcome of octogenarian patients undergoing transcatheter aortic valve implantation. Acta Cardiol. 2013;68(6):599–606.
17. Schoenenberger AW, Werner N, Bramlage P, Martinez-Selles M, Maggi S, Bauernschmitt R, Thoenes M, Kurucova J, Michel JP, Ungar A. Comprehensive geriatric assessment in patients undergoing transcatheter aortic valve implantation–rationale and design of the European CGA-TAVI registry. Eur Geriatr Med. 2014;5(1):8–13.
18. Katz S, Downs TD, Cash HR, Grotz RC. Progress in development of the index of ADL. The Gerontologist. 1970;10(1):20–30.
19. Katz S, Ford AB, Moskowitz RW, Jackson BA, Jaffe MW. Studies of illness in the aged. The index of ADL: a standardized measure of biological and psychosocial function. JAMA. 1963;185:914–9.
20. Lawton MP, Brody EM. Assessment of older people: self-maintaining and instrumental activities of daily living. The Gerontologist. 1969;9(3):179–86.
21. Pfeiffer E. A short portable mental status questionnaire for the assessment of organic brain deficit in elderly patients. J Am Geriatr Soc. 1975;23(10):433–41.
22. Conwell Y, Forbes NT, Cox C, Caine ED. Validation of a measure of physical illness burden at autopsy: the cumulative illness rating scale. J Am Geriatr Soc. 1993;41(1):38–41.
23. Linn BS, Linn MW, Gurel L. Cumulative illness rating scale. J Am Geriatr Soc. 1968;16(5):622–6.
24. Vellas B, Guigoz Y, Garry PJ, Nourhashemi F, Bennahum D, Lauque S, Albarede JL. The Mini Nutritional Assessment (MNA) and its use in grading the nutritional state of elderly patients. Nutrition (Burbank, Los Angeles County, Calif). 1999;15(2):116–22.
25. Bliss MR, McLaren R, Exton-Smith AN. Mattresses for preventing pressure sores in geriatric patients. Mon Bull Minist Health Public Health Lab Serv. 1966;25:238–68.
26. Di Bari M, Balzi D, Roberts AT, Barchielli A, Fumagalli S, Ungar A, Bandinelli S, De Alfieri W, Gabbani L, Marchionni N. Prognostic stratification of older persons based on simple administrative data: development and validation of the "Silver Code", to be used in emergency department triage. J Gerontol A Biol Sci Med Sci. 2010;65(2):159–64.
27. Guralnik JM, Simonsick EM, Ferrucci L, Glynn RJ, Berkman LF, Blazer DG, Scherr PA, Wallace RB. A short physical performance battery assessing lower extremity function: association with self-reported disability and prediction of mortality and nursing home admission. J Gerontol. 1994;49(2):M85–94.
28. Kappetein AP, Head SJ, Genereux P, Piazza N, van Mieghem NM, Blackstone EH, Brott TG, Cohen DJ, Cutlip DE, van Es GA, et al. Updated standardized endpoint definitions for transcatheter aortic valve implantation: the valve academic research Consortium-2 consensus document (VARC-2). Eur J Cardiothorac Surg. 2012;42(5):S45–60.
29. Kodali S, Thourani VH, White J, Malaisrie SC, Lim S, Greason KL, Williams M, Guerrero M, Eisenhauer AC, Kapadia S, et al. Early clinical and echocardiographic outcomes after SAPIEN 3 transcatheter aortic valve replacement in inoperable, high-risk and intermediate-risk patients with aortic stenosis. Eur Heart J. 2016;37(28):2252–62.

30. Wendler O, Schymik G, Treede H, Baumgartner H, Dumonteil N, Ihlberg L, Neumann FJ, Tarantini G, Zamarano JL, Vahanian A. SOURCE 3 registry: design and 30-day results of the European Postapproval registry of the latest generation of the SAPIEN 3 transcatheter heart valve. Circulation. 2017;135(12):1123–32.

31. Chieffo A, Petronio AS, Mehilli J, Chandrasekhar J, Sartori S, Lefèvre T, Presbitero P, Capranzano P, Tchetche D, Iadanza A, et al. Acute and 30-day outcomes in women after TAVR: results from the WIN-TAVI (Women's INternational Transcatheter Aortic Valve Implantation) real-world registry. J Am Coll Cardiol Intv. 2016;9(15):1589–600.

32. Wenaweser P, Stortecky S, Heg D, Tueller D, Nietlispach F, Falk V, Pedrazzini GB, Jeger RV, Reuthebuch O, Carrel T, et al. Short-term clinical outcomes among patients undergoing transcatheter aortic valve implantation in Switzerland: the Swiss TAVI registry. EuroIntervention. 2014;10(8):982–9.

33. Chieffo A, Van Mieghem NM, Tchetche D, Dumonteil N, Giustino G, Van der Boon RMA, Pierri A, Marcheix B, Misuraca L, Serruys PW, et al. Impact of mixed aortic valve stenosis on VARC-2 outcomes and postprocedural aortic regurgitation in patients undergoing transcatheter aortic valve implantation. Catheter Cardiovasc Interv. 2015;86(5):875–85.

34. Leon MB, Smith CR, Mack MJ, Makkar RR, Svensson LG, Kodali SK, Thourani VH, Tuzcu EM, Miller DC, Herrmann HC, et al. Transcatheter or surgical aortic-valve replacement in intermediate-risk patients. N Engl J Med. 2016;374(17):1609–20.

35. Cockburn J, Dooley M, Trivedi U, De Belder A, Hildick-Smith D. A comparison between surgical risk scores for predicting outcome in patients undergoing transcatheter aortic valve implantation. J Cardiovasc Surg (Torino). 2017;58(3):467-72. doi:https://doi.org/10.23736/S0021-9509.16.09339-3. Epub 2016 Mar 16.

36. Collas V, Chong YM, Rodrigus I, Vandewoude M, Bosmans J. Predictive mortality estimation in older patients undergoing TAVI comparison of the logistic EuroSCORE, EuroSCORE II and STS-score. Eur Geriatr Med. 2015;6(1):11–4.

37. Giantin V, Valentini E, Iasevoli M, Falci C, Siviero P, De Luca E, Maggi S, Martella B, Orrù G, Crepaldi G, et al. Does the Multidimensional Prognostic Index (MPI), based on a Comprehensive Geriatric Assessment (CGA), predict mortality in cancer patients? Results of a prospective observational trial. J Geriatr Oncol. 2013;4(3):208–17.

38. Pilotto A, Addante F, Ferrucci L, Leandro G, D'Onofrio G, Corritore M, Niro V, Scarcelli C, Dallapiccola B, Franceschi M. The multidimensional prognostic index predicts short- and long-term mortality in hospitalized geriatric patients with pneumonia. J Gerontol A Biol Sci Med Sci. 2009;64(8):880–7.

39. Pilotto A, Addante F, Franceschi M, Leandro G, Rengo G, D'Ambrosio P, Longo MG, Rengo F, Pellegrini F, Dallapiccola B, et al. Multidimensional prognostic index based on a comprehensive geriatric assessment predicts short-term mortality in older patients with heart failure. Circ Heart Fail. 2010;3(1):14–20.

40. Sancarlo D, Pilotto A, Panza F, Copetti M, Longo MG, D'Ambrosio P, D'Onofrio G, Ferrucci L, Pilotto A. A Multidimensional Prognostic Index (MPI) based on a comprehensive geriatric assessment predicts short- and long-term all-cause mortality in older hospitalized patients with transient ischemic attack. J Neurol. 2012;259(4):670–8.

41. Sundermann S, Dademasch A, Rastan A, Praetorius J, Rodriguez H, Walther T, Mohr FW, Falk V. One-year follow-up of patients undergoing elective cardiac surgery assessed with the comprehensive assessment of frailty test and its simplified form. Interact Cardiovasc Thorac Surg. 2011;13(2):119–23.

42. Arnold SV, Reynolds MR, Lei Y, Magnuson EA, Kirtane AJ, Kodali SK, Zajarias A, Thourani VH, Green P, Rodes-Cabau J, et al. Predictors of poor outcomes after transcatheter aortic valve replacement: results from the PARTNER (Placement of Aortic Transcatheter Valve) trial. Circulation. 2014;129(25):2682–90.

43. Arnold SV, Afilalo J, Spertus JA, Tang Y, Baron SJ, Jones PG, Reardon MJ, Yakubov SJ, Adams DH, Cohen DJ. Prediction of poor outcome after transcatheter aortic valve replacement. J Am Coll Cardiol. 2016;68(17):1868–77.

44. Afilalo J, Kim S, O'Brien S, Brennan JM, Edwards FH, Mack MJ, McClurken JB, Cleveland JC Jr, Smith PK, Shahian DM, et al. Gait speed and operative mortality in older adults following cardiac surgery. JAMA Cardiol. 2016;1(3):314–21.

45. Alfredsson J, Stebbins A, Brennan JM, Matsouaka R, Afilalo J, Peterson ED, Vemulapalli S, Rumsfeld JS, Shahian D, Mack MJ, et al. Gait speed predicts 30-day mortality after transcatheter aortic valve replacement: results from the Society of Thoracic Surgeons/American College of Cardiology Transcatheter Valve Therapy Registry. Circulation. 2016;133(14):1351–9.

46. Di Bari M, Salvi F, Roberts AT, Balzi D, Lorenzetti B, Morichi V, Rossi L, Lattanzio F, Marchionni N. Prognostic stratification of elderly patients in the emergency department: a comparison between the "Identification of Seniors at Risk" and the "Silver Code". J Gerontol A Biol Sci Med Sci. 2012;67(5):544–50.

18

Driving following defibrillator implantation: development and pilot results from a nationwide questionnaire

Jenny Bjerre[1]*[iD], Simone Hofman Rosenkranz[2], Anne Mielke Christensen[1], Morten Schou[3], Christian Jøns[3], Gunnar Gislason[1] and Anne-Christine Ruwald[1,4]

Abstract

Background: Implantable cardioverter defibrillator (ICD) implantation is associated with driving restrictions which may have profound effects on the patient's life. However, there is limited patient-reported data on the information given about driving restrictions, the adherence to the restrictions, the incidence of arrhythmic symptoms while driving, and the driving restrictions' effect on ICD patients' daily life and quality of life factors. A specific questionnaire was designed to investigate these objectives, intended for use in a nationwide ICD cohort.

Methods: The conceptual framework based on literature review and expert opinion was refined in qualitative semi-structured focus group interviews with ten ICD patients. Content validity was pursued through pre-testing, including expert review and 28 cognitive interviews with patients at all ICD implanting centres in Denmark. Finally, the Danish Pacemaker and ICD registry was used to randomly select 50 ICD patients with a first-time implantation between January 1, 2013 and November 30, 2016 for pilot testing, followed by a test-retest on 25 respondents. Test-retest agreement was assessed using kappa statistics or intraclass correlation coefficients.

Results: The pilot test achieved a response rate of 78%, whereof the majority were web-based (69%). Only 49% stated they had been informed about any driving restrictions after ICD implantation, whereas the number was 75% after appropriate ICD shock. Among respondents, 95% had resumed private driving, ranging from 1 to 90 days after ICD implantation. In those informed of a significant ($\geq$ 1 month) driving ban, 55% stated the driving restrictions had impeded with daily life, especially due to limitations in maintaining employment or getting to/from work and 25% admitted they had knowingly been driving during the restricted period. There were six episodes of dizziness or palpitations not necessitating stopping the vehicle. Test-retest demonstrated good agreement of questionnaire items, with 69% of Kappa coefficients above 0.60.

Conclusions: We have developed a comprehensive questionnaire on ICD patients' perspective on driving. Pre-testing and pilot testing demonstrated good content validity, feasible data collection methods, and a robust response rate. Thus, we believe the final questionnaire, distributed to almost 4000 ICD patients, will capture essential evidence to help inform driving guidelines in this population.

Keywords: Implantable cardioverter defibrillators, Driving restrictions, Traffic safety, Patient-reported outcomes, Questionnaire

* Correspondence: jennybjerre@gmail.com
[1]Department of Cardiology, Cardiovascular Research, Copenhagen University Hospital Herlev-Gentofte, Kildegaardsvej 28, 2900 Hellerup, Denmark
Full list of author information is available at the end of the article

Background

Implantable cardioverter defibrillators (ICDs) are effective in preventing sudden cardiac death, both in patients who have survived a life-threatening arrhythmia (secondary prevention) and in patients who are at increased risk of life-threatening arrhythmias (primary prevention) [1–3]. However, since the early days of ICD treatment, driving following ICD implantation and ICD therapy has been controversial. The concern is that the underlying heart condition may cause an arrhythmia, potentially incapacitating the patient while operating a motor vehicle and causing harm to the patient or others. Hence, scientific societies have developed statements on the issue [4, 5]: The current European recommendations advise a four-week driving restriction following primary prevention ICD implantation and three-months restriction following secondary prevention ICD implantation as well as after appropriate ICD therapy [5]. In Denmark, primary prevention patients can resume driving 1 week following implantation, granted home-monitoring is established [6]. Professional driving and driving of large vehicles (> 3.5 metric tonnes) is permanently restricted [5, 6].

There is an overall paucity of research involving patient-reported outcomes in this area. The few available studies date back to the 1990s and were performed in small and selected patient populations, predominantly including secondary prevention patients. Notably, authors have not reported their methods for developing and testing the questionnaires and rarely presented the questionnaires themselves. These studies reported that information given on driving restrictions is often either lacking or cannot be recalled by the patients [7, 8], and even when instructed not to drive, adherence to the instructions is minimal [7–11]. Moreover, evidence suggest that driving restrictions following ICD implantation negatively impacts the patients' quality of life (QoL) [12].

In questionnaire research, it is pivotal that the questions asked are both relevant and comprehensive for the objective of the study - a measure of content validity. Likewise, the questionnaire items should be understandable and unambiguous for the target population, warranting thorough pre-testing of the measure before final application. Lastly, data collection procedures should be evaluated through a pilot test, to secure sufficient and analyzable responses.

We aimed to develop a questionnaire investigating ICD patients' experiences with driving and driving restrictions. The intended use was for a cross-sectional investigation in a nationwide Danish ICD cohort. This paper describes the process of developing and pre-testing the questionnaire and ultimately presents selected results from a pilot test.

Methods

The International Society for Quality of Life Research (ISO-QOL) recommendations for patient-reported outcome measures were used as a manual to guide questionnaire development and testing [13]. These recommendations have been developed with the aim to define minimum measurement standards to promote appropriate use of patient-reported outcomes research. Figure 1 demonstrates a flow chart of questionnaire development.

Problem formulation

Initially, we defined four specific objectives for the questionnaire: (1) Quantify the amount of information given to ICD patients on driving restrictions following ICD implantation and/or ICD shock; (2) Investigate whether ICD patients adhere to driving restrictions and which factors are associated with adherence to driving restrictions; (3) Determine what proportion of Danish ICD patients have experienced an ICD shock or cardiac symptoms of possible arrhythmia while driving, and whether these symptoms resulted in a motor vehicle accident; and (4) Identify whether driving restrictions influence factors associated with patient QoL.

Conceptualization: Literature and experts

Based on expert opinion and following review of the existing literature on driving following ICD implantation, an

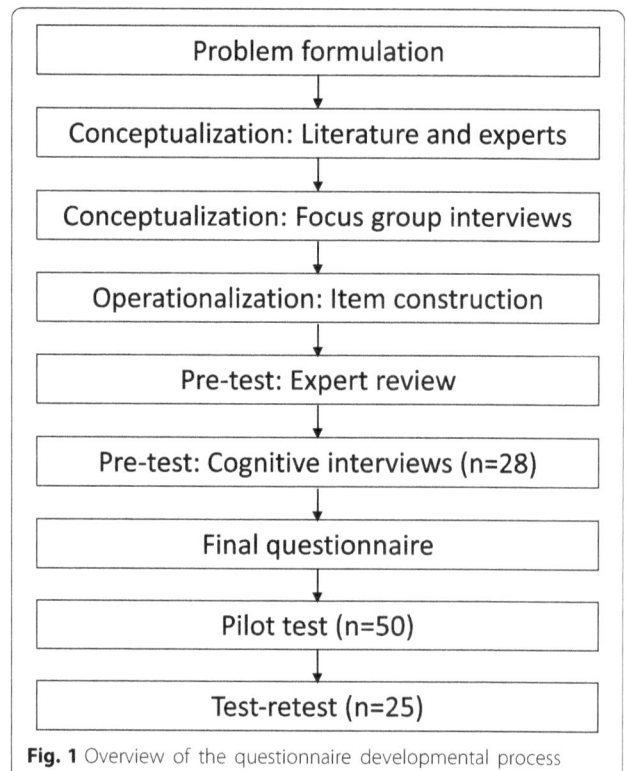

Fig. 1 Overview of the questionnaire developmental process

initial conceptual framework was developed which was successively refined in qualitative semi-structured focus group interviews. In summary, through conceptualization, specific variables were defined which could subsequently be transformed into items, thus connecting the research objectives with the content of the questionnaire. Additional file 1: Table S1 presents our research aims, hypotheses, concepts and their corresponding variable definitions as well as questionnaire item numbers. For example, the concept "Information about driving restrictions after ICD implantation" resulted in three variable definitions: (1) Whether the patient held a valid private driver's license (Group 1: car, motorcycle, tractor) during the 6 months leading up to ICD implantation; (2) Whether the patient held a valid Group 2 driver's license (Group 2: truck, bus or any vehicle for passenger transportation) during the 6 months leading up to ICD implantation; (3) Whether the patient was informed about driving restrictions following ICD implantation (for both Group 1 and Group 2) by health personnel (doctors, nurses and ICD technicians) during the hospitalization for ICD implantation.

A few concepts and variable definitions merit further elaboration: First, in order to compare questionnaire responses with current guideline recommendations, we chose to define private and professional driving based on the definitions in the European Heart Rhythm Association's recommendations for driving with ICDs and adapted by the Danish Society of Cardiology [5, 6]. For our aim of investigating the driving restrictions' influence on QoL factors, we were inspired by the World Health Organization's six proposed domains of QoL [14]. From the 24 facets of QoL proposed, we predicted that 10 could be affected by driving restrictions: negative feelings, positive feelings and self-esteem (psychological domain); mobility, activities of daily living and work capacity (level of independence domain); personal relationships and social support (social relationship domain); participation in and opportunities for recreation/leisure and transport (environment domain).

Conceptualization: Focus group interviews

To uncover unknown concepts related to driving following ICD implantation, we performed three focus group interviews with ten contemporary Danish ICD patients (20% female, median age 62 years, 50% primary prevention ICD indication). The participants were recruited from the outpatient clinic at a university hospital in The Capital Region of Denmark and purposive maximum sampling was used to achieve variation in pre-specified variables, including sex, age, ICD indication, previous ICD therapy and geographic residence. Briefly, the qualitative setting allowed ICD patients to elaborate on their perceptions and experiences with driving and the driving restrictions. Further, we could observe the social and cultural norms within groups of ICD patients and thus gain essential knowledge on what wording to use and how to approach certain delicate questions, such as adherence to driving restrictions [15].

Operationalization

We followed general technical rules for valid questionnaire design. Initially, the items were grouped into themes using a strategic order, taking into account spill over effects and placement of sensitive questions. Thus, the first questions were considered easy, whereas complexity increased throughout the questionnaire. Respondents were asked when they had resumed driving after ICD implantation or ICD shock, before the questions about what information on driving restrictions they had received. Intentionally, direct questions about adherence to driving restrictions were placed at the end of the questionnaire. Since not all questions were relevant for everyone, e.g. the majority of ICD patients have not experienced an ICD shock, branching methods were applied to guide the respondents through the questionnaire. For instance, following a few background questions (about self-assessed health, educational attainment, and employment status), respondents without a valid driver's license at time of ICD implantation were guided to the end of the questionnaire. Lastly, due to the sensitive nature of some of the questions, we chose to make all items voluntary including a possibility of skipping questions in the web-based questionnaire.

Question formulations were kept short and words with connotations were excluded. Help texts were included if deemed necessary. In order to minimize recall bias, we defined four distinct recall periods (which were confirmed realistic during focus groups) depending on the objective of the question: "the six months leading up to ICD implantation", "at the time of ICD implantation", "in periods with driving restrictions", and "during the previous month." Text including recall periods was underscored. Response categories were tailored to the question type: for factual questions, we particularly aimed for exhaustive and mutually exclusive response categories, whereas the focus for opinion questions was to achieve balance in the response categories. For potentially sensitive questions, including questions about driving behaviour and the driving restrictions' influence on factors related to QoL, we chose to express questions as opinions with corresponding Likert scale response categories (strongly agree to strongly disagree) [16], as opposed to factual questions with Yes/No response categories. Likert scale variation was kept minimal with either three- or five-point scales. Likewise, open response categories were generally avoided, but included in a few "other" response categories. Furthermore, the respondents were given the opportunity to leave comments after selected sections of the questionnaire.

Pre-test: Expert review

The first method used in evaluating the questionnaire was an informal, individually-based expert review. Four participating cardiologists or cardiology fellows (ACR, MS, JP and LS) and one device technician (JDP) each independently conducted a review and determined whether he/she found the items sufficient relative to the questionnaire's aims, or if a questionnaire item was problematic. Following adjustments based on these evaluations, the questionnaire was reviewed by a senior questionnaire expert (JC), independent from the study group. Adjustments following this expert review included minor modifications like introducing help texts to emphasize different recall periods, using continuous response categories for questions on time to resumption of driving following ICD implantation and/or shock, and strongly urging respondents to complete the questionnaire with a next of kin.

Pre-test: Cognitive interviews

Further examination of content validity and refinement of items was done by cognitive interviewing of 28 ICD patients in the outpatient clinic at all six ICD implanting centres in Denmark (range: 4–6 patients/centre). We chose to include ICD patients from all five regions of Denmark to capture any geographic variance potentially influencing questionnaire responses (Capital Region: 8 participants; Zealand Region: 4 participants; Southern Denmark: 5 participants; Central Jutland: 6 participants; Northern Jutland: 5 participants). On a given day, ICD patients visiting the outpatient clinic were approached in a random manner and were excluded only if they did not have a valid driver's licence at time of ICD implantation. A retrospective verbal probing approach was used, and the probe questions were asked following completion of each of the four sections of the questionnaire. Probes were both scripted (e.g. "What does the term ICD shock mean to you?") and spontaneous (e.g. "I noticed that you hesitated. Can you tell me what you were thinking?"). We utilized Tourangeau's 4-stage cognitive model, investigating: (1) comprehension of the question; (2) retrieval of information (recall strategy); (3) decision processes; and (4) response processes [17]. Another significant focus in these cognitive interviews was recognizing any reluctance in answering questions about adherence to driving restrictions and further, to identify what wording to use to make respondents trust that information on non-adherence would remain anonymous.

Head-investigator (JB) performed all the cognitive interviews over a period of 16 weeks as an iterative process with alterations of the questionnaire items where necessary after each interview session. The initial five rounds of cognitive interviews were conducted using the web-based questionnaire, while the patients in the last round of interviews were presented with the paper format questionnaire. After the cognitive interviews at each implanting centre were completed, JB reviewed and summarized the results and determined whether, for each tested item, significant problems had been detected. Throughout the interviewing process, the frequency of problems encountered per patient interviewed, declined (Additional file 2: Table S2).

Pilot test

The nationwide Danish Pacemaker and ICD registry was used to identify all individuals with a first-time ICD implantation in the period January 1, 2013 to November 30, 2016. Among these, 50 individuals were randomly selected to participate in the pilot test and were subsequently matched with up-to-date address data from the Danish Civil Person Register. Invitations to participate in the study were mailed on February 23, 2017. Participants were urged to complete the web-based questionnaire, however, an option to request a paper version was presented (Additional file 3, translated from Danish). Following 3 weeks, a reminder was mailed to all non-responders including a paper version of the questionnaire and a prepaid return envelope. The web-based questionnaire software SurveyXact, developed by Rambøll A/S and approved for research purposes by the Capital Region of Denmark and the Danish Data Protection Agency, was used for data collection [18]. The pilot test was terminated on April 13, 2017, after 7 weeks' data collection. All paper responses were entered into the web-based questionnaire software by double manual data entry to reduce the consequences of potential human errors.

Test-retest

To investigate the reproducibility of the questionnaire items, we invited the first 25 pilot test participants who responded to the questionnaire to complete the questionnaire again at 3 weeks after their first response. This timeframe was deemed appropriate as to avoid memory effects positively influencing the test-retest reliability. No reminders were distributed to test-retest participants.

Statistical analyses

Results of the pilot test were summarized by reporting responses on selected questionnaire items by available case analysis, thus, the number of responses to each question may vary. For descriptive analyses, categorical variables are reported as percentages and continuous variables are presented as medians with interquartile range. Test-retest agreement was investigated by kappa coefficients or weighted kappa coefficients for categorical variables and intraclass correlation coefficients for continuous variables. All analyses were performed using SAS (version 9.4, Cary, NC, USA).

Results

Focus group interviews

All concepts already identified from the literature were confirmed in the focus groups interviews, excluding the effect of driving restrictions on self-esteem. In addition, we discovered that many of the participants had changed their driving behaviour in some way after ICD implantation: For example, some patients reported being extra cautious when driving with children (e.g. driving at slower speed, avoiding the overtaking lane on highways) or avoiding highways altogether. Also, a significant proportion of primary prevention patients called for more information about potential driving restrictions in case of future ICD therapy and also being explained the rationale behind the driving restrictions, as they saw these as promoting factors for compliance with the restrictions. Generally, in an anonymous setting, the participants willingly volunteered information about not adhering to the driving restrictions.

Pilot test

Among the 50 ICD patients (9 women (18%)) invited to participate in the pilot test, 30 (60%) either responded electronically or requested a paper version of the questionnaire within 3 weeks. Following only one reminder, 39 participants (78%) completed the questionnaire (Fig. 2). Almost all web-based responses (85%) came within 1 week. Median time for completing the

questionnaire was 9.5 min for the web-based responses (IQR: 5.2–13.7 min).

Of the responders, 37 (97%) held a valid private driver's license for car, motorcycle or tractor (Group 1 drivers) prior to implantation and 11 (30%) held a valid driver's license for large vehicles or any professional driving (Group 2 drivers) (Fig. 3). However, only two responders had actively used their professional license during the 6 months prior to ICD implantation – both were truck drivers. The most common occasions (> 75%) for driving prior to ICD implantation included practical errands, visits to family and friends and in relation with leisure activities, while eight (22%) drove during work hours (Table 1).

Only half of the respondents remembered being informed of any driving restrictions for private driving. Of these, two thirds reported they had solely been informed verbally (Table 2). The information given by health personnel on driving following implantation as recalled by the patients ranged from resuming to drive immediately after ICD implantation to never to drive again. Still, patients were overall satisfied with the communication of the driving restrictions. Among the responders actively driving professionally prior to ICD implantation, only one (50%) could remember being told never to drive professionally again. Of the ICD patients having experienced an appropriate ICD shock, three out of four remembered having been verbally informed not to drive for 3 months.

Following ICD implantation, 35 (95%) of responders with a driver's license resumed private driving whereas professional driving was resumed by one responder (Fig. 3). Overall median time to resumption of driving was 14 days (interquartile range: 2–60) while professional

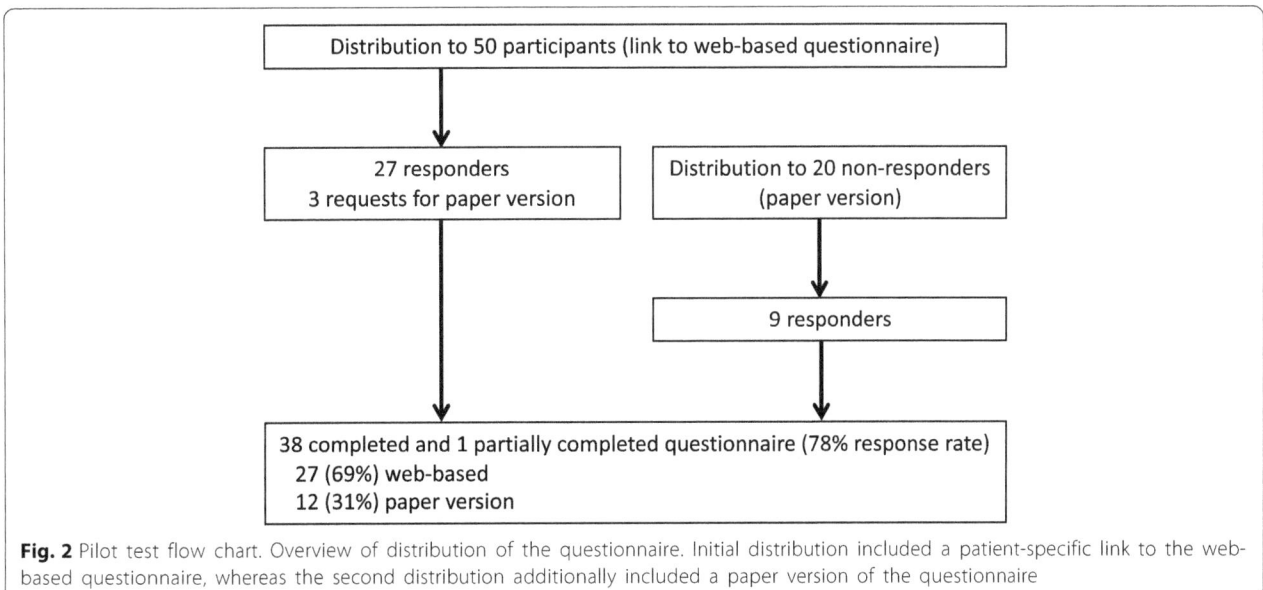

Fig. 2 Pilot test flow chart. Overview of distribution of the questionnaire. Initial distribution included a patient-specific link to the web-based questionnaire, whereas the second distribution additionally included a paper version of the questionnaire

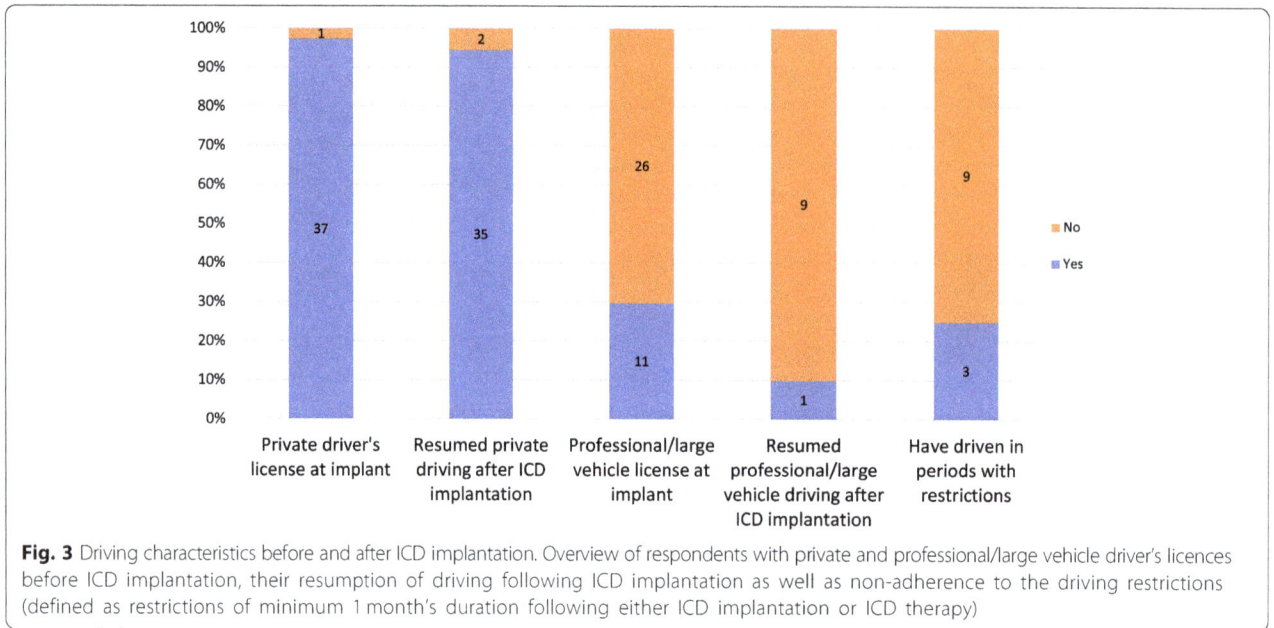

Fig. 3 Driving characteristics before and after ICD implantation. Overview of respondents with private and professional/large vehicle driver's licences before ICD implantation, their resumption of driving following ICD implantation as well as non-adherence to the driving restrictions (defined as restrictions of minimum 1 month's duration following either ICD implantation or ICD therapy)

Table 1 Driving characteristics before ICD implantation

Driving characteristics	No. of patients (%)
Private driver's license ($n = 38$)	37 (97%)
Professional/large vehicle driver's license ($n = 37$)	11 (30%)
Purpose of professional/large vehicle driver's licence ($n = 10$)	
Truck driver	4 (40%)
Bus driver	2 (20%)
Taxi driver	0
Other, including private use	4 (40%)
Use of professional/large vehicle driver's licence six months prior to implantation ($n = 10$)	2 (20%)
Other members of the household hold driver's license ($n = 37$)	26 (70%)
Typical occasions for driving six months prior to implantation ($n = 37$)	
Professional driving or driving of large vehicle during work hours	2 (5%)
During work hours	8 (22%)
To/from work/school	16 (43%)
In relation with practical errands	31 (84%)
To visit family and friends	33 (89%)
In relation with leisure activities	28 (76%)
Did not drive during the period	2 (5%)
Average hours/week driving prior to implantation ($n = 35$)	
< 1 h a week	0
1–3 h a week	12 (34%)
4–6 h a week	7 (20%)
7–9 h a week	7 (20%)
10 h a week or more	9 (26%)

driving was resumed at 8 months. Among patients being instructed of a minimum 1-month driving ban, either after ICD implantation or ICD shock, three patients (25%) admitted they had been driving although restricted. None had experienced an ICD shock or loss of consciousness while

Table 2 Information on driving restrictions following ICD implantation, as reported by patients

Variable	No. of patients (%)
Informed about driving restrictions ($n = 37$)	
Yes	18 (49%)
No	7 (19%)
Cannot remember	12 (32%)
Way information was given ($n = 18$)	
Only verbally	12 (67%)
Only in writing	–
Both verbally and in writing	6 (33%)
Information given ($n = 18$)	
Resume driving immediately	1 (6%)
Resume when I felt ready	1 (6%)
Resume after 1 week	4 (22%)
Resume after 1 month	3 (17%)
Resume after 3 months	8 (44%)
Resume after 6 months	–
Never to drive again	1 (6%)
Level of satisfaction with information given ($n = 18$)	
Very satisfied or satisfied	14 (78%)
Neutral	4 (22%)
Dissatisfied or very dissatisfied	–

driving, but two patients (6%) had experienced dizziness and four patients (11%) had experienced palpitations while driving. None of these events necessitated stopping the vehicle or resulted in a motor vehicle accident.

Overall, patients had not altered their driving behaviour after ICD implantation. Only four patients (12%) were afraid of having an ICD shock while driving, and only one patient was nervous about driving or tried to avoid highways as a consequence of ICD implantation. None avoided driving alone or driving with children in the car. Among the 11 patients with a significant driving restriction (defined as ≥1 month), six (55%) stated that the driving restrictions in some way had impeded with their daily life and 45 and 33% responded that they had been very limited in maintaining employment and getting to/from work, respectively.

Test-retest
Of the 25 responders invited to participate in a test-retest questionnaire, 19 (75%) responded within 3 weeks. Kappa statistics found that 69% of the analyzed questionnaire items had substantial agreement, with kappas or weighted kappas above 0.6, whereof 37.5% were above 0.8. (Additional file 4: Table S3). Generally, the kappas with moderate (0.4–0.6) and fair agreement (0.2–0.4) were found in the section on the driving restrictions' influence on factors associated with QoL. In one item, the only test-retest response was reverse, rendering a kappa of 0. The intraclass correlation coefficient for time to resumption of private driving following ICD implantation and appropriate ICD shock was 0.98 and 1.00, respectively, whereas the time to resumption of professional driving could not be analyzed as the item only had one test-retest response.

Discussion
Through a thorough developmental and testing process, we have constructed a questionnaire aimed to investigate ICD patients' perspective on driving, including the information received on driving following ICD implantation and/or ICD shock, adherence to the driving restrictions, episodes of cardiac symptoms while driving, the driving restrictions' influence on factors associated with QoL, and alterations of driving behaviour after ICD implantation. The pilot test administered to 50 randomly selected Danish ICD patients achieved a response rate of 78% over seven-week period with only one reminder. The high response rate confirms our understanding that this is an area of great importance to ICD patients and furthermore implies a high level of target population comprehension of the developed questionnaire.

Our pilot test results support previous research reporting poor communication between health professionals and ICD patients on the subject of driving [7, 9, 19]: 20% reported they had not received any information on driving restrictions after ICD implantation. However, in the final questionnaire it will be important to stratify these data on both ICD indication, as well as time since ICD implantation to account for time as a recall bias. In fact, 30% of responders reported they could not remember if they had been informed on any driving restrictions. Nevertheless, given that professional guidelines recommend driving restrictions after ICD implantation and ICD therapy, it is pivotal for patient compliance that these restrictions are communicated to the patients. A recent study found that a systematic counselling program before patient discharge had a positive impact on both patient compliance with treatment, as well as patient QoL [20]. Similar effects could be anticipated in terms of compliance with driving restrictions and our results will quantify the need for potential improvements in this area.

In the focus group interviews, some primary prevention ICD patients called for information at the time of ICD implantation on potential driving restrictions in case of future ICD shocks. However, to reduce respondent burden and because we considered the concepts would be more suitable for investigation in a qualitative method, we chose not to include these concepts in the final questionnaire.

Previous studies suggest many ICD patients resume driving earlier than instructed [7, 8, 10, 11]. Prior to developing the questionnaire, we had concerns regarding the patients' willingness to answer questions on sensitive matters such as non-adherence to driving restrictions. However, throughout the developmental process including both focus group and cognitive interviews, we found that this was not a substantial problem. Following recommendations from pre-test participants, we included multiple statements affirming that information would not be forwarded to the authorities. In the pilot test, 25% of responders with a significant driving ban admitted they had been driving while restricted. This is comparable to previously published results [8], thus, we feel assured that respondents not answering truthfully is not a major issue. To capture both ICD patients knowingly and unknowingly driving during the guideline-recommended restricted period, we also included questions about time to resumption of both private and professional driving after ICD implantation, as well as after ICD shock. For example, one Group 2 driver who believed he had not received information on restrictions for professional driving, stated that this had been resumed 8 months following implantation.

This questionnaire was not designed to measure overall QoL in an ICD population, but rather to investigate if the driving restrictions themselves had influenced factors associated with QoL. Particularly, the risk of losing the ability to earn an income as a professional driver has not been systematically investigated previously. Thus, we included a separate question to professional drivers on whether they had lost their job as a result of the driving restrictions. In the small pilot test sample, this was not the case for any of the two truck drivers. However, more than half of the respondents with a driving restriction longer than 1 month said the restrictions had impeded with their daily life, specifically maintaining employment and getting to/from work. Thus, the driving restrictions can definitely temporarily restrict ICD patients' ability to work and thus affect their household economic status, even if they are not professional drivers.

Focus groups revealed that some ICD patients alter their driving behaviour because of ICD implantation in other aspects than quantity of time spent driving. Consequently, we chose to include questions on this specific aim in the questionnaire. However, in the small pilot sample, only 12% expressed concerns about having an ICD shock while driving and only one respondent expressed avoidance behaviour with regards to driving on highways. By linking the final questionnaire with the ICD registry, the future results of the questionnaire can relevantly be stratified by ICD indication as well as history of ICD shocks.

The pilot test achieved a response rate of 78%, and impressively, more than two-thirds of the responses were web-based. This number was higher than anticipated in a population with a mean age around 62 years [21], and decreased the investigator's risk of making typing mistakes as well as the burden of manually entering paper responses into the web-based questionnaire database. Further, web-based questionnaires in general reduce respondent burden as the completed questionnaires do not need to be mailed. To capture a wide range of the target population and not exclude individuals with limited computer skills, we chose to move forward with both modalities of data collection.

Test-retest found almost perfect agreement in nearly 40% of the items and substantial agreement in 31% of all items [22]. The generally high reliability indicates that, despite the high mean age and disease burden in the population, the responses produced by the questionnaire are representative and stable over time. However, the limit for when kappa statistics are in sufficient agreement are both subjective and arbitrary, and furthermore, our small sample of 19 test-retest respondents should be considered. Besides, due to the branching of the questionnaire, we were unable to retest all items regarding rare events, for example the items on cardiac symptoms while driving.

Study limitations and future perspectives

Questionnaire studies pose some significant inherent limitations. Many relate to poor question design (e.g. problems with wording, leading questions, scale formats) or questionnaire design (e.g. formatting problems, too long or complex questionnaire) which we have tried to overcome by thorough pre-testing, but some questions will inevitably be misinterpreted. Moreover, though the focus group participants were generally good at recalling specific information from the time of ICD implantation, recall bias cannot be excluded. Also, social desirability may contribute to respondents giving untrue answers, particularly to the questions related to adherence, although focus group and cognitive interviews demonstrated the contrary. Lastly, we naturally only included patients who were alive at the time of questionnaire administration, introducing a healthy participant bias which, similarly to the non-response bias, covers the fact that responders (or survivors) could differ significantly from the non-responders.

The questionnaire was developed specifically for use in a nationwide cohort of Danish ICD patients and the final questionnaire has been administered to more than 3900 individuals. Due to the unique Danish administrative registries, we will be able to link the final questionnaire results with reliable clinical and demographic information, including indication for ICD implantation, socioeconomic status, and comorbidities. Importantly, linkage with the nationwide registries also allows comparison between responders and non-responders, a major strength in a questionnaire study.

In this pilot study, however, the results have not been linked with relevant clinical data and we were therefore not able to stratify results on important clinical information such as cardiac resynchronization status, pharmacological treatment and comorbidities such as diabetes. All of these will be relevant to include in the final questionnaire study when investigating factors associated with the risk of ICD therapy while driving, as they have been found to affect the risk of adverse clinical outcomes, including ICD therapy [21, 23–25]. Other limitations of the current study include lack of information on heart failure biomarker levels and home monitoring status which are also expected to affect clinical outcomes, especially in primary prevention patients with a cardiac resynchronization device [26–28].

Conclusion

In summary, we have developed a comprehensive questionnaire on the patient's perspective on driving and driving restrictions following ICD implantation, with good content validity and acceptable patient and investigator burden. From pilot test results, we anticipate that the final questionnaire, distributed to > 3900 ICD patients, will very likely reach a response rate above 60% and provide much-needed data about information on, adherence to and impact of driving restrictions in a large, nationwide, contemporary cohort of ICD patients. We believe these results will be valuable and potentially identify problematic areas in need of further focus or interventions.

Additional files

> **Additional file 1: Table S1.** Questionnaire Conceptualization Process: The research aims, hypotheses, concepts and corresponding variable definitions [7–12, 19, 29–33]. (DOCX 90 kb)
>
> **Additional file 2: Table S2.** Frequency of Problems Identified During Cognitive Interview Sessions. (DOCX 16 kb)
>
> **Additional file 3:** "Danish ICD Patients' Perspective on Driving – a Nationwide Survey. 2017". English version (translated from Danish) of the questionnaire specifically constructed for this research project. (PDF 927 kb)
>
> **Additional file 4: Table S3.** Test-Retest Agreement. (DOCX 19 kb)

Abbreviations
ICD: Implantable Cardioverter Defibrillator; QoL: Quality of Life

Acknowledgements
The authors are particularly grateful to all the ICD patients participating in the development of the questionnaire in either focus group interviews, cognitive interviews or the pilot test. Also, the authors would like to thank the ICD technicians and nurses at the six Danish implanting centres for valuable assistance in recruiting participants, particularly chief technician Jeanne Dahl Priess at the Pacemaker Outpatient Clinic, Copenhagen University Hospital Herlev and Gentofte who also provided valuable expert insights in the pre-testing phase. Lastly, the authors would like to thank cardiology fellows Lærke Smedegaard and Jannik Pallisgaard as well as senior questionnaire expert Jens Christiansen for participating in pre-test reviewing.

Funding
This work was supported by independent research grants from the Danish Heart Foundation (grant no. R107-A6633-B2258), The Arvid Nilsson Foundation and Eva & Henry Fraenkels Mindefond. None of the sponsors had any influence on the design, analysis or reporting of the study.

Authors' contributions
JB drafted the manuscript and was involved in study conception and design, data collection, analysis and interpretation of the data, and editing of the manuscript. SHR was involved in study conception and design, data collection and transcription, and editing of the manuscript. AM was involved in data collection, analysis and interpretation of the data, and editing of the manuscript. MS, CJ and GG were involved in study conception and design, and editing of the manuscript. AHR was involved in study conception, analysis and interpretation of the data, and design and editing of the manuscript. All authors have read and approved the final manuscript.

Ethics approval and consent to participate
The questionnaire study was reported to the Ethics Committee in the Capital Region of Denmark, which concluded that no ethical approval was needed (reference number: H-17002489). The study was approved by the Danish Data Protection Agency (J. no. 2007-58-0015; Local j. no. GEH-2014-013; I-suite no. 0273) and approval to obtain current addresses on the target population was granted by the Danish Health Data Authority (FSEID-2420). All participants in focus group interviews, cognitive interviews and pilot test were informed about the aim of the study and were assured that participation was voluntary, and the results would remain anonymous. We obtained written consent from all focus group participants and oral consent from all cognitive interview participants. Pilot test participants were informed that responding to the questionnaire would be considered providing consent.

Competing interests
The authors declare that they have no competing interests.

Author details
[1]Department of Cardiology, Cardiovascular Research, Copenhagen University Hospital Herlev-Gentofte, Kildegaardsvej 28, 2900 Hellerup, Denmark. [2]Research and Test Center for Health Technologies, Copenhagen University Hospital, Rigshospitalet-Glostrup, Valdemar Hansens Vej 1-23, 2600 Glostrup, Denmark. [3]Department of Cardiology, Copenhagen University Hospital Rigshospitalet-Glostrup, Blegdamsvej 9, 2100 Copenhagen Ø, Denmark. [4]Department of Medicine, Zealand University Hospital, Sygehusvej 10, 4000 Roskilde, Denmark.

References
1. Connolly SJ, Hallstrom AP, Cappato R, Schron EB, Kuck KH, Zipes DP, Greene HL, Boczor S, Domanski M, Follmann D, et al. Meta-analysis of the implantable cardioverter defibrillator secondary prevention trials. AVID, CASH and CIDS studies. Antiarrhythmics vs implantable defibrillator study. Cardiac arrest study Hamburg . Canadian implantable defibrillator study. Eur Heart J. 2000;21(24):2071–8.
2. Moss AJ, Zareba W, Hall WJ, Klein H, Wilber DJ, Cannom DS, Daubert JP, Higgins SL, Brown MW, Andrews ML. Prophylactic implantation of a defibrillator in patients with myocardial infarction and reduced ejection fraction. N Engl J Med. 2002;346(12):877–83.
3. Bardy GH, Lee KL, Mark DB, Poole JE, Packer DL, Boineau R, Domanski M, Troutman C, Anderson J, Johnson G, et al. Amiodarone or an implantable cardioverter-defibrillator for congestive heart failure. N Engl J Med. 2005; 352(3):225–37.
4. Epstein AE, Baessler CA, Curtis AB, Estes NA 3rd, Gersh BJ, Grubb B, Mitchell LB, American Heart A, Heart Rhythm S. Addendum to "personal and public safety issues related to arrhythmias that may affect consciousness: implications for regulation and physician recommendations: a medical/scientific statement from the American Heart Association and the north American Society of Pacing and Electrophysiology": public safety issues in patients with implantable defibrillators: a scientific statement from the American Heart Association and the Heart Rhythm Society. Circulation. 2007;115(9):1170–6.
5. Vijgen J, Botto G, Camm J, Hoijer CJ, Jung W, Le Heuzey JY, Lubinski A, Norekval TM, Santomauro M, Schalij M, et al. Consensus statement of the European heart rhythm association: updated recommendations for driving by patients with implantable cardioverter defibrillators. Europace. 2009;11(8):1097–107.
6. Dansk Cardiologisk Selskab. Retningslinjer for udstedelse af kørekort hos patienter med hjertelidelser. 2nd ed; 2012. p. 13–4.
7. Conti JB, Woodard DA, Tucker KJ, Bryant B, King LC, Curtis AB. Modification of patient driving behavior after implantation of a cardioverter defibrillator. Pacing Clin Electrophysiol. 1997;20(9 Pt 1):2200–4.
8. Mylotte D, Sheahan RG, Nolan PG, Neylon MA, McArdle B, Constant O, Diffley A, Keane D, Nash PJ, Crowley J, et al. The implantable defibrillator and return to operation of vehicles study. Europace. 2013;15(2):212–8.
9. Akiyama T, Powell JL, Mitchell LB, Ehlert FA, Baessler C. Resumption of driving after life-threatening ventricular tachyarrhythmia. N Engl J Med. 2001;345(6):391–7.
10. Craney JM, Powers MT. Factors related to driving in persons with an implantable cardioverter defibrillator. Prog Cardiovasc Nurs. 1995;10(3):12–7.
11. Finch NJ, Leman RB, Kratz JM, Gillette PC. Driving safety among patients with automatic implantable cardioverter defibrillators. Jama. 1993;270(13):1587–8.

12. James J, Albarran JW, Tagney J. The experiences of ICD patients and their partners with regards to adjusting to an imposed driving ban: a qualitative study. Coron Health Care. 2001;5(2):80–8.

13. Reeve BB, Wyrwich KW, Wu AW, Velikova G, Terwee CB, Snyder CF, Schwartz C, Revicki DA, Moinpour CM, McLeod LD, et al. ISOQOL recommends minimum standards for patient-reported outcome measures used in patient-centered outcomes and comparative effectiveness research. Qual Life Res. 2013;22(8):1889–905.

14. Division of Mental Health and Prevention of Substance Abuse. World Health Organization: WHOQOL Measuring Quality of Life; 1997. p. 1–13.

15. Mason J. Qualitative researching. 2nd ed. Thousand Oaks, CA: SAGE; 2002.

16. Likert R. A technique for the measurement of attitudes. Arch Psychology. 1932;140:1–55.

17. Tourangeau R. Cognitive science and survey methods: A cognitive perspective. In: Jabine T, Straf M, Tanur J, Tourangeau R, editors. Cognitive aspects of survey methodology: Building a bridge between disciplines. Washington D.C: National Academy Press; 1984. p. 73–100.

18. Rambøll A/S: SurveyXact by Ramboll [https://www.surveyxact.com]. Accessed May 30 2018.

19. Baessler C, Murphy S, Gebhardt L, Tso T, Ellenbogen K, Leman R. Time to resumption of driving after implantation of an automatic defibrillator (from the dual chamber and VVI implantable defibrillator [DAVID] trial). Am J Cardiol. 2005;95(5):665–6.

20. Biscaglia S, Tonet E, Pavasini R, Serenelli M, Bugani G, Cimaglia P, Gallo F, Spitaleri G, Del Franco A, Aquila G, et al. A counseling program on nuisance bleeding improves quality of life in patients on dual antiplatelet therapy: a randomized controlled trial. PLoS One. 2017;12(8):e0182124.

21. Ruwald AC, Vinther M, Gislason GH, Johansen JB, Nielsen JC, Petersen HH, Riahi S, Jons C. The impact of co-morbidity burden on appropriate implantable cardioverter defibrillator therapy and all-cause mortality: insight from Danish nationwide clinical registers. Eur J Heart Fail. 2017;19(3):377–86.

22. Landis JR, Koch GG. The measurement of observer agreement for categorical data. Biometrics. 1977;33(1):159–74.

23. Moss AJ, Hall WJ, Cannom DS, Klein H, Brown MW, Daubert JP, Estes NA 3rd, Foster E, Greenberg H, Higgins SL, et al. Cardiac-resynchronization therapy for the prevention of heart-failure events. N Engl J Med. 2009; 361(14):1329–38.

24. Sardu C, Santamaria M, Funaro S, Sacra C, Barbieri M, Paolisso P, Marfella R, Paolisso G, Rizzo MR. Cardiac electrophysiological alterations and clinical response in cardiac resynchronization therapy with a defibrillator treated patients affected by metabolic syndrome. Medicine (Baltimore). 2017;96(14):e6558.

25. Ruwald AC, Gislason GH, Vinther M, Johansen JB, Nielsen JC, Philbert BT, Torp-Pedersen C, Riahi S, Jons C. Importance of beta-blocker dose in prevention of ventricular tachyarrhythmias, heart failure hospitalizations, and death in primary prevention implantable cardioverter-defibrillator recipients: a Danish nationwide cohort study. Europace. 2018;20(Fi2):f217–24.

26. Sardu C, Marfella R, Santamaria M, Papini S, Parisi Q, Sacra C, Colaprete D, Paolisso G, Rizzo MR, Barbieri M. Stretch, injury and inflammation markers evaluation to predict clinical outcomes after implantable cardioverter defibrillator therapy in heart failure patients with metabolic syndrome. Front Physiol. 2018;9:758.

27. Hindricks G, Taborsky M, Glikson M, Heinrich U, Schumacher B, Katz A, Brachmann J, Lewalter T, Goette A, Block M, et al. Implant-based multiparameter telemonitoring of patients with heart failure (IN-TIME): a randomised controlled trial. Lancet. 2014;384(9943):583–90.

28. Sardu C, Santamaria M, Rizzo MR, Barbieri M, di Marino M, Paolisso G, Santulli G, Marfella R. Telemonitoring in heart failure patients treated by cardiac resynchronisation therapy with defibrillator (CRT-D): the TELECART study. Int J Clin Pract. 2016;70(7):569–76.

29. Johansson I, Stromberg A. Experiences of driving and driving restrictions in recipients with an implantable cardioverter defibrillator--the patient perspective. J Cardiovasc Nurs. 2010;25(6):E1–e10.

30. Tagney J, James JE, Albarran JW. Exploring the patient's experiences of learning to live with an implantable cardioverter defibrillator (ICD) from one UK centre: a qualitative study. Eur J Cardiovasc Nurs. 2003;2(3):195–203.

31. Curtis AB, Conti JB, Tucker KJ, Kubilis PS, Reilly RE, Woodard DA. Motor vehicle accidents in patients with an implantable cardioverter-defibrillator. J Am Coll Cardiol. 1995;26(1):180–4.

32. Trappe HJ, Wenzlaff P, Grellman G. Should patients with implantable cardioverter-defibrillators be allowed to drive? Observations in 291 patients from a single center over an 11-year period. J Interv Card Electrophysiol. 1998;2(2):193–201.

33. Ruwald MH, Okumura K, Kimura T, Aonuma K, Shoda M, Kutyifa V, Ruwald AC, McNitt S, Zareba W, Moss AJ. Syncope in high-risk cardiomyopathy patients with implantable defibrillators: frequency, risk factors, mechanisms, and association with mortality: results from the multicenter automatic defibrillator implantation trial-reduce inappropriate therapy (MADIT-RIT) study. Circulation. 2014;129(5):545–52.

19

Lipomatous hypertrophy of the atrial septum – a benign heart anomaly causing unexpected surgical problems

Grzegorz Bielicki[1], Marceli Lukaszewski[2]* ⓘ, Kinga Kosiorowska[1], Jacek Jakubaszko[1], Rafal Nowicki[1] and Marek Jasinski[1,2]

Abstract

Background: Lipomatous hypertrophy of the atrial septum (LHAS) is an anomaly of the heart. It is characterized by an infiltration of adipocytes into myocytes of the interatrial septum, sparing the fossa ovalis, which gives a characteristic hourglass-shaped image. Due to the progress in imaging techniques, it can be recognized more frequently, but it is still often misdiagnosed.

Case presentation: We present a case of 65-year-old woman with an incidentally discovered lipomatous hypertrophy of the atrial septum during cardiac surgery, which has caused the technical problems for surgeons with bicaval cannulation and visualization of the operated structures of the heart. Due to the unclear shadow in the lung parenchyma, the patient had preoperative computed tomography (CT) done, but the study report focused only on the lung description, neglecting visible changes in the structure of the heart. Based on the standardly performed intra-operative transesophageal echocardiography (TEE), as well as by analyzing the chest X-ray and CT scans, the diagnosis of LHAS was made. It allowed the surgeon to leave the mass intact, thus not increasing the risk of the baseline surgery.

Conclusions: LHAS is a rare but increasingly recognized anomaly of the heart. Contemporary diagnostic methods allow to diagnose and make the right therapeutic decisions. The utility of TEE and analysis of X-ray images, in this case, allowed the surgeon to recognize LHAS, and because of its histologically benign nature and asymptomatic course, to leave this change intact. Surgical treatment should be limited only to cases of patients with life-threatening cardiovascular complications.

Keywords: Lipomatous hypertrophy, Interatrial septum, TEE, Computered tomography

Background

Heart tumors are often underestimated by professionals in the field. Being relatively rare, secondary neoplasms are mostly the result of advanced malignant melanoma, lymphoma, and leukemia. Benign tumors such as myxomas, lipomas, papillary fibroelastomas, angiomas, and fibromas represent about 75% of primary cardiac tumors [1, 2]. A separate non-neoplastic benign cardiac lesion, that may be mistaken for various heart tumors, is lipomatous hypertrophy of the atrial septum (LHAS), first described by Prior in 1964, based on autopsy study [3]. The etiology of LHAS has not been recognized. It is presumed that due to the involvement of embryonic mesenchymal cells in the primary formation of atria, the atrial septum cells may differentiate into adipocytes with appropriate stimuli [4]. In the histological image analysys, no mitoses are observed, hence the change does not represent a malignancy [5]. Morphologically, it is presented as a non-encapsulated excessive epicardial fat deposition in the septum secundum, that infiltrates the area of the interatrial septum that spares the fossa ovalis

* Correspondence: marceliluk@gmail.com
[2]Department of Anaesthesiology and Intensive Therapy, Wroclaw Medical University, Borowska 213, 50-556 Wroclaw, Wroclaw, Poland
Full list of author information is available at the end of the article

[6]. The thickness of the septum can reach 20 mm and more [7]. Accumulation of adipose tissue can also be observed in subepicardium, crista terminalis, endocardium, and mediastinum. In differential diagnostics, it is required to take into account possible adipose tissue neoplasms. Unlike LHAS, lipomas are encapsulated, round, homogeneous and do not infiltrate myocardium fibers. Lipomatous hypertrophy is associated with obesity and is seen more frequently in elderly and female patients [8, 9]. Development of imaging techniques has enabled more frequent recognition of usual asymptomatic masses [10]. In a prospective study using computed tomography, lipomatous hypertrophy was identified in 2.2% of the patients [11]. Extremely rare infiltration of adipocytes, causing distortion of the septum, may pose life-threatening cardiovascular complications requiring urgent cardiac surgery intervention [12]. The rare complications of LHAS include superior vena cava syndrome, severe cardiac arrhythmias (sick sinus syndrome, arrhythmias, changes in P waveform morphology in ECG), pericardial effusion, heart failure and sudden cardiac death [13, 14]. However, the majority of cases are clinically silent and are detected accidentally during routine chest X-ray, echocardiography, surgery or autopsy [15].

Case presentation

We present a case of a 65-year-old female patient admitted to the Cardiac Surgery Department in Wroclaw in January 2018 with severe mitral regurgitation (MR) and the history of ischemic heart disease, after elective percutaneous coronary intervention of the circumflex branch of left coronary artery with two drug-eluting stents (DES) implantation 4 years earlier. Furthermore, the patient diagnosed with many chronic conditions, such as metabolic syndrome, obesity with BMI 33 and gastroesophageal reflux disease. Currently, with an exercise dyspnoea for about 2 years, intensifying in recent weeks, she was hospitalized in the Cardiology Department for further diagnostics. The transthoracic echocardiography (TTE) revealed non dilated left ventricle with a normal systolic ejection fraction of 60%, and no evidence of segmental wall motion abnormalities, severe MR with the prolapse of the A2 segment and systolic restriction of the posterior leaflet. Colour Doppler showed a highly distinctive eccentric turbulent jet directed towards the lateral wall and the base of the left atrium with ERO 0.6cm^2 and regurgitant volume of 60 ml. Additionally, in the performed coronary angiography, hemodynamically significant narrowing was found in the area of the previously implanted DES. The patient was then consulted by the cardiac surgeon and qualified for surgery. After admission to the Cardiac Surgery Department, as part of the pre-operative preparation, TTE was again performed, in which the severe MR was confirmed and no pathological structures in

the right atrium were described. Due to the unclear image in the right pulmonary field, described by the radiologist in the chest X-ray (Fig. 1), diagnostics was extended by performing a computed tomography of the chest, which excluded the presence of pathological shadow in the lung parenchyma. There was no referral to the atrial septum in the CT report. The patient was scheduled for mitral valve repair surgery and coronary artery bypass grafting (CABG) with the use of saphenous vein graft to the circumflex artery. During the standard procedure of commencing the cardiopulmonary bypass (CPB) and bicaval cannulation, it was found difficult to insert the cannulas from the atrium into both vena cavas. Therefore the cannulation was performed using the smaller cannula sizes, which eventually allowed to go on bypass. On the free wall of the atrial septum, there was a thickening and an excess of adipose tissue with a firm consistency and the size of a walnut, significantly impeding access to the operated mitral valve through the left atrium, and probably completely preventing surgery by the transseptal approach. In the transesophageal echocardiography (TEE), a characteristic image of LHAS was confirmed by the presence of hypertrophy of the septum, up to 2.7 cm, an hourglass shape with a characteristic indentation at the place of the fossa ovalis (Figs. 2 and 3). Based on the intra-operative TEE, as well as by analyzing the chest X-ray and CT scans, the diagnosis of LHAS was made. Due to the asymptomatic course of the LHAS and the complexity of the scheduled operation, the decision was made to leave the change intact. The mitral valve was replaced through the left atrial approach. The surgery was completed in a standard manner and the weaning from the CBP went uneventfully. The patient's early postoperative period was a routine.

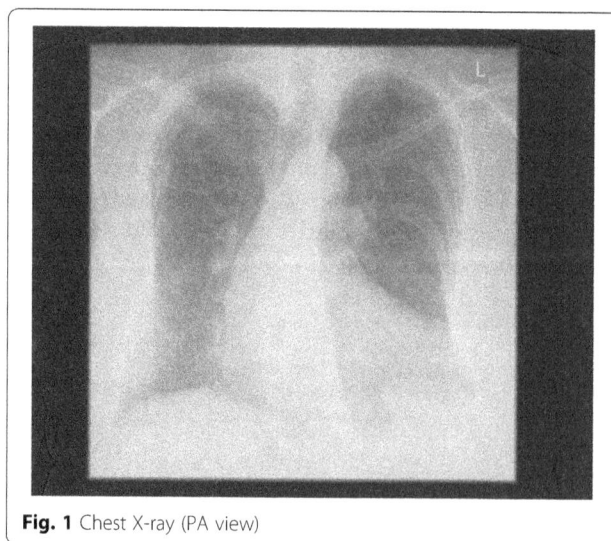

Fig. 1 Chest X-ray (PA view)

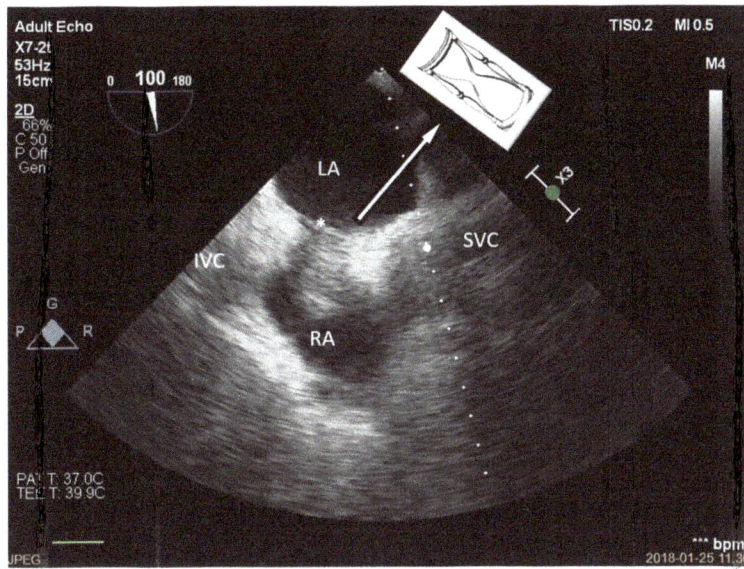

Fig. 2 TEE. ME view at the level of fossa ovalis (*) demonstrates lipomatous tissue, with a characteristic hourglass (dumbbell) shape, infiltrating the septum between the right (RA) and left atria (LA) with sparing of the fossa ovalis. The change is located very close to the ostium of the inferior vena cava (IVC)

Discussion and conclusions

Lipomatous hypertrophy of the atrial septum is a rare but increasingly recognized non-neoplastic benign abnormality of the heart. Since the first mention in literature in 1964, fewer than 300 cases of LHAS have been described, most of which were based on autopsy studies. Lipomatous lesion derives entirely from the upper and/or lower part of the atrial septum, typically sparing the fossa ovalis, giving a characteristic, considered by some to be pathognomonic, an hourglass-shaped image, with a tendency to bulge into the right atrium, which may be related with a thickening of crista terminalis (Fig. 3). The first descriptions of LHAS in vivo were made on the basis of echocardiography, and in 1983 Fyke et al. published the first diagnostic guidelines [16]. Currently, TTE, TEE, CT (preferred multislice CT - MSCT) and MRI are used for diagnostics. Transthoracic echocardiography, usually performed first, is not a

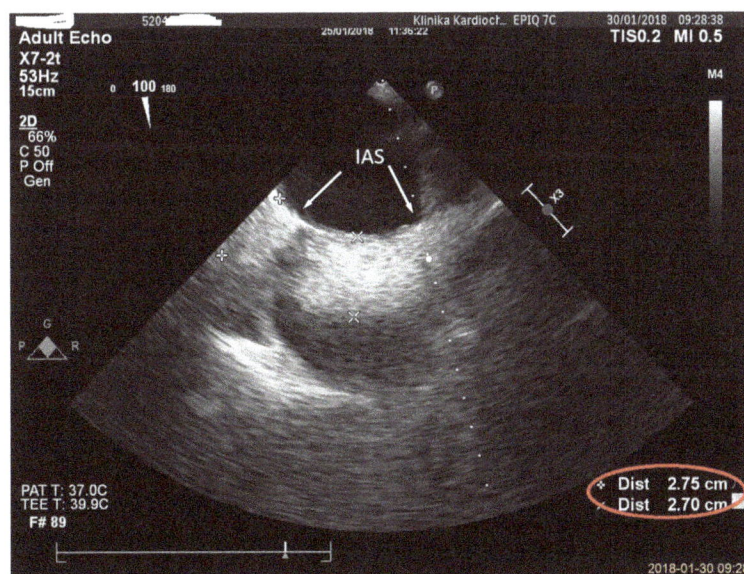

Fig. 3 TEE. ME view demonstrates clearly visible boundaries of the interatrial septum (IAS) with intense hyperechogenic, measuring 2.75 cm and 2.7 cm, lipomatous tissue, respecting the fossa ovalis

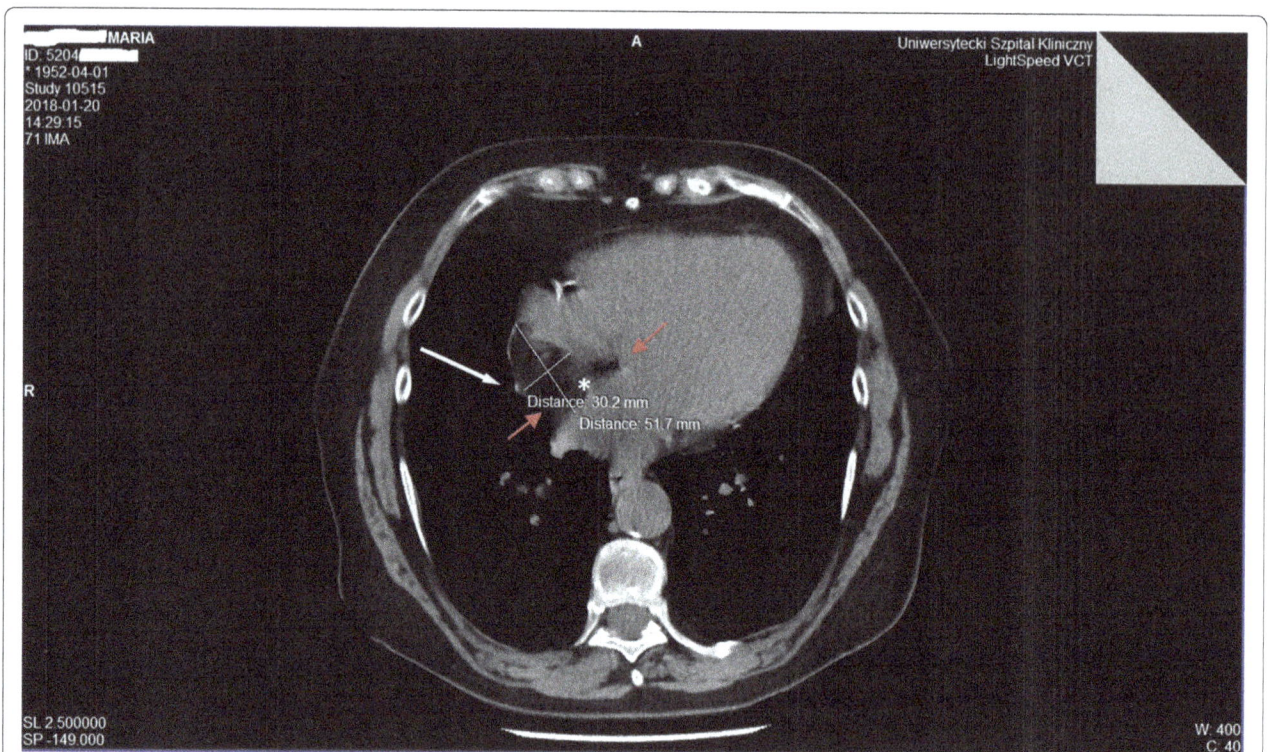

Fig. 4 CT scan. Visible lipomatous tissue surrounding the fossa ovalis (*) with the characteristic hourglass shape (between the red arrows). The marked mass, measuring 30.2 mm × 51.7 mm, extends to the back wall of the right atrium (RA) and crista terminalis (white arrow)

very accurate diagnostic tool with limited imaging of the heart structures, however, transesophageal examination (TEE) is much more precise and shows the pathological mass quite well. CT scans enable the visualization of adipose tissue. Lipomatous changes also demonstrate minimal contrast enhancement, which allows us to exclude the other suspected pathologies. The typical localization, shape, and image, including the density of changes in CT, allows to differentiate LHAS from heart tumors and make a diagnosis without first confirming in histopathological examination [8, 17]. The actual incidence of LHAS in the population is not known. This is due to its asymptomatic course, and the lack of well-targeted diagnostics. Previously described in the literature cases were based on autopsy, surgery and clinical imaging incidental findings or were associated with the symptomatic course of the disease. Among the rare risk factors of LHAS are emphysema with steroid therapy, in which the predisposition to the mediastinal and intracardiac deposition of adipose tissue is observed, cereberotendinous xantomatosis, mediastino-abdominal lipomatosis and long-term parenteral nutrition [1, 11]. Arrhythmia, rarely associated with LHAS, was first observed in 1969 by Kluge [18]. The mechanism of its formation has not been explained, however, it seems to be related with the infiltration of adipocytes interfering with the structure of

the atrial myocytes, and thus the normal conduction pathways are interrupted [11, 19]. Arrhythmia manifests mainly in atrial fibrillation, atrial premature complexes, supraventricular arrhythmias, ectopic and junctional rhythm. It is also presumed that the incidence of atrial arrhythmia is related to septal thickness [20]. Dickerson et al. presented a case of the patient with symptomatic LHAS who had atrial flutter, and following complete resection of the lesion, the symptoms completely resolved [21]. The mechanism in which the removal of LHAS resulted in the return of the sinus rhythm is unclear, although the authors speculate that the area of arrhythmogenic foci involved the right atrial wall with the crista terminalis, and as a result of resection, the pathological path between the superior vena cava (SVC) and the right atrium was discontinued, just like in the Cox-Maze procedure.

LHAS can cause undesirable consequences due to its size and localization. An abundant volume causing atrial septum bulging into the atrial cavities may cause symptoms, but most importantly may render some surgical and percutaneous interventions particularly challenging. Therefore, while pre-interventional recognition of LHAS in certainly important for cardiac surgery, this is even more important for invasive cardiological interventions involving transseptal catheterization access. This approach is commonly used in interventional cardiology,

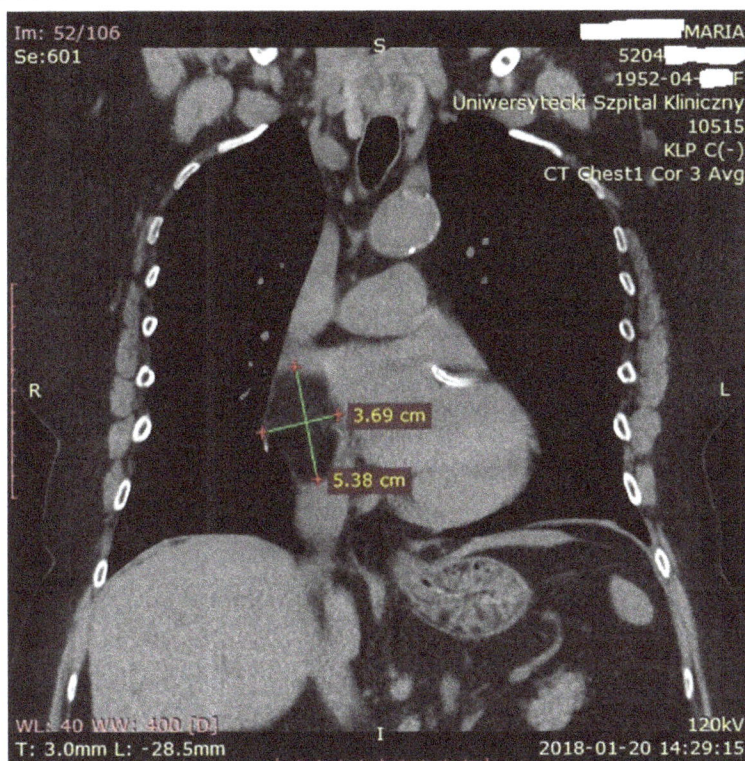

Fig. 5 CT scan. Lipomatous mass in the interatrial septum (IVS) bulging to the right atrium (RA), in the axis of the SVC and IVC, measuring 3.69 cm × 5.38 cm

to treat number of anatomical defects of the heart, such as closure of atrial septal defects (ASDs), patent foramen ovales (PFO) or correction of the functional mitral regurgitation through percutaneous "edge-to-edge" mitral valve repair, as well as in interventional electrophysiology to treat left atrial arrhythmias through commonly used transseptal puncture [6]. A very rare problem related to the size of the mass and the anatomy of the right atrium are technical difficulties, as described above, during the bicaval cannulation, when commencing the CPB and difficulties in accessing the operated heart structures. In the presented case, resistance was encountered while inserting the venous cannulas. Based on the standardly performed intraoperatively TEE, as well as by analyzing the chest X-ray (Fig. 1) and CT scans, a diagnosis of LHAS was made (Figs. 4 and 5). Choosing the smaller cannula sizes allowed for an effective cannulation and transition to cardiopulmonary bypass in order to perform the surgery. Access from the left atrium to the operated mitral valve was significantly impeded, and the transseptal approach, without disturbing the LHAS structure, could not be possible.

In the presented case, a complex cardiac surgery was successfully performed. Asymptomatic LHAS does not require cardiac surgery. Surgical treatment of LHAS should be limited only to cases of patients with marginal obstruction of the SVC or the right atrium, which is an indication for a resection of the lesion with simultaneous interatrial septum plasty. The performed procedure may be a beneficial therapeutic option in patients with arrhythmia [1, 9, 21]. Long-term benefits of the surgery and the risk of recurrence have not been investigated [2].

Abbreviations

BMI: Body mass index; CABG: Coronary artery bypass grafting; CPB: Cardiopulmonary bypass; CT: Computed tomography; DES: Drug-eluting stents; ECG: Electrocardiogram; ERO: Effective regurgitant orfice; IAS: Interatrial septum; IVC: Inferior vena cava; LA: Left atrium; LHAS: Lipomatous hypertrophy of the atrial septum; MR: Mitral regurgitation; MRI: Magnetic resonance imaging; MSCT: Multislice computered tomography; RA: Right atrium; SVC: Superior vena cava; TEE: Transesophageal echocardiogram; TTE: Transthoracic echocardiography

Authors' contributions

GB Concept/design, Data analysis/interpretation, Data collection. MŁ Concept/design, Data analysis/interpretation, Drafting article. KK Data collection, Drafting article. JJ Data collection, Critical revision of article. RN Data collection, Critical revision of article. MJ Critical revision of article, Approval of article. All authors read and approved the final manuscript.

Competing interests

The authors declare that they have no competing interests.

Author details
[1]Department of Cardiac Surgery, Wroclaw Medical University, Wroclaw, Poland. [2]Department of Anaesthesiology and Intensive Therapy, Wroclaw Medical University, Borowska 213, 50-556 Wroclaw, Wroclaw, Poland.

References

1. Heyer C, Kagel T, Lemburg S, Bauer T, Nicolas V. Lipomatous hypertrophy of the interatrial septum. Chest. 2003;124(6):2068–73.
2. Cohn L, Bryne J. Cardiac surgery in the adult, fourth edition. 4th ed. Blacklick: McGraw-Hill Publishing; 2012. p. 1245–76.
3. Prior JT. Lipomatous hypertrophy of cardiac interatrial septum: a lesion resembling hibernoma, lipoblastomatosis and infiltrating lipoma. Arch Pathol. 1964;78:11–5.
4. Nadra I. Lipomatous hypertrophy of the ineratrial septum; a commonly misdiagnosed mass often leading to unnecessary cardiac surgery. Heart. 2004;90(12):66.
5. O'Connor S, Recavarren R, Nichols LC, Parwani AV. Lipomatous hypertrophy of the interatrial septum: an overview. Arch Pathol Lab Med. 2006;130:397–9.
6. Laura DM, Donnino RM, Kim EE, Benenstein RJ, Freedberg RS, Sarić M. Lipomatous atrial septal hypertrophy: a review of its anatomy, pathophysiology, multimodality imaging, and relevance to percutaneous interventions. J Am Soc Echocardiogr. 2016;29(8):717–23.
7. Burke AP, Litovsky S. Virmani R. Lipomatous hypertrophy of the atrial septum presenting as a right atrial mass m J Surg Pathol. 1996;20:678–85.
8. Rojas C, Jaimes C, El-Sherief A, Medina H, Chung J, Ghoshhajra B, Abbara S. Cardiac CT of non-shunt pathology of the interatrial septum. Journal of Cardiovascular Computed Tomography. 2011;5(2):93–100.
9. Cheezum M, Jezior M, Carbonaro S, Villines T. Lipomatous hypertrophy presenting as superior vena cava syndrome. Journal of Cardiovascular Computed Tomography. 2014;8(3):250–1.
10. López-Candales A. Massive Lipomatous hypertrophy of the right atria. Heart Views : The Official Journal of the Gulf Heart Association. 2013;14(2):85–7.
11. Xanthos T, Giannakopoulos N, Papadimitriou L. Lipomatous hypertrophy of the interatrial septum: a pathological and clinical approach. Int J Cardiol. 2007;121:4–8.
12. Strecker T, Weyand M, Agaimy A. Lipomatous hypertrophy of the atrial septum in a patient undergoing coronary artery bypass surgery. Case Reports in Pathology. 2016;2016:1–4.
13. Ak K, Isbir S, Kepez A, Turkoz K, Elci E, Arsan S. Large Lipomatous hypertrophy of the interventricular septum. Tex Heart Inst J. 2014;41(2):231–3.
14. Sato Y, Matsuo S, Kusama J, et al. Lipomatous hypertrophy of the interatrial septum presenting a sick sinus syndrome. Int J Cardiol. 2006; https://doi.org/10.1016/j.ijcard.2006.07.161.
15. Cannavale G, Francone M, Galea N, Vullo F, Molisso A, Carbone I, Catalano C. Fatty images of the heart: Spectrum of normal and pathological findings by computed tomography and cardiac magnetic resonance imaging. Biomed Res Int. 2018; https://doi.org/10.1155/2018/5610347.
16. Fyke FE, Tajik AJ, Edwards WD, Seward JB. Diagnosis of lipomatous hypertrophy of the atrial septum by two-dimensional echocardiography. J Am Coll Cardiol. 1983;1(5):1352–7.
17. Meaney JF, Kazerooni EA, Jamadar DA, Korobkin M. CT appearance of lipomatous hypertrophy of the interatrial septum. AJR Am J Roentgenol. 1997;168:1081–4.
18. Kluge WF. Lipomatous hypertrophy of the interatrial septum. Northwest Med. 1969;68:25–30.
19. Erhardt LR. Abnormal electrical activity in lipomatous hy-pertrophy of the interatrial septum. Am Heart J. 1974;87:571–6.
20. Abarello P, Maiese A, Bolino G. Case study of sudden cardiac death caused by lypomatous hypertrophy of the interatrial septum. Med Leg J. 2012;80:102–4.
21. Dickerson J, Smith M, Kalbfleisch S, Firstenberg M. Lipomatous hypertrophy of the Intraatrial septum resulting in right atrial inflow obstruction and atrial flutter. Ann Thorac Surg. 2010;89(5):1647–9.

20

High-sensitivity troponin T release profile in off-pump coronary artery bypass grafting patients with normal postoperative course

Wen Ge[1†], Chang Gu[2†], Chao Chen[3†], Wangwang Chen[3], Zhengqiang Cang[3], Yuliang Wang[4], Chennan Shi[3] and Yangyang Zhang[5,6*] (iD)

Abstract

Background: The aim of the study was to investigate the high-sensitivity troponin T (hs-TnT) release profile in off-pump coronary artery bypass grafting (OPCABG) patients with normal postoperative course.

Methods: From January 2015 to October 2016, 398 consecutive OPCABG patients who had normal postoperative courses were enrolled. Blood samples for hs-TnT were collected at several time points and the comparisons among different time points grouped by various factors were further analyzed.

Results: There were 317 male and 81 female patients, with a median age of 64. For 66.1% of the patients, peak hs-TnT occurred at the 24th hour after OPCABG, regardless of the groups divided by different factors. In total, the hs-TnT values were much higher in male group ($P = 0.035$), in patients who need 5 or more bypass grafts ($P = 0.035$) and in patients with high-risk EuroSCORE II assessment ($P = 0.013$). However, we failed to find any significant differences between different age groups ($P = 0.129$) or among different coronary heart disease classifications ($P = 0.191$).

Conclusions: The hs-TnT values were affected by various factors and culminated around the first 24 h following OPCABG. It may provide some useful information for future clinical studies of myocardial biomarkers after OPCABG.

Keywords: High-sensitivity troponin T, Off-pump coronary artery bypass grafting, Release profile

Background

Myocardial cell injury is inevitable after cardiac surgery, leading to the elevation of various cardiac biomarkers. Myocardial infarction (MI), caused by myocardial injury or coronary artery anomaly, is a major cause of disability and death around the world. Perioperative MI may cause adverse events such as reoperation, longer intensive care unit (ICU)/hospital stay or even hospital deaths after cardiac surgery [1–4]. Currently, MI can be defined by many clinical characteristics including elevated values of biomarkers of myocardial ischemia necrosis, myocardial contrast echocardiography and electrocardiography (ECG) results [5].

It has been proved that postoperative serum cardiac troponin T (TnT) level is correlated with increased morbidity and mortality after coronary artery bypass grafting (CABG) [6–8]. Compared with postoperative TnT, preoperative serum TnT does not offer an additional predictive value [9]. Nevertheless, preoperative troponins, with low cut-off value, could provide better predictive value than postoperative values after preoperative percutaneous coronary intervention (PCI) [10]. Nowadays, the new generation hs-TnT could detect minor myocardial injury with higher sensitivity and has been widely used in cardiac surgery.

Postoperative MI has been well recognized and the consensus on MI has been developed for many revisions. Understanding of release profiles after different cardiac procedures helps clinicians perceive perioperative MI and take measures to avoid relevant adverse events [1]. Previous studies have reported the release profile of hs-TnT after cardiac surgery [1, 11]. However, the number of enrolled patients who underwent OPCABG in previous researches

---

* Correspondence: zhangyangyang_wy@vip.sina.com
†Wen Ge, Chang Gu and Chao Chen contributed equally to this work.
5Department of Cardiovascular Surgery, East Hospital, Tongji University School of Medicine, 150 Jimo Road, Shanghai 200120, China
6Key Laboratory of Arrhythmias of the Ministry of Education of China, East Hospital, Tongji University School of Medicine, Shanghai 200120, China
Full list of author information is available at the end of the article

was relatively small and the release profile is of significance for CABG patients with normal postoperative courses. Therefore, we undertook an investigation of the release profile following OPCABG in 398 patients who had normal postoperative courses.

Methods

Patients

From January 2015 to October 2016, we consecutively enrolled OPCABG patients who had normal postoperative courses. The exclusion criteria were as follows: (1) emergency operation; (2) postoperative MI; (3) postoperative renal failure; (4) severe postoperative complications; (5) perioperative death; (6) the interval between preoperative MI and surgery less than 3 weeks in patients with preoperative MI. According to the third universal definition of myocardial infarction, CABG-related MI can be defined by the high postoperative troponin level (above $10 \times$ 99th percentile upper reference limit (URL)) in patients with normal baseline troponin values within the first 48 h after surgery. Besides, one of the following occurred can also be recognized as CABG related MI: (1) new pathological Q wave or new left bundle branch block; (2) angiographically detected new graft or native coronary artery occlusion; (3) imaging evidence of new regional wall motion abnormality or new loss of viable myocardium [5].

The study was approved by the ethics committees of Shanghai East Hospital (ID2018097). All clinical procedures were performed in accordance with current clinical guidelines and regulations. All patients included in the study, or their legal representatives, signed written informed consents to participate in the study and for all surgical procedures. We reviewed the medical records for all the patients. All the corresponding clinical data including age, sex, body mass index (BMI), coronary artery disease (CAD) classification, New York Heart Association (NYHA) class, comorbidity, preoperative atrial fibrillation, history of PCI, numbers of bypass grafts and the results of serological examination were collected.

Twenty-four hours before surgery, blood samples were obtained for hs-TnT from venous puncture for the first time. Thereafter, blood samples were collected from the end time of surgery at 6, 12, 24, 48, 72, 96 and 120 h postoperatively. Samples were measured in the central laboratory of hospital by standard techniques. Plasma levels of cardiac hs-TnT were measured on Roche CARDIAC reader (Roche cobas E 411). The detection limit is 0 ng/L to 10,000 ng/L. The normal limit is 0 ng/L to 14 ng/L.

Statistics

All the clinical data were analyzed by using SPSS 19.0 software package (SPSS Inc., Chicago, IL). Variables among patients include gender, age, number of bypass grafts, EuroSCORE II, and CAD classification. If continuous variables conform to the normal distribution, then variables will be expressed as mean ± standard deviation, else variables will be expressed as median and interquartile range (IQR). The distributions of hs-TnT classified by these factors were estimated by using Prism 5.0 (Graph Pad Software Inc., La Jolla, CA) and the last observation carried forward (LOCF) method was used to deal with dropout data of hs-TnT [12]. The difference of hs-TnT at different points was compared by repeated measurements. All P values were two-sided and statistical significance was set at 0.05.

Results

Overall, there were 3184 monitoring points and 99 of them had incomplete hs-TnT data (99/3184, 3.11%). Every patient had their pre-operative data. At 6, 12, 24, 48, 72, 96 and 120 h after surgery, the number of patients who failed in data collection was 14, 14, 16, 17, 9, 14 and 15 respectively. Missing rate at each time point was less than 5%. Three hundred ninety-eight OPCABG patients with normal postoperative course were enrolled in our study. There were 317 male and 81 female, with a median age of 64(11). Of the 398 patients, there were 244 (61.3%) patients with stable angina pectoris, 109 (27.4%) patients with unstable angina pectoris and 45 (11.3%) patients with acute myocardial infarction, respectively. All the 45 patients with acute MI received surgery after 3 weeks. As for NYHA class, patients with class II accounted for the

Table 1 Baseline clinical characteristics of OPCABG patients

Variables	Total ($N = 398$)
Age (y)	$^{\triangle}$64(11)
Female (n, %)	81(20.4)
Weight (kg)	69.03 ± 10.46(37–125)
Height (cm)	166.79 ± 7.18(144–184)
BMI (kg/m^2)	24.75 ± 2.90(15.60–38.58)
Diabetes (n, %)	106(26.6)
Hypertension (n, %)	218(54.8)
Stroke (n, %)	3(0.8)
Peripheral vascular disease (n, %)	10(2.5)
Previous PCI (n, %)	15(3.8)
Atrial flutter and fibrillation (n, %)	6(1.5)
Pulmonary hypertension (n, %)	108(27.1)
Acute myocardial infarction (n, %)	45(11.3)
Unstable angina pectoris (n, %)	109(27.4)
NYHA class II (n, %)	248(62.3)
LVEF (%)	60.56 ± 8.01(32.7–72.8)
Number of grafts (n)	3.92 ± 1.05(1–6)

$^{\triangle}$Values of variables stand for median and interquartile range (IQR)
Abbreviations: *BMI* body mass index, *COPD* chronic obstructive pulmonary disease, *Scr* Serum creatinine, *Ccr* endogenous creatinine clearance rate, *LVEF* left ventricular ejection fraction

Table 2 Comparisons among different time points grouped by various factors

	24 h before OP	PO 6 h	PO12h	PO 24 h	PO 48 h	PO 72 h	PO 96 h	PO 120 h
Total	81.98 ± 367.60	142.27 ± 11,208	186.12 ± 145.36	207.13 ± 176.81	165.30 ± 149.34	134.06 ± 123.41	103.74 ± 100.68	72.34 ± 79.52
Group by gender								
Male (n = 317)	92.92 ± 407.98	150.75 ± 112.65	190.64 ± 141.43	213.76 ± 176.88	170.57 ± 151.19	137.99 ± 124.17	108.40 ± 106.46	76.19 ± 83.69
Female (n = 81)	39.14 ± 103.83	109.08 ± 103.97	168.45 ± 159.53	181.18 ± 175.21	144.65 ± 140.91	118.69 ± 119.91	85.48 ± 71.50	57.30 ± 58.54
Group by grafts								
G1 (n = 279)	89.39 ± 424.06	129.51 ± 104.26	173.99 ± 143.33	193.35 ± 169.58	153.56 ± 146.50	124.67 ± 123.86	100.44 ± 103.31	72.31 ± 84.31
G2 (n = 119)	64.58 ± 174.74	172.18 ± 123.97	214.18 ± 146.72	239.45 ± 189.54	192.82 ± 152.92	156.07 ± 120.01	111.48 ± 94.21	72.44 ± 67.28
Group by EuroSCORE II								
HRG (n = 62)	87.46 ± 176.87*	169.09 ± 125.95**	219.53 ± 169.83***	262.19 ± 275.68****	213.12 ± 230.94*****	171.18 ± 191.37******	135.39 ± 148.29*******	95.81 ± 113.85********
LRG (n = 336)	80.96 ± 392.99	137.32 ± 108.81	179.96 ± 140.89	196.97 ± 150.14	156.47 ± 127.35	127.19 ± 105.25	97.90 ± 88.26	68.01 ± 70.80
Group by age								
Elderly (n = 105)	89.60 ± 420.82	137.04 ± 105.12	178.56 ± 138.02	196.92 ± 149.48	156.27 ± 124.11△	128.52 ± 106.91	98.69 ± 88.02	65.83 ± 62.79△△
Young (n = 293)	60.97 ± 139.73	156.66 ± 128.78	206.96 ± 162.79	235.27 ± 234.91	190.16 ± 201.97	149.33 ± 159.97	117.65 ± 128.80	90.18 ± 111.98
Group by CAD								
SAP (n = 244)	65.21 ± 368.34▲	140.13 ± 97.59	187.26 ± 145.49	187.26 ± 145.49	210.96 ± 192.52	168.01 ± 163.61	104.99 ± 105.93	71.13 ± 80.48
USAP (n = 109)	54.09 ± 142.57	142.55 ± 131.44	179.22 ± 135.21	190.28 ± 134.15	158.48 ± 113.69	125.45 ± 87.68	96.70 ± 72.59	73.07 ± 69.93
AMI (n = 45)	240.38 ± 625.21	153.19 ± 134.88	196.69 ± 169.23	227.18 ± 178.92	167.10 ± 146.69	134.42 ± 113.17	113.97 ± 127.76	77.16 ± 96.16

Abbreviations:G1 group1, number grafts ≤4; G2 group2, number grafts ≥5, HRG high risk group (EuroSCORE II > =2.00%), LRG low risk group (EuroSCORE II < 2.00%), CAD coronary atherosclerotic heart disease, SAP Stable angina pectoris, USAP Unstable angina pectoris, AMI acute myocardial infarction, OP operation, PO postoperative

* $P = 0.003$; ** $P = 0.040$; *** $P = 0.049$; **** $P = 0.007$; ***** $P = 0.006$; ****** $P = 0.010$; ******* $P = 0.007$; ******** $P = 0.011$; △ $P = 0.045$; △△ $P = 0.007$; ▲ $P = 0.008$

majority (248, 62.3%). Fifteen patients had PCI operations before. Besides, during the operation, the mean numbers of bypass grafts were 3.9 (range from 1 to 6) (Table 1).

Hs-TnT profiles

The hs-TnT profiles and comparisons are shown in Table 2 and Figs. 1, 2, 3, 4 and 5 according to different factors including gender, age, number of bypass grafts, EuroSCORE II, and CAD classification. Values of TnT stand for means±standard deviation (SD). During perioperative period (24 h before surgery to 120 h after surgery), the profiles all experienced wide variability. Peak hs-TnT value occurred at the 24th hour after OPCABG, regardless of the groups divided by different factors.

When grouped by gender, the hs-TnT values were much higher in male group in total ($P = 0.035$). Besides, when compared at each time point, the values were all higher in men, and only at the 6th hour after surgery did the hs-TnT value have statistical discrepancy ($P = 0.003$) (Fig. 1).

When grouped by number of bypass grafts, the hs-TnT values were much higher in patients who need 5 or more bypass grafts ($P = 0.035$). In addition, when compared at each time point, the hs-TnT values in patients with 5 or more bypass grafts were much higher at 6 ($P < 0.001$), 12 ($P = 0.011$), 24 ($P = 0.017$), 48 ($P = 0.016$) and 72 ($P = 0.020$) hours after surgery, respectively (Fig. 2).

When grouped by EuroSCORE II, there was statistical difference between high-risk group (EuroSCORE II,> = 2.00) and low risk group (EuroSCORE II,< 2.00) ($P = 0.013$). Furthermore, when compared at each time point, the hs-TnT values were all higher in high-risk group and all had significant differences after surgery (Fig. 3).

When grouped by age, in total, although the hs-TnT values in elderly patients (> = 70 y) were higher, we failed to find any significant differences between the two groups ($P = 0.129$). However, when compared at each time point, there were significant differences at 48 ($P = 0.045$) and 120 ($P = 0.007$) hours after the surgery (Fig. 4).

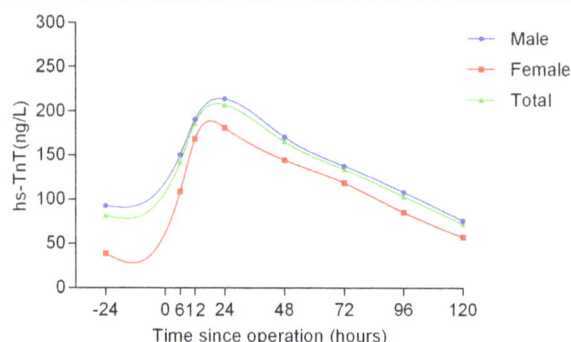

Fig. 2 Comparisons among different time points grouped by the number of grafts. The blue curve represented patients who need less than 5 bypass grafts and the red curve represented patients who need 5 or more bypass grafts, while the total population curve was in green

When grouped by CAD classification, this factor did not have significant impact on the variability of hs-TnT values ($P = 0.191$). Interestingly, when compared at each time point, only preoperative values had significant differences ($P = 0.008$) (Fig. 5).

Discussion

Elevation of cardiac biomarkers was a common phenomenon following CABG, which was ascribed to a number of causes including, though not limited to, cardiomyocyte death from insufficient myocardial protection, embolism, regional or/and global ischemia and surgical procedure injuries. Of all the covariates predictive of mortality, the elevation of troponins in the first 24 h following CABG is one of the strongest correlative factors [13]. Therefore, it is worthy to identify postoperative MI and differentiate expected elevation of troponins from unexpected suspicious perioperative MI in order to guide clinical decisions. Carmona et al. [14] indicated that both CABG and OPCABG are safe and there were no statistically significant differences in terms of long-term all-cause

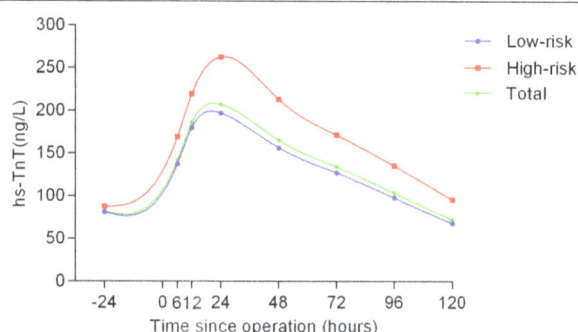

Fig. 1 Comparisons among different time points grouped by gender. The blue curve represented male and the red curve represented female, while the total population curve was in green

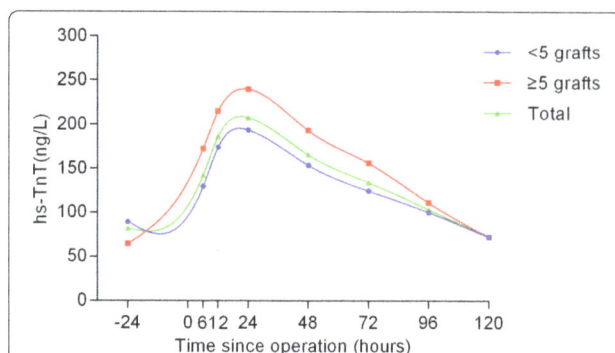

Fig. 3 Comparisons among different time points grouped by EuroSCORE. The blue curve represented low risk group (EuroSCORE II, < 2.00) and the red curve represented high-risk group (EuroSCORE II, > = 2.00), while the total population curve was in green

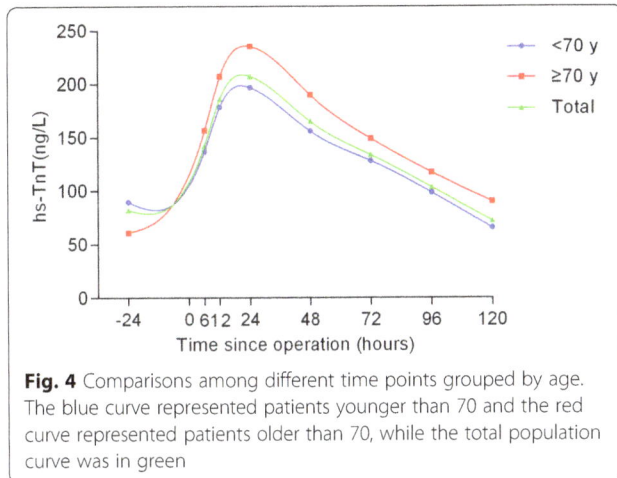

Fig. 4 Comparisons among different time points grouped by age. The blue curve represented patients younger than 70 and the red curve represented patients older than 70, while the total population curve was in green

mortality. However, they found OPCABG was related with less postoperative morbidity and shorter ICU and hospital stay. Currently, there is no consensus on hs-TnT release profile after OPCABG. When compared with conventional TnT, hs-TnT has higher sensitivity especially when measured early after symptom onset and has the advantage in early diagnosis of acute MI [15–17]. The present study showed that, in OPCABG patients with normal postoperative course, the hs-TnT could sensitively reflect the extent of myocardial damage and its value peaks around the 24th hour after surgery.

With normal postoperative course, the release of hs-TnT differed among individuals undergoing OPCABG. Various factors contributed to the variation in hs-TnT release. The serum hs-TnT level can be influenced by patient factors and perioperative factors. Gore et al. [18] demonstrated that the uniform 14 ng/l cut-off value for hs-TnT may lead to over-diagnosis of perioperative MI in male or elderly patients because men and the elderly have higher normal URL. In our series, although high level (more than 10 times of URL) of hs-TnT has been found in some patients, they did not have concomitant symptoms

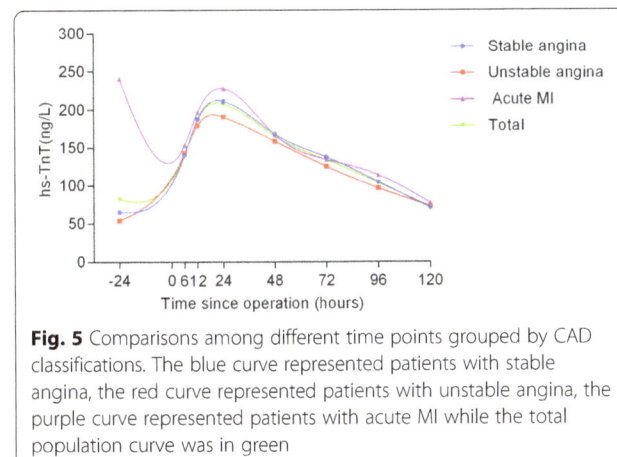

Fig. 5 Comparisons among different time points grouped by CAD classifications. The blue curve represented patients with stable angina, the red curve represented patients with unstable angina, the purple curve represented patients with acute MI while the total population curve was in green

like (1) new pathological Q wave; (2) angiographically detected new graft or native coronary artery occlusion (3) imaging evidence of new regional wall motion abnormality or new loss of viable myocardium [5]. Therefore, they could not be defined as postoperative MI, but could suggest a certain degree of myocardial damage. Besides, some comorbidities like hypertension, diabetes mellitus, ventricular hypertrophy and the efficacy of plasma troponin clearance can also affect hs-TnT level [1, 19, 20]. Perioperative factors like cardiotonic drug usage and cardiac arrhythmia are proved to have an impact on the hs-TnT values [21].

In our series, there was an interesting phenomenon that values of postoperative hs-TnT were much greater than URL. Jorgensen et al. reported that they observed 99 patients undergoing CABG and the cardiac troponin (cTnI) levels were far above the cut-off point of guideline. The median peak value in normal postoperative course was 7675 ng/L, which was 255 times the URL [22]. Another literature also reported the same results [23–25]. The possible explanation for this phenomenon was that the complexity and multi-factors of cardiac surgery led to myocardial damage, which was more serious than PCI.

As for patient factors, increased age and impaired renal function contributed to high level of serum hs-TnT, and thus affecting diagnostic accuracy for acute MI [26]. Elderly age (> 70 years) has been considered as a significant risk factor for elevated hs-TnT. As previous study reported, regardless of the final diagnosis, hs-TnT concentrations in elderly patients were much higher than that in younger patients (20.9 ng/L versus 3.9 ng/L) [26]. These results were basically consistent with ours. In our study, the hs-TnT values in elderly patients were higher. Furthermore, when compared at each time point, there were significant differences at 48 ($P = 0.045$) and 120 ($P = 0.007$) hours after the surgery. The reason would be that when renal function declined from age, elderly patients will have low estimated glomerular filtration rate. As a result, hs-TnT could not be eliminated in time, leading to relatively high hs-TnT level in peripheral blood.

Among patients with different CAD types, there were significant differences when comparing the data of the 24th hour before operation, which were in accordance with patients' condition. Postoperatively, there were no statistical differences among them and the results indirectly reflected the effectiveness of surgery. As for EuroSCORE II, the score itself has included comprehensive assessments of patients. High-risk patients had more risk factors than low-risk ones. The chances for myocardial damage increase. As a result, the hs-TnT level was higher in high-risk group.

There are some limitations in our study. First, although this study contains 398 OPCABG patients, the sample size is still relatively small. Second, this is a retrospective designed study, which may cause a certain degree of selection bias. Third, there would be interaction among different perioperative factors, which may affect hs-TnT level, leading to the exclusion of patients with false positive perioperative MI.

Conclusions

Our study demonstrated that the hs-TnT release profile in OPCABG patients who had normal postoperative courses and the hs-TnT values were affected by various factors and often peak around the 24th hour following OPCABG. It may provide some useful information for future clinical studies of myocardial biomarkers after OPCABG.

Abbreviations

BMI: Body mass index; CABG: Coronary artery bypass grafting; CAD: Coronary artery disease; cTnI: Cardiac troponin; ECG: Electrocardiography; hs-TnT: High-sensitivity troponin T; ICU: Intensive care unit; IQR: Interquartile range; LOCF: Last observation carried forward; MI: Myocardial infarction; NYHA: New York Heart Association; OPCABG: Off-pump coronary artery bypass grafting; PCI: Percutaneous coronary intervention; SD: means±standard deviation; TnT: Troponin T; URL: Upper reference limit

Acknowledgements

We wish to thank the help in surgeries given by Prof. Yongfeng Shao, Prof. Xiaowei Wang, Dr. Lei Wei, Dr. Sheng Zhao, Dr. Xiangxiang Zheng, Dr. Haoliang Sun. Dr. Luyao Ma, and Dr. Wei Zhang.

Funding

This work was supported by the practice innovation training program projects for the Jiangsu students in college (201510312043Y to C. C) (201510312073Z to Z. C) (201710312024Z to Y. W) (201710312063X to C. S).

Authors' contributions

Y.Z. made substantial contributions to conception and design. Acquisition of funding owe to C.C., Z.C., Y.W. and C.S. W.C., Y.W. and C.S. were involved in acquisition of data. C.G., C.C. and Z.C. were responsible for analysis and interpretation of data. W.G., C.G. and C.C. were major contributors in writing and revising the manuscript. W.G. and Y.Z. gave final approval of the version to be published. All authors read and approved the final manuscript.

Competing interests

The authors declare that they have no competing interests.

Author details

[1]Department of Cardiothoracic Surgery, Shuguang Hospital, affiliated to Shanghai University of TCM, Shanghai 200021, China. [2]Department of Thoracic Surgery, Shanghai Chest Hospital, Shanghai Jiao Tong University, Shanghai 200030, China. [3]The First Clinical Medical College of Nanjing Medical University, Nanjing 210029, China. [4]Department of Hygiene Analysis and Detection School of Public Health Nanjing Medical University, Nanjing 210029, China. [5]Department of Cardiovascular Surgery, East Hospital, Tongji University School of Medicine, 150 Jimo Road, Shanghai 200120, China. [6]Key Laboratory of Arrhythmias of the Ministry of Education of China, East Hospital, Tongji University School of Medicine, Shanghai 200120, China.

References

1. Markman PL, Tantiongco JP, Bennetts JS, et al. High-sensitivity troponin release profile after cardiac surgery [J]. Heart Lung Circ. 2016;22(6):475.
2. Chaitman BR, Alderman EL, Sheffield LT, et al. Use of survival analysis to determine the clinical significance of new Q waves after coronary bypass surgery. Circulation. 1983;67(2):302–9.
3. Force T, Hibberd P, Weeks G, et al. Perioperative myocardial infarction after coronary artery bypass surgery. Clinical significance and approach to risk stratification. Circulation. 1990;82(3):903–12.
4. Mahaffey KW, Roe MT, Kilaru R, et al. Creatine kinase-MB elevation after coronary artery bypass grafting surgery in patients with non-ST-segment elevation acute coronary syndromes predict worse outcomes: results from four large clinical trials. Eur Heart J. 2007;28(4):425–32.
5. Thygesen K, Alpert JS, Jaffe AS, et al. Third universal definition of myocardial infarction. Eur Heart J. 2012;33(20):2551–67.
6. Søraas CL, Friis C, Engebretsen KVT, et al. Troponin T is a better predictor than creatine kinase-MB of long-term mortality after coronary artery bypass graft surgery. Am Heart J. 2012;164(5):779–85.
7. Muehlschlegel JD, Perry TE, Liu KY, et al. Troponin is superior to electrocardiogram and creatinine kinase MB for predicting clinically significant myocardial injury after coronary artery bypass grafting. Eur Heart J. 2009;30(13):1574–83.
8. Mohammed AA, Agnihotri AK, van Kimmenade RRJ, et al. Prospective, comprehensive assessment of cardiac troponin T testing after coronary artery bypass graft surgery. Circulation. 2009;120(10):843–50.
9. Lehrke S, Steen H, Sievers HH, et al. Cardiac troponin T for prediction of short-and long-term morbidity and mortality after elective open heart surgery. Clin Chem. 2004;50(9):1560–7.
10. Petäjä L, Røsjø H, Mildh L, et al. Predictive value of high-sensitivity troponin T in addition to EuroSCORE II in cardiac surgery. Interact Cardiovasc Thorac Surg. 2016;23(1):133–41.
11. De Mey N, Brandt I, Van Mieghem C, et al. High-sensitive cardiac troponins and CK-MB concentrations in patients undergoing cardiac surgery. Crit Care. 2015;19(1):P158.
12. Saha C, Jones MP. Bias in the last observation carried forward method under informative dropout. J Statist Plann Inference. 2009;139(2):246–55.
13. Domanski MJ, Mahaffey K, Hasselblad V, et al. Association of myocardial enzyme elevation and survival following coronary artery bypass graft surgery. JAMA. 2011;305(6):585–91.
14. Carmona P, Paredes F, Mateo E, Mena-Durán AV, Hornero F, Martínez-León J. Is off-pump technique a safer procedure for coronary revascularization? A propensity score analysis of 20 years of experience. Interact Cardiovasc Thorac Surg. 2016;22:612–9.
15. Morrow DA, Cannon CP, Rifai N, et al. Ability of minor elevations of troponins I and T to predict benefit from an early invasive strategy in patients with unstable angina and non-ST elevation myocardial infarction: results from a randomized trial. JAMA. 2001;286(19):2405–12.
16. Keller T, Zeller T, Peetz D, et al. Sensitive troponin I assay in early diagnosis of acute myocardial infarction. N Engl J Med. 2009;361(9):868–77.
17. Ndrepepa G, Braun S, Schulz S, et al. Comparison of prognostic value of high-sensitivity and conventional troponin T in patients with non-ST-segment elevation acute coronary syndromes. Clin Chim Acta. 2011; 412(15):1350–6.
18. Gore MO, Seliger SL, Nambi V, et al. Age-and sex-dependent upper reference limits for the high-sensitivity cardiac troponin T assay. J Am Coll Cardiol. 2014;63(14):1441–8.
19. de Lemos JA, Drazner MH, Omland T, et al. Association of troponin T detected with a highly sensitive assay and cardiac structure and mortality risk in the general population. JAMA. 2010;304(22):2503–12.
20. Apple FS, Collinson PO, IFCC task force on clinical applications of cardiac biomarkers. Analytical characteristics of high-sensitivity cardiac troponin assays. Clin Chem. 2012;58(1):54–61.
21. Katus HA, Schoeppenthau M, Tanzeem A, et al. Non-invasive assessment of perioperative myocardial cell damage by circulating cardiac troponin T. Br Heart J. 1991;65(5):259–64.
22. Jorgensen PH, Nybo M, Jensen MK, Mortensen PE, Poulsen TS, Diederichsen ACP, et al. Optimal cut-off value for cardiac troponinI in ruling out type 5 myocardial infarction. Interact Cardiovasc Thorac Surg. 2014;18:544–50.

23. Thielmann M, Massoudy P, Schmermund A, Neuhäuser M, Marggraf G, Kamler M, et al. Diagnostic discrimination between graft-related and non-graft-related perioperative myocardial infarction with cardiac troponin I after coronary artery bypass surgery. Eur Heart J. 2005;26:2440–7.
24. Noora J, Ricci C, Hastings D, Hill S, Cybulsky I. Determination of troponin I release after CABG surgery. J Card Surg. 2005;20:129–35.
25. Peivandi AA, Dahm M, Opfermann UT, Peetz D, Doerr F, Loos A, et al. Comparison of cardiac troponin I versus T and creatine kinase MB after coronary artery bypass grafting in patients with and without perioperative myocardial infarction. Herz. 2004;29:658–64.
26. Chenevier-Gobeaux C, Meune C, Freund Y, et al. Influence of age and renal function on high-sensitivity cardiac troponin T diagnostic accuracy for the diagnosis of acute myocardial infarction. Am J Cardiol. 2013;111(12):1701–7.

21

Safety and efficacy of ultrathin strut biodegradable polymer sirolimus-eluting stent versus durable polymer drug-eluting stents

Ping Zhu, Xin Zhou, Chenliang Zhang, Huakang Li, Zhihui Zhang* and Zhiyuan Song* (ORCID)

Abstract

Background: The Orsiro biodegradable polymer sirolimus-eluting stent (O-SES) is a new-generation biodegradable polymer drug-eluting stent with the thinnest strut thickness to date developed to improve the percutaneous treatment of patients with coronary artery disease. We perform a meta-analysis of randomized clinical trials (RCTs) comparing the efficacy and safety of an ultra-thin, Orsiro biodegradable polymer sirolimus-eluting stent (O-SES) compared with durable polymer drug-eluting stents (DP-DESs).

Methods: Medline, Embase, and CENTRAL databases were searched for randomized controlled trials comparing the safety and efficacy of O-SES versus DP-DES. Paired reviewers independently screened citations, assessed risk of bias of included studies, and extracted data. We used the Mantel-Haenszel method to calculate risk ratio (RR) by means of a random-effects model.

Results: Six RCTs with a total of 6949 patients were selected. All included trials were rated as low risk of bias. The O-SES significantly reduced the risk of myocardial infarction (RR 0.78, 95% confidence interval [CI] 0.62–0.98; $I^2 = 0\%$; 10 fewer per 1000 [from 1 fewer to 18 fewer]; high quality) compared with the DP-DES. There was no significant difference between O-SES and DP-DES in the prevention of stent thrombosis (RR: 0.75; 95% CI: 0.52–1.08), cardiac death (RR: 0.93; 95% CI: 0.63–1.36), target lesion revascularization (RR 1.10, 95% CI 0.86–1.42) and target vessel revascularization (RR 0.97, 95% CI 0.78–1.21).

Conclusion: Among patients undergoing percutaneous coronary intervention, O-SES resulted in significantly lower rates of myocardial infarction than DP-DES and had a trend toward reduction in stent thrombosis.

Keywords: Meta-analysis, Biodegradable polymer, Durable polymer, Percutaneous coronary intervention

Background

The implantation of a drug-eluting stent (DES) that prevent restenosis by the release of antiproliferative agents from polymers is considered the standard approach for percutaneous coronary intervention [1]. After DES implantation, however, the lifelong presence of a durable polymer (DP) might induce chronic inflammation, cell proliferation, delay arterial healing, long-term endothelial dysfunction, and occasionally cause cardiovascular events such as myocardial infarction (MI) and stent thrombosis (ST) [2, 3]. Raising

awareness of this risk motivated the improvements of stents with biodegradable polymer (BP) allowing elimination of the polymer by degradation. Despite these iterations, the potential benefits for BP-DES remain largely unproven. BP-DES has shown superior profiles over bare-metal stents and first-generation DP-DES [4–6] but shares a similar efficacy and safety profile compared with second-generation DP-DES [7, 8].

The Orsiro biodegradable polymer sirolimus-eluting stent (O-SES; Biotronik, Bülach, Switzerland) is a novel DES consisting of an ultrathin strut cobalt chromium design with a bioresorbable, poly-Llactic acid polymer coating that releases sirolimus [9]. Furthermore, O-SES

* Correspondence: xyzpj@126.com; zysong2010@126.com
Department of Cardiology, Southwest Hospital, Third Military Medical University (Army Medical University), Chongqing, China

has the thinnest strut thickness to date (60 μm), and thus provides good flexibility and deliverability. Preclinical study has reported that thin struts reduced both intimal proliferation and thrombus formation [10]. Evidence in the bare-metal stent era suggested reduced arterial injury and angiographic restenosis with low stent strut thickness [11]. The reduced strut thickness of 40% has been reported to improve outcomes compared with early generation drug-eluting stents [12]. Thus, the use of thin struts might reduce the risk of potentially fatal complications, such as ST and MI [10].

Recently, the safety and efficacy of O-SES compared with contemporary DP-DES has been assessed in randomized controlled trials (RCTs) [13–18]. However, the results of these trials were controversial. Early, modest-sized studies in this field failed individually to prove that O-SES was super to DP-DES [13–15, 17, 18]. In late 2017, a new trial has endorsed the safety and effectiveness of O-SES compared with DP-everolimus-eluting stents (EES) [16]. Therefore, we conducted a meta-analysis to compare the efficacy and safety of O-SES to DP-DES.

Methods

The registered study protocol is available on PROSPERO (CRD42017081107). The findings of the meta-analysis was reported according to the Preferred Reporting Items for Systematic Reviews and Meta-Analyses (PRISMA) [19].

Eligibility criteria
Inclusion criteria

1) Population: adult participants (≥18 years) with percutaneous coronary intervention.
2) Intervention: percutaneous coronary intervention with O-SES.
3) Comparison intervention: percutaneous coronary intervention with DP-SES.
4) Outcome: Primary outcome was MI, as defined by the individual trials. Secondary outcomes were definite or probable ST, cardiac death, target vessel revascularization (TVR), and target lesion revascularization (TLR).
5) Study design: RCT.

Exclusion criteria

We excluded duplicate reports and post hoc analyses.

Search strategy

Medline, EMBASE, and the Cochrane Library at the CENTRAL Register of Controlled Trials were searched with the assistance of a professional librarian. The last electronic search was performed on October 20, 2017. We also reviewed the reference lists of the original trials, prior meta-analysis, and review articles. There were no restrictions on language. For the search strategy, we used, in various relevant combinations, MeSH terms and keywords pertinent to the intervention of interest: "biodegradable polymer", "Orsiro", "drug-eluting stent", "sirolimus", "durable polymer", "controlled trials" and "randomized controlled trial." (Table 3 in Appendix 1).

Study selection

Two investigators performed the study selection independently. They screened titles and abstracts for initial study inclusion. They screened the full text of potentially relevant trials. Disagreements were resolved by consensus with a senior author. Follow-up of all outcomes was at 12 months.

Data collection process

Two investigators independently extracted data from the included RCTs using a standardized electronic form. Disagreements between the two investigators were resolved by consensus with a third investigator. Authors of studies were contacted when suitable data were not available.

Assessment of risk of bias and quality of evidence

Two investigators assessed the risk of bias of the trials by using the risk of bias tool of The Cochrane Collaboration [20]. Disagreements were discussed with a third author. Trials with more than two high-risk components were considered as a moderate risk of bias, and trials with more than four high-risk components as having a high risk of bias.

We used the GRADE approach to rate the quality of evidence and generate absolute estimates of effect for the outcomes [21]. We used detailed GRADE guidance to assess the overall risk of bias, indirectness, inconsistency, imprecision and publication bias and summarized results in an evidence profile.

Outcomes

The safety outcomes of the analysis included MI, definite or probable ST, and cardiac death, and the efficacy outcomes included TVR and TLR. The primary outcome was MI, which was defined by the individual trials.

Data synthesis

Computations were performed with RevMan- v 5.3.3 (a freeware available from The Cochrane Collaboration). Analyses for all outcomes were done on an intention-to-treat basis. The meta-analysis was done using random effect models regardless of the level of heterogeneity. The risk ratios (RR) along with 95% confidence intervals (CI) was calculated for dichotomous data. We assessed heterogeneity with the Chi^2 test (threshold $p = 0.10$) and the I^2 tests, I^2 values lower than 25%, 25–50%, and higher than 75% represented low, moderate, and high heterogeneity, respectively [22]. A 2-tailed P value of < 0.05 was set for statistical significance.

We conducted trial sequential analysis (TSA) for primary outcome (MI) using TSA software (version 0.9.5.9; Copenhagen Trial Unit, Copenhagen, Denmark) [23]. We used the O'Brien-Fleming approach to compute the trial sequential monitoring boundaries. An optimal information size was set to a two-sided alpha of 0·05, beta 0·80, relative risk reduction of 20%.

If a pooled analysis included 10 or more studies, we planned to use a funnel plot to explore the possibility of published bias.

We performed a subgroup analysis according to the different types of DP-DES (Everolimus versus Zotarolimus).

We planned sensitivity analyses:1. by performing meta-analysis using both fixed-effect models; 2. using alternative imputation methods; 3 using odds ratios instead of risk ratios;

Results

Study selection and characteristics

The search strategy yielded 331 manuscript abstracts (Fig. 1). Excluding 316 non-pertinent titles or abstracts,

15 studies were assessed according to the selection criteria. Six trials [13–18] were included in the meta-analysis.

Study characteristics

The baseline characteristics of included trials have been summarized in Table 1 and Tables 4 and 5 in Appendices 2 and 3. All trials published from 2015 to 2017. A total of 3120 patients receiving DP-SES compared with 3829 patients treated with O-SES. The types of DP-DES included zotarolimus-eluting stents (ZES, 2 trials) and everolimus-eluting stents (EES, 4 trials). All trials reported outcomes at 12-months follow-up, whereas one [15] of them even reported outcomes at 24-months follow-up. To decrease heterogeneity, we included only outcomes at 12-months follow-up in the meta-analysis.

Risk of bias and quality of evidence

All six trials were at low risk of bias (Fig. 2). The greatest risk of bias came from blinding. The nature of the trial

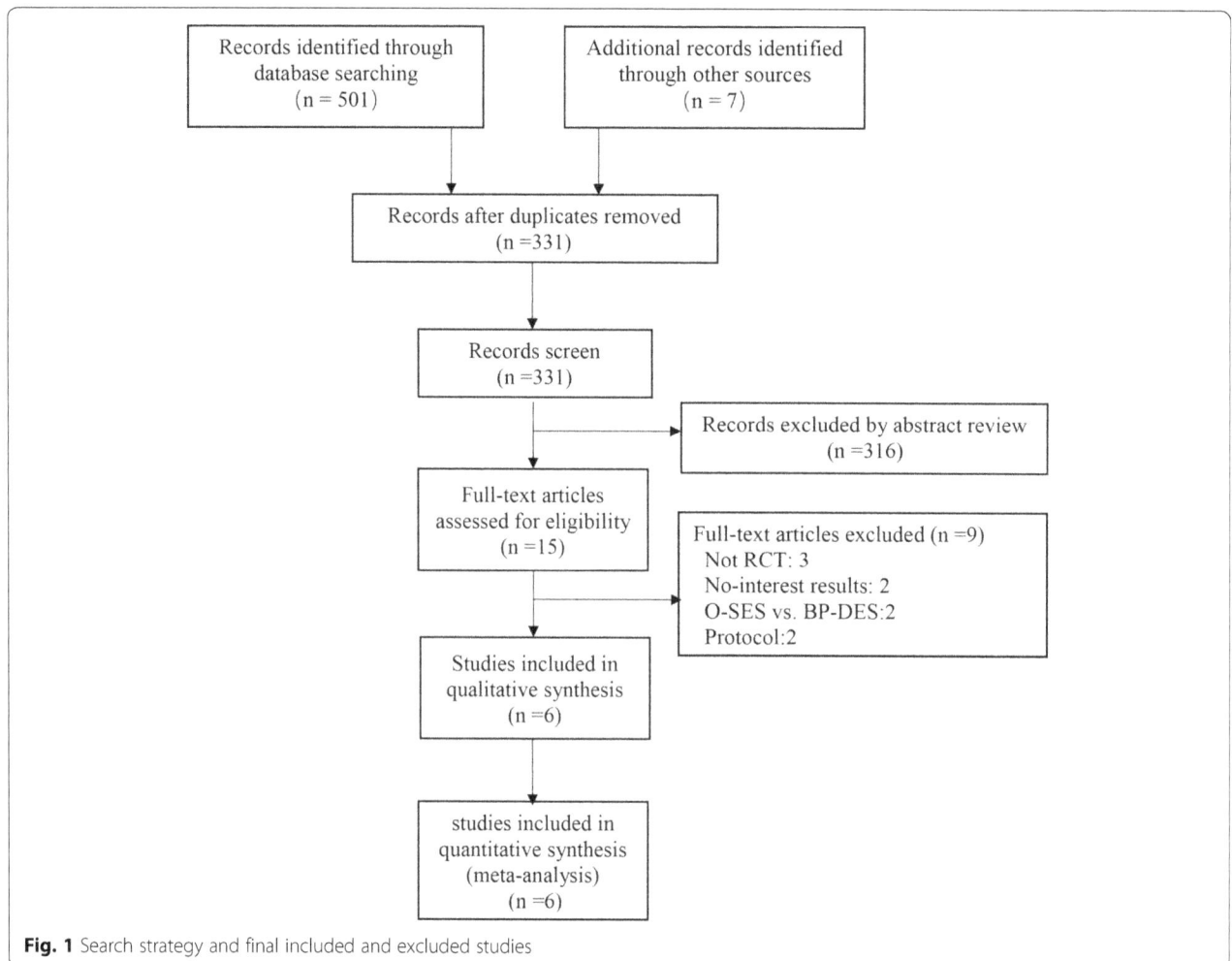

Fig. 1 Search strategy and final included and excluded studies

Table 1 Characteristics of patients in eligible studies

Trial	Year	No. of Patients		Follow-up (months)	DAPT (Months)	O-DES Characteristics			DP-DES Characteristics		
		O-SES	DP-DES			Stent	Thickness	Drug	Stent	Thickness	Drug
BIO-RESORT	2016	1169	1173	12	6	Orsiro	60	Sirolimus	Resolute Integrity	91	zotarolimus
BIOFLOW II	2015	298	154	12	> 6	Orsiro	60	Sirolimus	Xience Prime	81	Everolimus
BIOFLOW V	2017	884	450	12	> 6	Orsiro	60	Sirolimus	Xience Prime	81	Everolimus
BIOSCIENCE	2016	1063	1056	12	12	Orsiro	60	Sirolimus	Xience Prime	81	Everolimus
ORIENT	2017	250	122	12	> 12	Orsiro	60	Sirolimus	Resolute Integrity	91	zotarolimus
PRISON IV	2017	165	165	12	> 12	Orsiro	60	Sirolimus	Xience Prime	81	Everolimus

interventions precluded blinding of their physicians; whereas five of trials stated that blinding of outcome assessment was used and the other one was unclear. GRADE summary findings for all outcomes is showed in Table 2. We did not use funnel plots to assess the existence of possible publication bias because there were only six trials included in our meta-analysis.

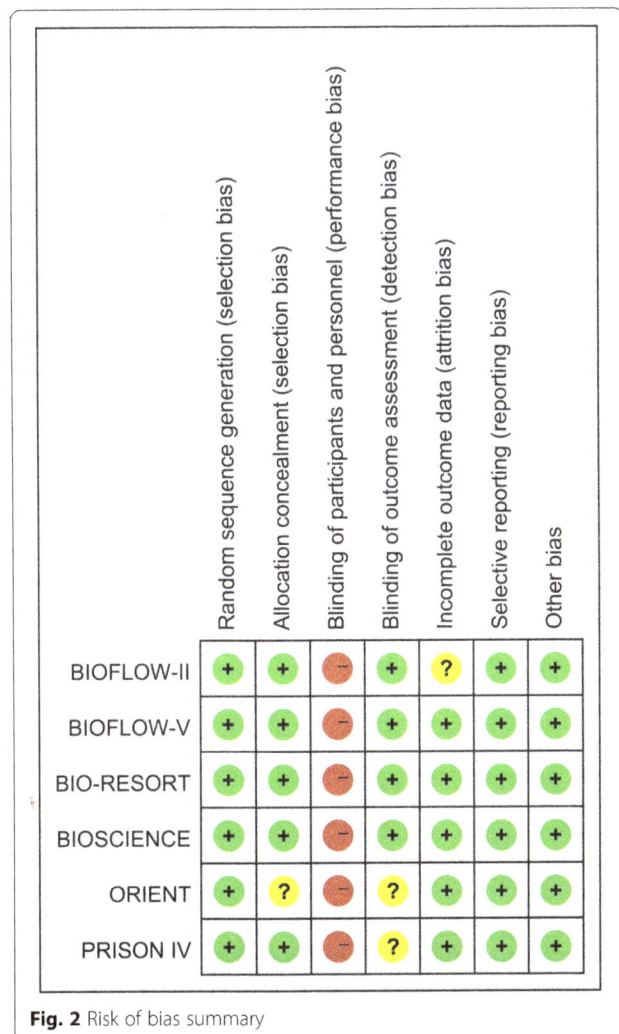

Fig. 2 Risk of bias summary

Safety endpoints: MI, ST, and cardiac mortality

The associations between O-SES versus DP-DES and safety outcomes are shown in Fig. 3. All six trials reported safety outcomes. MI occurred in 142 of 3777(3.8%) participants randomized to the O-SES group and 147 of 3095(4.8%) participants randomized to the medical therapy group. The risk ratio (RR) for MI also confer an advantage of O-SES over DP-DES (RR 0.78, 95% CI 0.62–0.98; I^2 = 0%; 10 fewer per 1000 [from 1 fewer to 18 fewer]; high quality). Sensitivity analyses using an alternative statistical method (Inverse Variance; RR 0.78, 95% CI 0.62–0.97; I^2 = 0%), effect measure (Odds Ratio 0.77, 95% CI 0.60–0.97; I^2 = 0%), and analysis model showed similar results of MI (Fixed; RR 0.78, 95% CI 0.62–0.98; I^2 = 0%). TSA confirmed that the required information size was not met (Fig. 5 in Appendix 4).

The meta-analysis showed no significant difference between O-SES and DP-SES on ST (RR: 0.75; 95% CI: 0.52–1.08; I^2 = 0%) or cardiac mortality (RR: 0.93; 95% CI: 0.63–1.36; I^2 = 0%).

Efficacy outcomes: TVR and TLR

All the included studies presented outcomes of TVR and TLR, showing that there was no statistically significant difference between O-SES and DP-DES regarding TVR (RR 0.97, 95% CI 0.78–1.21) and TLR (RR 1.10, 95% CI 0.86–1.42). (Fig. 4).

Subgroup analysis

We performed a subgroup analysis based on various DES types (everolimus and zotarolimus). Like the overall analysis, this subgroup analysis showed that O-SES has certain benefit in reducing risk of MI compared to DP-EES (RR 0.75, 95% CI 0.58–0.96; I^2 = 0%, Fig. 6 in Appendix 5) but this benefit did not show in cardiac mortality, ST, TVR, or TLR. There is no significant difference between O-SES and DP-ZES in the risks of MI, cardiac mortality, TVR, or TLR.

Table 2 GRADE evidence profile of outcomes, O-SES versus DP-DES

Outcome	No. of patients (Studies)		Study results (95% CI) and measurements	Absolute effect estimates (per 1000)			Quality	Importance
	O-SES	DP-DES		O-SES	DP-DES	Absolute Risk (95% CI)		
Myocardial infarction	142/3777 (3.8%)	147/3095 (4.7%)	RR 0.78 (0.62 to 0.98)	37	47	10 fewer (from 1 fewer to 18 fewer)	⊕⊕⊕⊕ High	Critical
Stent thrombosis	50/3767 (1.3%)	63/3095 (2%)	RR 0.75 (0.52 to 1.08)	15	20	5 fewer (from 10 fewer to 2 more)	⊕⊕⊕⊖ Moderate[a]	Important
Cardiac death	50/3777 (1.3%)	50/3095 (1.6%)	RR 0.93 (0.63 to 1.36)	15	16	1 fewer (from 6 fewer to 6 more)	⊕⊕⊕⊖ Moderate[a]	Important
Target vessel revascularization	166/3778 (4.4%)	141/3092 (4.6%)	RR 0.97 (0.78 to 1.21)	45	46	1 fewer (from 10 fewer to 10 more)	⊕⊕⊕⊕ High	Important
Target lesion revascularization	129/3777 (3.4%)	101/3094 (3.3%)	RR 1.1 (0.86 to 1.42)	36	33	3 more (from 5 fewer to 14 more)	⊕⊕⊕⊕ High	Important

CI Confidence interval, RR Risk ratio, O-SES Orsiro biodegradable polymer sirolimus-eluting stent, DP-DES Durable polymer drug-eluting stents;

High quality: Further research is very unlikely to change our confidence in the estimate of effect. Moderate quality: Further research is likely to have an important impact on our confidence in the estimate of effect and may change the estimate. Low quality: Further research is very likely to have an important impact on our confidence in the estimate of effect and is likely to change the estimate. Very low quality: We are very uncertain about the estimate

[a]Serious imprecision

A   Myocardial infarction

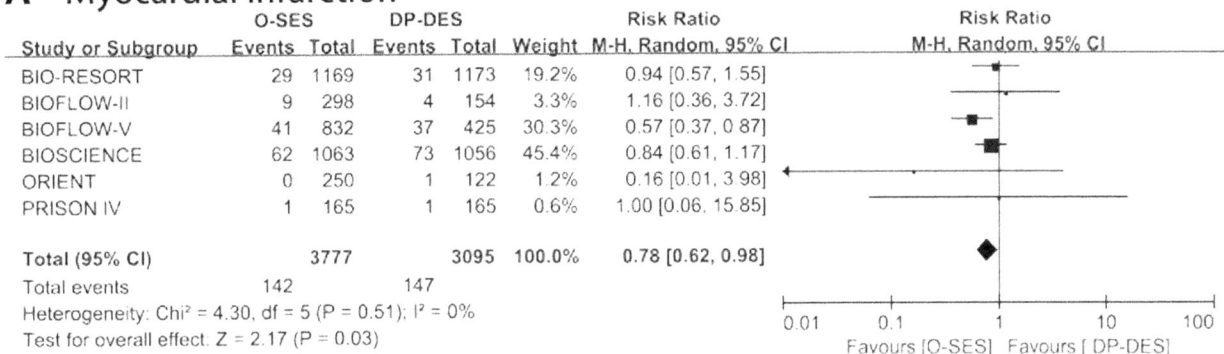

Study or Subgroup	O-SES Events	O-SES Total	DP-DES Events	DP-DES Total	Weight	Risk Ratio M-H, Random, 95% CI
BIO-RESORT	29	1169	31	1173	19.2%	0.94 [0.57, 1.55]
BIOFLOW-II	9	298	4	154	3.3%	1.16 [0.36, 3.72]
BIOFLOW-V	41	832	37	425	30.3%	0.57 [0.37, 0.87]
BIOSCIENCE	62	1063	73	1056	45.4%	0.84 [0.61, 1.17]
ORIENT	0	250	1	122	1.2%	0.16 [0.01, 3.98]
PRISON IV	1	165	1	165	0.6%	1.00 [0.06, 15.85]
Total (95% CI)		3777		3095	100.0%	0.78 [0.62, 0.98]
Total events	142		147			

Heterogeneity: Chi² = 4.30, df = 5 (P = 0.51); I² = 0%
Test for overall effect: Z = 2.17 (P = 0.03)

Risk Ratio M-H, Random, 95% CI
0.01   0.1   1   10   100
Favours [O-SES]   Favours [DP-DES]

B   Stent thrombosis

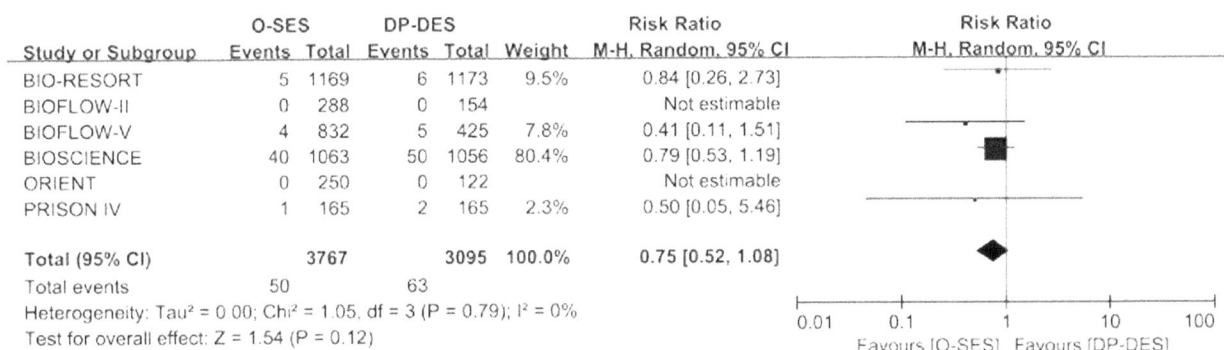

Study or Subgroup	O-SES Events	O-SES Total	DP-DES Events	DP-DES Total	Weight	Risk Ratio M-H, Random, 95% CI
BIO-RESORT	5	1169	6	1173	9.5%	0.84 [0.26, 2.73]
BIOFLOW-II	0	288	0	154		Not estimable
BIOFLOW-V	4	832	5	425	7.8%	0.41 [0.11, 1.51]
BIOSCIENCE	40	1063	50	1056	80.4%	0.79 [0.53, 1.19]
ORIENT	0	250	0	122		Not estimable
PRISON IV	1	165	2	165	2.3%	0.50 [0.05, 5.46]
Total (95% CI)		3767		3095	100.0%	0.75 [0.52, 1.08]
Total events	50		63			

Heterogeneity: Tau² = 0.00; Chi² = 1.05, df = 3 (P = 0.79); I² = 0%
Test for overall effect: Z = 1.54 (P = 0.12)

Risk Ratio M-H, Random, 95% CI
0.01   0.1   1   10   100
Favours [O-SES]   Favours [DP-DES]

C   Cardiac death

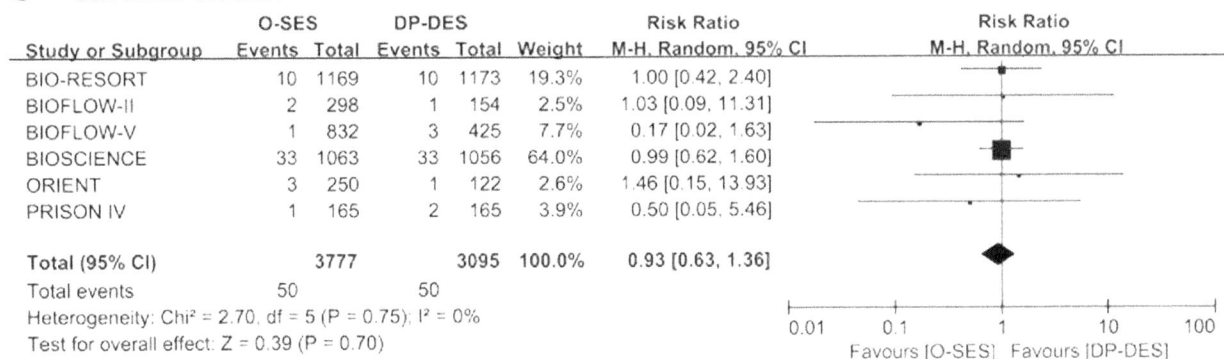

Study or Subgroup	O-SES Events	O-SES Total	DP-DES Events	DP-DES Total	Weight	Risk Ratio M-H, Random, 95% CI
BIO-RESORT	10	1169	10	1173	19.3%	1.00 [0.42, 2.40]
BIOFLOW-II	2	298	1	154	2.5%	1.03 [0.09, 11.31]
BIOFLOW-V	1	832	3	425	7.7%	0.17 [0.02, 1.63]
BIOSCIENCE	33	1063	33	1056	64.0%	0.99 [0.62, 1.60]
ORIENT	3	250	1	122	2.6%	1.46 [0.15, 13.93]
PRISON IV	1	165	2	165	3.9%	0.50 [0.05, 5.46]
Total (95% CI)		3777		3095	100.0%	0.93 [0.63, 1.36]
Total events	50		50			

Heterogeneity: Chi² = 2.70, df = 5 (P = 0.75); I² = 0%
Test for overall effect: Z = 0.39 (P = 0.70)

Risk Ratio M-H, Random, 95% CI
0.01   0.1   1   10   100
Favours [O-SES]   Favours [DP-DES]

Fig. 3 Forest plot assessing safety outcomes. A: myocardial infarction, B: definite or probable stent thrombosis, C: cardiac death. CI = confidence interval; M-H = Mantel-Haenszel; SE = standard error

Discussion

In this meta-analysis of 6 RCTs, we found that MI was significantly lower in patients with O-SES than in patients with DP-DES. There was no evidence of a difference between groups concerning cardiac mortality, ST, TLR, and TVR.

Possibly our most important finding was the significant risk reduction for MI in patients with O-SES compared with DP-DES. Contrary to our meta-analysis, however, recent meta-analyses showed that BP-DES were similar regarding cardiovascular outcomes including MI compared to second-generation DP-DES [8, 24].

Similarly, a meta-analysis comparing BP-SES with DP-DES found there was no significant difference in the risk of MI [25]. The different results regarding MI between our meta-analysis and previous meta-analyses may be explained by the different eligibility criteria. Our meta-analysis included trials comparing O-SES with DP-DES rather than BP-DES (or BP-SES) with DP-DES. O-SES has the thinnest strut thickness to date. It is probable that the thinner stent struts of the O-SES (60 μm) compared with DP-DES (81–91 μm) lead to the lower risk of MI. The effect of stent strut thickness has been well established. In fact, compared to the thicker struts, thinner struts have been

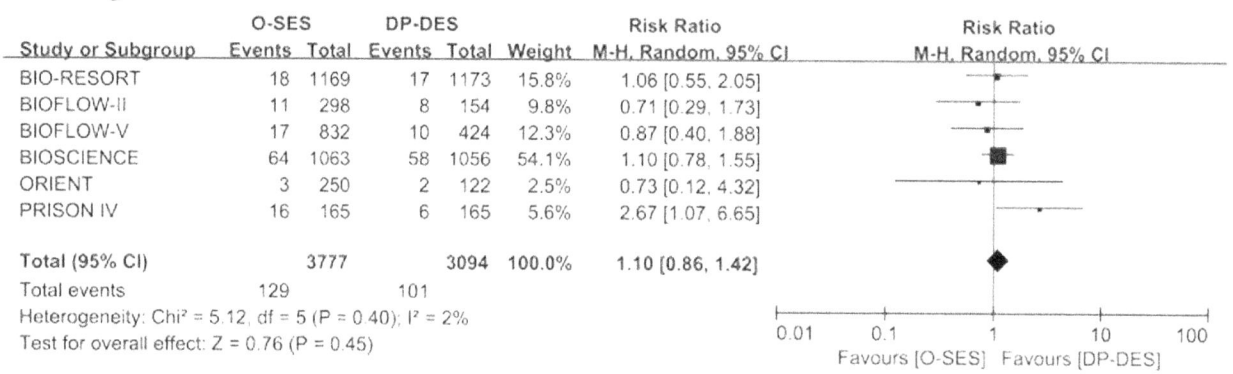

Fig. 4 Forest plot assessing efficacy outcomes. A: target vessel revascularization, B: target lesion revascularization (TLR). CI = confidence interval; M-H = Mantel-Haenszel; SE = standard error

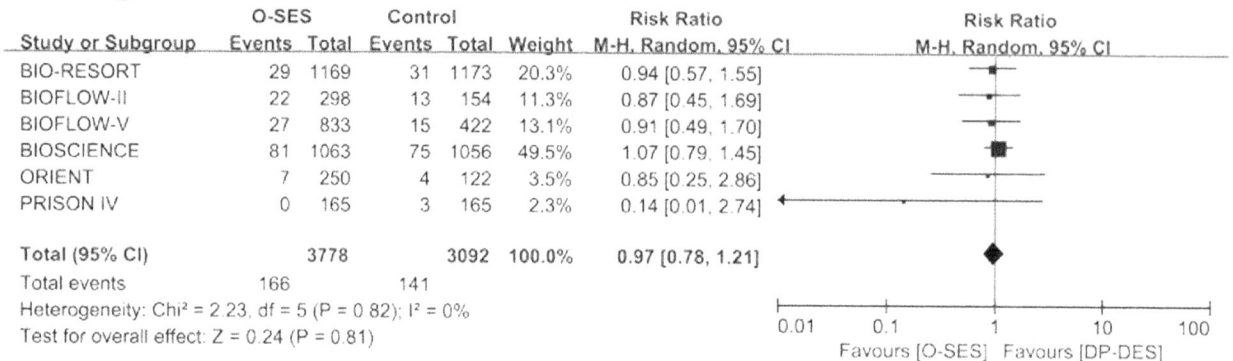

shown to reduce vessel injury, inflammation, neointimal proliferation, and thrombus formation [10, 11, 26, 27]. Reduction in strut thickness from stainless steel (132–140 μm) to chromium alloys (81–91 μm) contributed to a decreased risk of MI by about 40–80% [28–31].

Our meta-analysis has reported results suggestive of a protective effect of O-SES on ST compared with DP-DSE but failed to show the statistical significance of this association. One explanation for this fail was the small number of events during the follow-up. New generation DES have the most favourable safety and efficacy outcomes to date, adverse events have become less frequent in the past decade. Thus, to find a significant difference in management strategy, additional RCTs needs to follow patients for a long duration or enrol substantial numbers.

Our study did not show a significant decrease of TVR or TLR in O-SES compared with DP-DES. Indeed, two prior network meta-analyses have demonstrated a reduced risk of TVR and TLR of BP-DES compared to DP-DES [4, 32]. But, BP-SES were not included in the two network meta-analyses. A meta-analysis comparing BP-SES with DP-DES found similar efficacy profiles between those groups [25].

Strengths and limitations

Strengths of our meta-analysis included duplicate assessment of risk of bias, eligibility, and data abstraction. The meta-analysis included a rigorous assessment of the quality of evidence. We have evaluated relative and absolute risks, which are crucial for making decisions between O-SES and DP-DES.

First, different DP-DES platforms were used for comparison in the RCTs included in our meta-analysis. However, authors attempted to overcome these differences by performing a subgroup analysis based on DP-DES. We found O-SES significantly decreased MI compared to DP-EES but not to DP-ZES.

Second, a small number (6 RCTs, 6949 patients) and short follow-up duration (12 months) of included trials might afford insufficient ability to detect differences in rare events. For example, our results might suggest a reduced ST in O-SES but failed to show the statistical significance of this association. Thus, longer duration of follow-up and larger populations are required for further research.

Third, the limited number of included RCTs lead to insufficiently detect the presence of publication bias. However, publication bias is unlikely as most included RCTs had negative results.

Fourth, previous meta-analysis suggested a possible increased midterm risk for ST and MI with BP-DES [33]. However, we did not report mid- and long-term outcomes in this topic, because follow-up data of longer than 1 year is limited. Thus, the mid- and long-term safety and efficacy of O-SES vs. DP-DES is not clealy established.

Fifth, although the statistical heterogeneity was very low in most outcomes ($I^2 = 0$), there may be substantially clinical heterogeneity, which was driven by differences in methodological and clinical features between trials. For example, the duration and the type of dual antiplatelet therapy may have an influence on outcomes; however, we cannot perform a subgroup analyses on dual antiplatelet therapy because of lack of data from included trials. Sixth, TSA found that the required information size was not met. Thus, this review mirrors the lack of quantity of the included trials. The results of ongoing and future well designed, large randomized clinical trials are needed.

Conclusions

Compared with DP-DES, O-SES showed a significantly reduced risk of MI and a trend toward reduction in ST.

Appendix 1

Table 3 Search strategy on PubMed

#1	"Percutaneous Coronary Intervention"[Mesh]
#2	"Coronary Disease"[Mesh]
#3	"PCI"
#4	"CAD"
#5	(#1) OR (#2) OR (#3) OR (#4)
#6	"biodegradable"[tiab]
#7	"degradable"[tiab]
#8	"bioabsorbable"[tiab]
#9	"absorbable"[tiab]
#10	"absorptive"[tiab]
#11	" orsiro"[tiab]
#12	"O-SES"[tiab]
#13	"dissolvable"[tiab]
#14	(#6) OR (#7) OR (#8) OR (#9) OR (#10) OR (#11) OR (#12) OR (#13)
#15	"Polymers"[Mesh] OR "Polymer"[tiab] OR "coating"[tiab]
#16	(#14) AND (#15)
#17	"BioMatrix" OR "NOBORI" OR "Axxess" OR "Supralimus" OR "Infinnium" OR "BioMime" OR "Orsiro" OR "DESyne" OR "SYNERGY" OR "MiStent" OR "Excel" OR "Firehawk" OR "NOYA" OR "Inspiron" OR "Tivoli" OR "BuMA" OR "Svelte" OR "Custom" OR "NEVO" OR "Elixir" OR "JACTAX" OR "CORACTO"
#18	(#16)) OR (#17)
#19	"randomized controlled trial"[pt] OR "controlled clinical trial"[pt] OR "randomized"[tiab] OR "randomly"[tiab] OR "trial"[tiab] OR " clinical trials as topic"[sh]
#20	# (5) AND # (18) AND # (19)

Appendix 2

Table 4 Characteristics of patients in eligible studies

	Age	Male sex (%)	Hypertension (%)	Diabetes mellitus (%)	Smoker (%)	Previous MI (%)	ACS (%)	Stable angina (%)
BIO-RESORT	64 ± 11	72	46	18	30	19	70	30
BIOFLOW II	63 ± 10	77	78	28	27	27	NR	NR
BIOFLOW V	65 ± 10	74	80	35	23	27	51	48
BIOSCIENCE	66 ± 12	77	68	23	29	20	53	31
ORIENT	65 ± 11	72	65	26	27	NR	45	55
PRISON IV	63 ± 10	78	56	20	33	30	17	70

Appendix 3

Table 5 Primary and second outcomes of the Included Trials

	Primary outcome	Second outcomes
BIO-RESORT	target vessel failure at 12 months	target lesion failure, death, myocardial infarction, coronary revascularization, major adverse cardiac events, patient-oriented composite endpoint, definite or probable stent thrombosis
BIOFLOW II	in-stent late lumen loss at 9 months	in-segment late lumen loss and in-stent and in-segment minimal luminal diameter, percent diameter stenosis, and binary restenosis. Cardiac death, procedure-related deaths, myocardial infarction, target-lesion revascularization.
BIOFLOW V	target lesion failure at 12 months	major adverse cardiac events (all-cause death, myocardial infarction or ischemia-driven target lesion revascularization), target vessel failure, the individual components of the composite endpoints at 30 days and 12 months, and definite or probable stent thrombosis according to academic research consortium (arc) criteria.
BIOSCIENCE	target-lesion failure at 12 months	all-cause death, cardiac death, myocardial infarction, target vessel mi, coronary revascularization, major adverse cardiac events, patient-oriented composite endpoint, stent thrombosis, target lesion revascularization, target vessel revascularization, repeat revascularization, target vessel failure, cerebrovascular event
ORIENT	in-stent late lumen loss at 9 months,	in-segment late lumen loss, percentage diameter stenosis, and binary restenosis at 9 months; all-cause death, cardiac death, myocardial infarction, repeat revascularization, ischemic stroke, hemorrhagic stroke, bleeding, stent thrombosis, target lesion failure, target vessel failure
PRISON IV	in-segment late lumen loss at 9 months	in-stent late lumen loss, in-stent and in-segment percentage of diameter stenosis, binary restenosis, and re-occlusions at 9 months; clinically indicated target lesion, revascularization or target vessel revascularization, myocardial infarction, death (cardiac and noncardiac), stent thrombosis, target vessel failure, and major adverse cardiac events.

Appendix 4

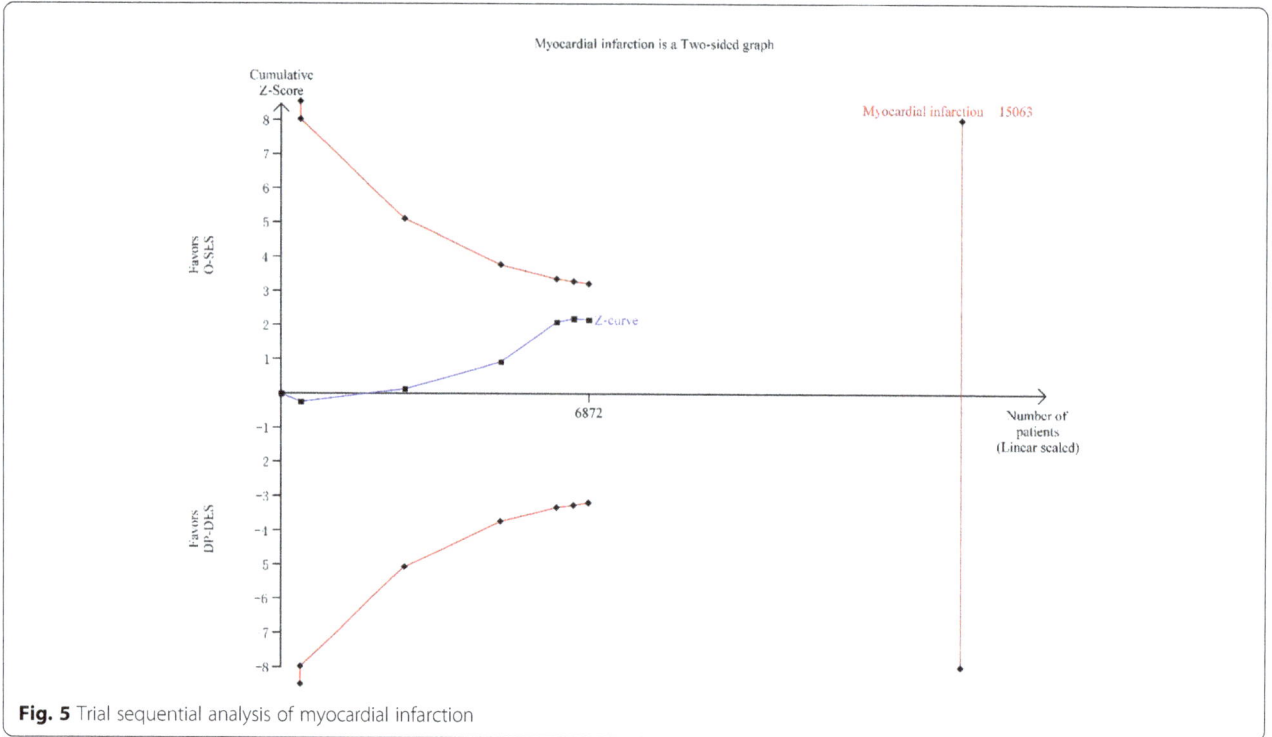

Fig. 5 Trial sequential analysis of myocardial infarction

Appendix 5

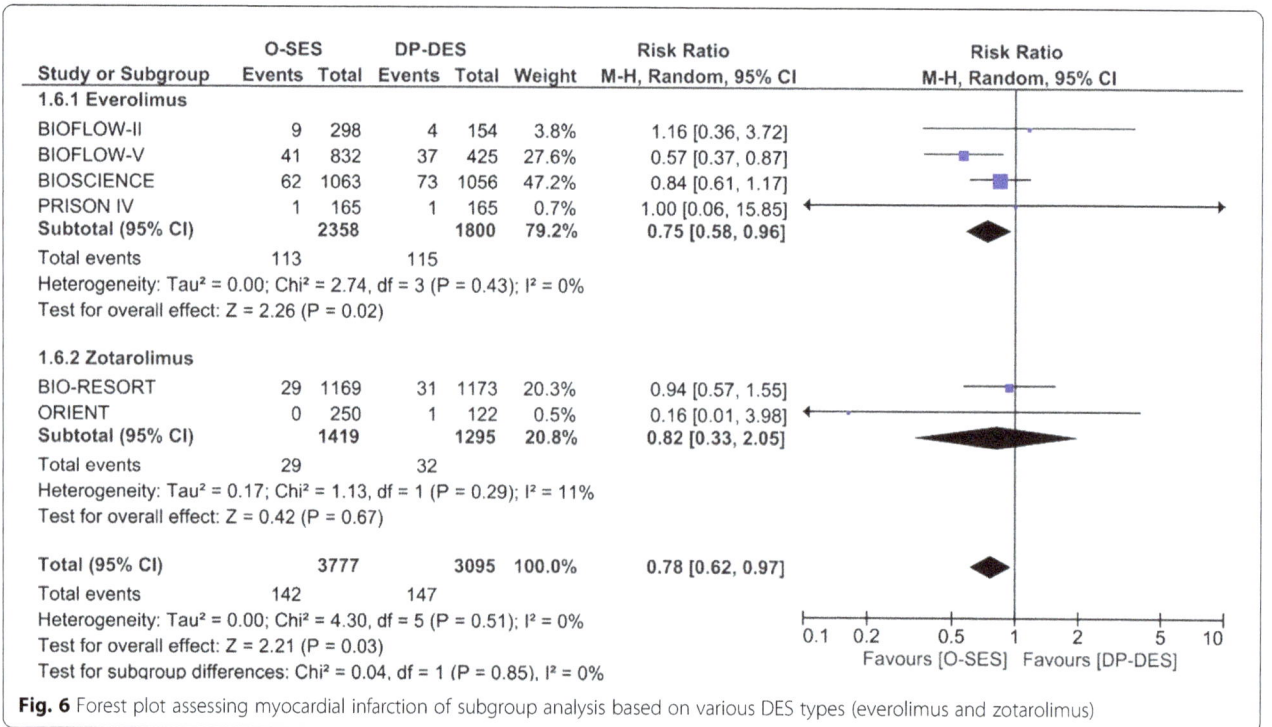

Fig. 6 Forest plot assessing myocardial infarction of subgroup analysis based on various DES types (everolimus and zotarolimus)

Abbreviations
BP: Biodegradable polymer; CI: Confidence intervals; DES: Drug-eluting stent; DP: Durable polymer; EES: Everolimus-eluting stents; MI: Myocardial infarction; O-SES: Orsiro biodegradable polymer sirolimus-eluting stent; RCTs: Randomized controlled trials; RR: Risk ratios; ST: Stent thrombosis; TLR: Target lesion revascularization; TVR: Target vessel revascularization; ZES: Zotarolimus-eluting stents

Funding
This work is supported by Southwest Hospital Project: SWH2016JSTSZD-09.

Authors' contributions
PZ and ZS had the idea for the review, and PZ and XZ managed the literature search and data extraction. PZ, XZ, CZ, HL, ZZ and ZS developed the analysis plan. PZ and XZ conducted the analysis and developed the figures. HL, PZ, and ZS wrote the original draft of the manuscript. PZ, XZ, and ZS determined the study approach, interpreted the results, and critically reviewed the manuscript. All authors read and approved the final manuscript.

Competing interests
The authors declare that they have no competing interests.

References
1. Byrne RA, Stone GW, Ormiston J, Kastrati A. Coronary balloon angioplasty, stents, and scaffolds. Lancet. 2017;390(10096):781–92.
2. Joner M, Finn AV, Farb A, Mont EK, Kolodgie FD, Ladich E, Kutys R, Skorija K, Gold HK, Virmani R. Pathology of drug-eluting stents in humans: delayed healing and late thrombotic risk. J Am Coll Cardiol. 2006;48(1):193–202.
3. Finn AV, Nakazawa G, Joner M, Kolodgie FD, Mont EK, Gold HK, Virmani R. Vascular responses to drug eluting stents: importance of delayed healing. Arterioscler Thromb Vasc Biol. 2007;27(7):1500–10.
4. Navarese EP, Tandjung K, Claessen B, Andreotti F, Kowalewski M, Kandzari DE, Kereiakes DJ, Waksman R, Mauri L, Meredith IT, et al. Safety and efficacy outcomes of first and second generation durable polymer drug eluting stents and biodegradable polymer biolimus eluting stents in clinical practice: comprehensive network meta-analysis. BMJ. 2013;347:f6530.
5. Kang SH, Park KW, Kang DY, Lim WH, Park KT, Han JK, Kang HJ, Koo BK, Oh BH, Park YB, et al. Biodegradable-polymer drug-eluting stents vs. bare metal stents vs. durable-polymer drug-eluting stents: a systematic review and Bayesian approach network meta-analysis. Eur Heart J. 2014;35(17):1147–58.
6. Palmerini T, Benedetto U, Biondi-Zoccai G, Della Riva D, Bacchi-Reggiani L, Smits PC, Vlachojannis GJ, Jensen LO, Christiansen EH, Berencsi K, et al. Long-term safety of drug-eluting and bare-metal stents: evidence from a comprehensive network meta-analysis. J Am Coll Cardiol. 2015;65(23): 2496–507.
7. Stefanini GG, Holmes DR Jr. Drug-eluting coronary-artery stents. N Engl J Med. 2013;368(3):254–65.
8. El-Hayek G, Bangalore S, Casso Dominguez A, Devireddy C, Jaber W, Kumar G, Mavromatis K, Tamis-Holland J, Samady H. Meta-analysis of randomized clinical trials comparing biodegradable polymer drug-eluting stent to second-generation durable polymer drug-eluting stents. JACC Cardiovasc Interv. 2017;10(5):462–73.
9. Stefanini GG, Taniwaki M, Windecker S. Coronary stents: novel developments. Heart. 2014;100(13):1051–61.
10. Kolandaivelu K, Swaminathan R, Gibson WJ, Kolachalama VB, Nguyen-Ehrenreich KL, Giddings VL, Coleman L, Wong GK, Edelman ER. Stent thrombogenicity early in high-risk interventional settings is driven by stent design and deployment and protected by polymer-drug coatings. Circulation. 2011;123(13):1400–9.
11. Kastrati A, Mehilli J, Dirschinger J, Dotzer F, Schuhlen H, Neumann FJ, Fleckenstein M, Pfafferott C, Seyfarth M, Schomig A. Intracoronary stenting and angiographic results: strut thickness effect on restenosis outcome (ISAR-STEREO) trial. Circulation. 2001;103(23):2816–21.
12. Windecker S, Stortecky S, Stefanini GG, da Costa BR, Rutjes AW, Di Nisio M, Silletta MG, Maione A, Alfonso F, Clemmensen PM, et al. Revascularisation versus medical treatment in patients with stable coronary artery disease: network meta-analysis. BMJ. 2014;348:g3859.
13. Windecker S, Haude M, Neumann FJ, Stangl K, Witzenbichler B, Slagboom T, Sabate M, Goicolea J, Barragan P, Cook S, et al. Comparison of a novel biodegradable polymer sirolimus-eluting stent with a durable polymer everolimus-eluting stent: results of the randomized BIOFLOW-II trial. Circ Cardiovasc Interv. 2015;8(2):e001441.
14. von Birgelen C, Kok MM, van der Heijden LC, Danse PW, Schotborgh CE, Scholte M, Gin R, Somi S, van Houwelingen KG, Stoel MG, et al. Very thin strut biodegradable polymer everolimus-eluting and sirolimus-eluting stents versus durable polymer zotarolimus-eluting stents in allcomers with coronary artery disease (BIO-RESORT): a three-arm, randomised, non-inferiority trial. Lancet. 2016;388(10060):2607–17.
15. Zbinden R, Piccolo R, Heg D, Roffi M, Kurz DJ, Muller O, Vuilliomenet A, Cook S, Weilenmann D, Kaiser C, et al. Ultrathin strut biodegradable polymer Sirolimus-eluting stent versus durable-polymer Everolimus-eluting stent for percutaneous coronary revascularization: 2-year results of the BIOSCIENCE trial. J Am Heart Assoc. 2016;5(3):e003255.
16. Kandzari DE, Mauri L, Koolen JJ, Massaro JM, Doros G, Garcia-Garcia HM, Bennett J, Roguin A, Gharib EG, Cutlip DE, et al. Ultrathin, bioresorbable polymer sirolimus-eluting stents versus thin, durable polymer everolimus-eluting stents in patients undergoing coronary revascularisation (BIOFLOW V): a randomised trial. Lancet. 2017;390(10105):1843–52.
17. Kang SH, Chung WY, Lee JM, Park JJ, Yoon CH, Suh JW, Cho YS, Doh JH, Cho JM, Bae JW, et al. Angiographic outcomes of Orsiro biodegradable polymer sirolimus-eluting stents and resolute integrity durable polymer zotarolimus-eluting stents: results of the ORIENT trial. EuroIntervention. 2017;12(13):1623–31.
18. Teeuwen K, van der Schaaf RJ, Adriaenssens T, Koolen JJ, Smits PC, Henriques JP, Vermeersch PH, Joe T, Gin RM, Scholzel BE, Kelder JC, et al. Randomized multicenter trial investigating angiographic outcomes of hybrid Sirolimus-eluting stents with biodegradable polymer compared with Everolimus-eluting stents with durable polymer in chronic Total occlusions: the PRISON IV trial. JACC Cardiovasc Interv. 2017;10(2):133–43.
19. Liberati A, Altman DG, Tetzlaff J, Mulrow C, Gotzsche PC, Ioannidis JP, Clarke M, Devereaux PJ, Kleijnen J, Moher D. The PRISMA statement for reporting systematic reviews and meta-analyses of studies that evaluate healthcare interventions: explanation and elaboration. BMJ. 2009;339:b2700.
20. Shinichi A. Cochrane handbook for systematic reviews of interventions. Online Kensaku. 2014;35(3):154–5.
21. Guyatt GH, Oxman AD, Vist GE, Kunz R, Falck-Ytter Y, Alonso-Coello P, Schunemann HJ. GRADE: an emerging consensus on rating quality of evidence and strength of recommendations. BMJ. 2008;336(7650):924–6.
22. Higgins JP, Thompson SG. Quantifying heterogeneity in a meta-analysis. Stat Med. 2002;21(11):1539–58.
23. Brok J, Thorlund K, Gluud C, Wetterslev J. Trial sequential analysis reveals insufficient information size and potentially false positive results in many meta-analyses. J Clin Epidemiol. 2008;61(8):763–9.
24. Pandya B, Gaddam S, Raza M, Asti D, Nalluri N, Vazzana T, Kandov R, Lafferty J. Biodegradable polymer stents vs second generation drug eluting stents: a meta-analysis and systematic review of randomized controlled trials. World J Cardiol. 2016;8(2):240–6.
25. Yang Y, Lei J, Huang W, Lei H. Efficacy and safety of biodegradable polymer sirolimus-eluting stents versus durable polymer drug-eluting stents: a meta-analysis of randomized trials. Int J Cardiol. 2016;222:486–93.
26. Soucy NV, Feygin JM, Tunstall R, Casey MA, Pennington DE, Huibregtse BA, Barry JJ. Strut tissue coverage and endothelial cell coverage: a comparison between bare metal stent platforms and platinum chromium stents with and without everolimus-eluting coating. EuroIntervention. 2010;6(5):630–7.
27. Pache J, Kastrati A, Mehilli J, Schuhlen H, Dotzer F, Hausleiter J, Fleckenstein M, Neumann FJ, Sattelberger U, Schmitt C, et al. Intracoronary stenting and angiographic results: strut thickness effect on restenosis outcome (ISAR-STEREO-2) trial. J Am Coll Cardiol. 2003;41(8):1283–8.
28. Kandzari DE, Leon MB, Popma JJ, Fitzgerald PJ, O'Shaughnessy C, Ball MW, Turco M, Applegate RJ, Gurbel PA, Midei MG, et al. Comparison of zotarolimus-eluting and sirolimus-eluting stents in patients with native coronary artery disease: a randomized controlled trial. J Am Coll Cardiol. 2006;48(12):2440–7.

29. Stone GW, Midei M, Newman W, Sanz M, Hermiller JB, Williams J, Farhat N, Mahaffey KW, Cutlip DE, Fitzgerald PJ, et al. Comparison of an everolimus-eluting stent and a paclitaxel-eluting stent in patients with coronary artery disease: a randomized trial. Jama. 2008;299(16):1903–13.

30. Leon MB, Mauri L, Popma JJ, Cutlip DE, Nikolsky E, O'Shaughnessy C, Overlie PA, McLaurin BT, Solomon SL, Douglas JS Jr, et al. A randomized comparison of the Endeavor zotarolimus-eluting stent versus the TAXUS paclitaxel-eluting stent in de novo native coronary lesions 12-month outcomes from the ENDEAVOR IV trial. J Am Coll Cardiol. 2010;55(6):543–54.

31. Stone GW, Rizvi A, Newman W, Mastali K, Wang JC, Caputo R, Doostzadeh J, Cao S, Simonton CA, Sudhir K, et al. Everolimus-eluting versus paclitaxel-eluting stents in coronary artery disease. N Engl J Med. 2010;362(18):1663–74.

32. Bangalore S, Toklu B, Amoroso N, Fusaro M, Kumar S, Hannan EL, Faxon DP, Feit F. Bare metal stents, durable polymer drug eluting stents, and biodegradable polymer drug eluting stents for coronary artery disease: mixed treatment comparison meta-analysis. *BMJ*. 2013;347:f6625.

33. Cassese S, Byrne RA, Ndrepepa G, Kufner S, Wiebe J, Repp J, Schunkert H, Fusaro M, Kimura T, Kastrati A. Everolimus-eluting bioresorbable vascular scaffolds versus everolimus-eluting metallic stents: a meta-analysis of randomised controlled trials. *Lancet*. 2016;387(10018):537–44.

22

Three-dimensional thoracic aorta principal strain analysis from routine ECG-gated computerized tomography: feasibility in patients undergoing transcatheter aortic valve replacement

Alessandro Satriano[1,2] (iD), Zachary Guenther[1,3], James A. White[1,2], Naeem Merchant[1,3], Elena S. Di Martino[4], Faisal Al-Qoofi[2], Carmen P. Lydell[1,3†] and Nowell M. Fine[2*†]

Abstract

Background: Functional impairment of the aorta is a recognized complication of aortic and aortic valve disease. Aortic strain measurement provides effective quantification of mechanical aortic function, and 3-dimenional (3D) approaches may be desirable for serial evaluation. Computerized tomographic angiography (CTA) is routinely performed for various clinical indications, and offers the unique potential to study 3D aortic deformation. We sought to investigate the feasibility of performing 3D aortic strain analysis in a candidate population of patients undergoing transcatheter aortic valve replacement (TAVR).

Methods: Twenty-one patients with severe aortic valve stenosis (AS) referred for TAVR underwent ECG-gated CTA and echocardiography. CTA images were analyzed using a 3D feature-tracking based technique to construct a dynamic aortic mesh model to perform peak principal strain amplitude (PPSA) analysis. Segmental strain values were correlated against clinical, hemodynamic and echocardiographic variables. Reproducibility analysis was performed.

Results: The mean patient age was 81±6 years. Mean left ventricular ejection fraction was 52±14%, aortic valve area (AVA) 0.6±0.3 cm^2 and mean AS pressure gradient (MG) 44±11 mmHg. CTA-based 3D PPSA analysis was feasible in all subjects. Mean PPSA values for the global thoracic aorta, ascending aorta, aortic arch and descending aorta segments were 6.5±3.0, 10.2±6.0, 6.1±2.9 and 3.3±1.7%, respectively. 3D PSSA values demonstrated significantly more impairment with measures of worsening AS severity, including AVA and MG for the global thoracic aorta and ascending segment (p<0.001 for all). 3D PSSA was independently associated with AVA by multivariable modelling. Coefficients of variation for intra- and inter-observer variability were 5.8 and 7.2%, respectively.

Conclusions: Three-dimensional aortic PPSA analysis is clinically feasible from routine ECG-gated CTA. Appropriate reductions in PSSA were identified with increasing AS hemodynamic severity. Expanded study of 3D aortic PSSA for patients with various forms of aortic disease is warranted.

Keywords: Computerized tomography, Strain, 3-dimensional, Aortic valve stenosis, Transcatheter aortic valve replacement

* Correspondence: nmfine@ucalgary.ca
†Equal contributors
[2]Division of Cardiology, Department of Cardiac Sciences, Libin Cardiovascular Institute of Alberta, University of Calgary, South Health Campus, 4448 Front Street SE, Calgary, Alberta T3M 1M4, Canada
Full list of author information is available at the end of the article

Background

Alterations in aortic biomechanical properties are recognized to occur with advancing age and in patients with primary and secondary forms of aortopathy [1, 2]. The resultant impairment in aortic function is an important contributor to global cardiovascular performance [3–5], and has been shown to have prognostic implications in specific patient cohorts, such as those with calcific degenerative aortic valve stenosis (AS) [6–8]. Indeed, associations between AS and increased aortic stiffness have been reliably demonstrated, leading to a theory that aortic disease may contribute to both symptom burden and clinical outcomes in this population [6, 8, 9]. However, optimal methods for assessing thoracic aorta biomechanics remains uncertain.

ECG-gated, contrast-enhanced computerized tomographic angiography (CTA) offers unique advantages for the study of aortic deformation. With complete 3-dimensional (3D) visualization at high isotropic spatial resolution, small displacements of the aortic wall can be resolved throughout the complex architecture. Multiphase reconstruction of such imaging has previously been used to derive 2-dimensional (2D) strain, [10–12]. A methodology exists to perform in-vivo 3D aortic strain analysis requiring a single segmentation at end-diastole, optically and automatically tracked in 3 dimensions throughout the cardiac cycle relying on a velocity-field reconstructed for the whole dataset by means image-based feature tracking, described by Satriano et al. [13]. Another approach exists leveraging on segmentations performed throughout the cardiac cycle, described by Pasta et al. [14]. In this approach, the point cloud obtained for the end-diastolic aortic luminal surface is projected normally onto the surfaces reconstructed for other cardiac phases [14]. However, the application of the single-segmentation approach [13] specifically to multi-phase CTA is previously undescribed. The latter is of interest given an emerging desire to serially and reproducibly evaluate regional patterns of disease across specific clinical populations [15]. Furthermore, the 3D optical tracking throughout the cardiac cycle [13] allows reconstruction of the full displacement field of the mesh, beyond the displacement of each node perpendicularly to the mesh. This allows for a comprehensive quantification of deformation [13]. Facilitating such an ability to evaluate 3D deformation, Principal strain analysis has been identified as an ideal deformation measure as it endeavors to measure tissue expansion without requirement for a pre-established axis of reference, describing the dominant (or principal) direction which strain is occurring within the tissue. This establishes a geometry-independent marker that may better represent vessel wall fiber orientation [16].

Exploiting the combined advantages of ECG-gated CTA and principal strain analysis, this study aimed to assess both the clinical feasibility and reproducibility of performing 3D principal aortic strain analysis in a clinical referral population. Among patients referred for transcatheter aortic valve replacement (TAVR), a population recognized for their burden of aortic disease and routinely referred for ECG-gated CTA, we identify the capacity of this technique to visualize and quantify global values and regional patterns of aortic deformation. Internal validation of aortic strain measures against expected influences of AS severity was also explored.

Methods

Study population

Twenty-one consecutive patients with severe, symptomatic AS referred for TAVR were included [17]. All patients underwent pre-operative assessment with ECG-gated CTA and transthoracic echocardiography prior to TAVR. Patients with atrial fibrillation, contraindications to receiving iodinated contrast dye, and those having prior aortic or cardiac surgery were excluded. Clinical and demographic data and systemic blood pressure (measured by brachial artery cuff sphygmomanometer) were obtained at the time of echocardiography. This study was reviewed and approved by the University of Calgary Research Ethics Board, and a waiver of consent was granted for access to patient health information due to the retrospective nature of the analysis.

Computed tomography imaging protocol

A routine pre-TAVR protocol CTA was performed with retrospective ECG gating (10 phases throughout the cardiac cycle) and dose modulation in all cases [18]. CT examinations were performed on two 64-slice CT scanners (Discovery C750 HD, GE Healthcare, Milwaukee Wisconsin). A volume of 80-100 mL of commercially available intravenous ioversol 320 mg/mL contrast was injected at 5 mL/sec followed by 50 mL of normal saline. The CT scanner detector collimation width was 0.625 mm, detector coverage was 40 mm, and the slice thickness was 0.625 mm. Gantry rotation time was 0.35 sec and the scan pitch was 0.16-0.2 depending on heart rate. The tube voltage was fixed at 100 kVp and 120 kVp for patients with a body mass index of ≤30 and >30, respectively. Maximum tube current ranged from 400 and 700 mA with ECG-gated dose modulation reducing the tube current to 20% maximum between 80-20% of the R-R interval. Images were reconstructed using a standard algorithm at 10% intervals throughout the cardiac cycle, with a slice thickness of 0.625 mm. This protocol resulted in a mean radiation exposure of 13.0 ± 1.7 mSv. Data sets were transferred offline to stand-alone workstations for further analysis.

CTA strain analysis

Three-dimensional strain analysis was performed as previously described, using a single segmentation of the aorta [13]. Briefly, an active-contour based segmentation of the thoracic aorta was performed from an end-diastolic CTA image series according to the approach described by Caselles et al.,[19] and implemented within a commercially available software platform ITK-SNAP [20]. No resampling of the obtained contouring was performed. The resultant 3D mesh model of the aorta was down-sampled and smoothed with a volume preserving approach,[21] using the commercially available software Meshlab [22]. Within the custom-built Matlab-based software that was previously described and validated, a velocity field was determined displacing the mesh from every n-th phase to the (n+1)-th phase for every phase from a single end-diastolic segmentation,[13] and the mean peak systolic maximum principal strain for the region of interest was computed [13]. Strain calculations were performed for each mesh element and then resolved for both the global thoracic aorta, and for each of the following segmental regions: ascending aorta (sino-tubular junction to the brachiocephalic artery), aortic arch (brachiocephalic artery to the left subclavian artery) and descending thoracic aorta (left subclavian artery to the level of the diaphragm) [23]. All measurements were calculated in the form of peak principal strain amplitude (PPSA), from the Green-Lagrange strain tensor. The choice of computing strain over computing displacement allows quantification of aortic deformation without this being affected by rigid motion. This measurement describes the dominant direction of tissue lengthening, and is therefore expressed as a positive value [16].

Echocardiographic imaging protocol

Echocardiography was performed using a standardized clinical protocol with an iE33 system (Philips Medical Systems, Andover, Maryland) and an S5-1 transducer (1–5 MHz). Measurements were made from an average of 3 cardiac cycles. Assessment of left ventricular (LV) geometry and function and aortic valve (AV) function were performed according to published guidelines [24, 25]. LV volumes and ejection fraction (EF) were measured using the biplane Simpson method, and volumes were indexed to body surface area (BSA). Peak AV pressure gradient was calculated as: ($4 \times$ [peak AV velocity^2]), while mean pressure gradient was calculated by tracing the velocity-time integral (VTI) of the systolic transvalvular continuous-wave Doppler imaging signal. The LV outflow tact (LVOT) diameter was measured 5 mm proximal to the AV annulus. LV stroke volume was calculated according to the continuity equation as: (LVOT diameter)$^2 \times 0.785 \times$ (LVOT VTI), and indexed to BSA, while the AV area was calculated as: (LVOT diameter)^2

$\times 0.785 \times$ (LVOT VTI/AV VTI). The presence and severity of aortic valve regurgitation (AR) was graded based on multiple parameters as previously described [26]. Systemic vascular resistance was calculated as: $80 \times$ mean arterial pressure (MAP)/cardiac output (CO), where MAP is the diastolic blood pressure + (pulse pressure/3) and CO is the LV stroke volume × heart rate [27]. Systemic arterial compliance was calculated as LV stroke volume index/pulse pressure, and systemic arterial elastance as (systolic blood pressure $\times 0.9$)/LV stroke volume index [8]. Valvulo-arterial impedance was calculated as: (systolic blood pressure + mean aortic valve pressure gradient)/LV stroke volume index, representing the valvular and arterial factors opposing LV ejection by absorption of LV mechanical energy [8].

Statistical analysis

Categorical variables are presented as counts with percentages, while continuous variables are expressed as the mean±standard deviation. Comparisons for continuous data were performed using 2-sample Student's t-test. Multiple comparisons of CTA-based 3D aortic PPSA between aortic segments were performed using one-way ANOVA. Relationships between 3D aortic PPSA and clinical, hemodynamic and echocardiographic parameters were evaluated using univariable linear regression analysis. A multivariable linear regression model was performed to assess the independent correlates of global thoracic aorta and ascending aorta 3D PPSA; including age, gender, history of hypertension, stroke, LVEF, AV area, and valvulo-arterial impedance. The amount of variance accounted for by these correlates was derived from the global r^2 of the model. CTA-based 3D aortic PPSA intraobserver variability was evaluated by having one experienced observer perform the analysis on 10 randomly selected patients and then blindly repeating the analysis one week later. Interobserver variability assessment was conducted by having a second experienced and blinded observer perform the analysis on the same 10 patients. Intraobserver and interobserver variability testing was evaluated by Bland Altman analysis, and coefficients of variation were calculated. Additionally, both intra- and interobserver agreement were analyzed by calculating intra-class correlation (ICC) coefficient with 95% confidence intervals (CI). All statistical analysis was performed using commercially available software (Matlab R2015b, The MathWorks, Inc., Natick, Massachusetts). A two-sided p-value of ≤0.05 was considered statistically significant.

Results

Study subjects

Among the 21 patients studied, all had adequate CTA image quality for 3D aortic PPSA analysis. Baseline clinical characteristics are shown in Table 1. There was a high prevalence of hypertension, with a minority of patients having prior myocardial infarction, heart failure and stroke.

Echocardiographic characteristics

Baseline echocardiographic characteristics are presented in Table 2. The mean LVEF was 52.6±14.2%. Five patients (24%) had a reduced LVEF of <45%. Four patients (19%) showed echocardiographic findings consistent with low-flow, low-gradient AS (defined as mean systolic transvalvular Doppler gradient <40 mmHg, with concomitant LV stroke volume index <35 mL/m^2) [28]. No patient had greater than mild aortic valve regurgitation. Significantly elevated systemic vascular resistance and arterial compliance, arterial elastance and valvulo-arterial impedance were demonstrated. This is consistent with highly elevated valvular and arterial opposition to LV ejection coupled with a low stroke volume, characteristics consistent with chronic and severe AS.

Table 1 Baseline patient characteristics (N=21)

Parameter	Value
Clinical	
Age (years)	81 ± 6
Female, N (%)	6 (29%)
Height (m)	1.7 ± 0.1
Weight (kg)	80.7 ± 17.2
Body mass index (kg/m^2)	24.8 ± 4.1
Body surface area (m^2)	1.9 ± 0.2
Hypertension, N (%)	12 (57%)
Diabetes mellitus	3 (14%)
Hyperlipidemia	10 (48%)
Coronary artery disease, N (%)	12 (57%)
Prior myocardial infarction, N (%)	6 (29%)
Congestive heart failure, N (%)	8 (38%)
Stroke, N (%)	3 (14%)
Hemodynamic	
Heart rate (bpm)	61 ± 10
Systolic blood pressure (mmHg)	124 ± 16
Diastolic blood pressure (mmHg)	63 ± 12
Mean arterial pressure (mmHg)	87 ± 12
Pulse pressure (mmHg)	56 ± 14
Laboratory	
Hemoglobin (g/L)	129 ± 19
Creatinine (mcgmol/L)	106 ± 46
Estimated glomerular filtration rate (mL/min)	57 ± 17

Data are expressed as mean ± SD for continuous data and count (percentage) for categorical data

Table 2 Baseline echocardiographic characteristics (N=21)

Parameter	Value
Left ventricular ejection fraction (%)	52 ± 14
Left ventricular end-diastolic volume index (ml/m^2)	53 ± 16
Left ventricular end-systolic volume index (ml/m^2)	26 ± 15
Left ventricular stroke volume index (ml/m^2)	26 ± 7
Aortic valve annulus diameter (mm)	23 ± 3
Aortic valve area (cm^2)	0.6 ± 0.3
Aortic valve mean pressure gradient (mmHg)	44 ± 11
Aortic valve peak pressure gradient (mmHg)	76 ± 18
Systemic vascular resistance (mmHg min/L)	28.9 ± 8
Systemic arterial compliance (ml/mmHg/m^2)	1.0 ± 0.4
Systemic arterial elastance (mmHg/mL))	2.3 ± 0.7
Valvulo-arterial impedance (mmHg/mL/m^2)	6.7 ± 2.1

Data are expressed as mean ± SD for continuous data and count (percentage) for categorical data. SD, standard deviation

CTA 3D aortic strain

Three-dimensional aortic PPSA values for the global thoracic aorta, and for the ascending aorta, aortic arch and descending aorta segments were 6.5±3.0, 10.2±6.0, 6.1±2.9 and 3.3±1.7%, respectively, with a statistically significant difference observed between each aortic segment (p<0.0001). An example of 3D aortic PPSA from a patient with AS awaiting TAVR is provided in Fig. 1 (Additional file 1), demonstrating the typical spatial distribution of 3D PPSA observed in this population with greater strain along the greater curve of the ascending aorta segment (consistent with AS jet directionality) followed by respective reductions in strain amplitude in the aortic arch and descending aorta segments. Fig. 1 demonstrates increased strain in the following regions 1) the ascending aorta, where the aortic valve outflow jet is present, 2) in proximity of the aortic branch vessels (where either a change in curvature or concave curvature is present), and 3) in regions of relatively greater curvature, such as the aortic arch, its branches, and regions of the descending aorta.

Correlation of 3D aortic PSSA, patient characteristics and echocardiographic measures

As reported in Table 3, neither global thoracic aortic 3D PPSA nor ascending aorta 3D PPSA were associated with any baseline clinical or hemodynamic variables in this patient population, inclusive of LV function, with the exception of prior stroke. In contrast, significant associations were observed between 3D aortic PPSA and echocardiographic measures of AS severity (Table 3). Specifically, significant correlations were observed for both global thoracic aorta and ascending aorta 3D PPSA measurements and AV area, and mean and peak AV pressure gradients, demonstrating more impaired strain

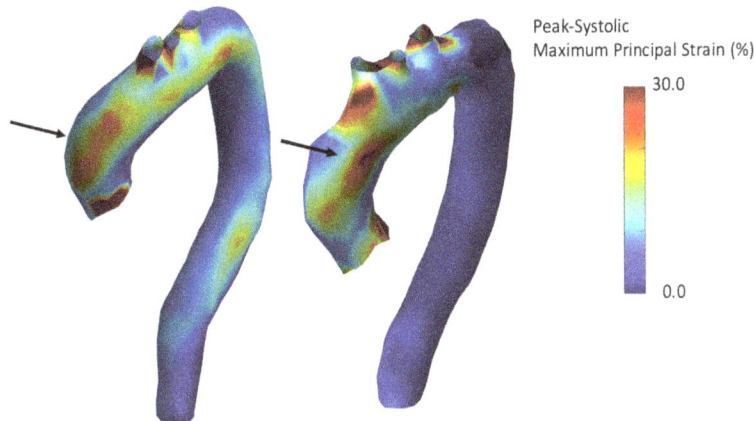

Fig. 1 Thoracic aorta 3-dimensional peak principal strain amplitude (PPSA) calculations using ECG-gated CTA from two patients with severe aortic valve stenosis awaiting transcatheter aortic valve replacement. These images demonstrate regional heterogeneity of 3D aortic PPSA with greater amplitude strain along the ascending aorta greater curvature (arrow, consistent with AS jet directionality) and relatively reduced strain amplitude in the aortic arch and descending aorta segments. The two patients demonstrate consistent regional strain patterns

with worsening AS severity. Linear regression plots describing this relationship between ascending aorta 3D PPSA and both AV area and mean AV gradient are presented in Fig. 2a and b, respectively. Corresponding plots for global thoracic aorta 3D PPSA are presented in Fig. 2c and d, respectively.

Multivariable linear regression analyses, performed separately for global thoracic aorta and ascending aorta 3D PPSA, and clinical, hemodynamic and echocardiographic variables are reported Table 4, and again demonstrate that measures of AS severity were the most significantly correlated to reduced aortic strain. The percentage of variance of 3D aortic PPSA accounted for by the variables included in the model are reported as the global r^2 (Table 4).

Reproducibility

Bland-Altman plots documenting high intra- and inter-observer reproducibility for 3D global thoracic aorta PPSA are presented in Figs. 3 and 4, respectively. The coefficients of variation for intra- and inter-observer variability were 5.8 and 7.2%, respectively. ICC values were significant for both intra- and interobserver reproducibility ($p < 0.0001$ for both). The intraobserver reproducibility value for 3D global thoracic aorta PSSA was 0.98 (0.92-0.99), while the interobserver reproducibility value was 0.96 (0.86-0.99).

Discussion

This study demonstrates the clinical feasibility and reproducibility of 3D thoracic aorta wall principal strain mapping using routine ECG-gated CTA. Assessments of global and regional aortic biomechanics showed significantly greater strain impairment with worsening hemodynamic measures of AS severity, consistent with

findings demonstrated previously by 2D aortic strain techniques [12, 29]. Accordingly, this study establishes the potential of routine ECG-gated CTA to provide reproducible measures of 3D global and regional aortic tissue health, and seeds interest for exploring such postprocessing techniques across a broad range of patients with aortic disease currently evaluated by CTA.

Multiple factors are recognized to contribute to increased aortic stiffness that are well expressed in our sentinel cohort of patients with AS, including advanced age, comorbidities such as hypertension, and underlying atherosclerotic disease that affects both the AV and the arterial vascular system [9, 30]. The resultant impairment in thoracic aorta function has important biomechanical consequences on both ventricular performance and adverse remodeling, particularly among patients with AS due to impaired ventricular-arterial coupling given that both aortic stiffness and distensibility directly influence ventricular afterload incremental to that caused by valvular obstruction [3, 31]. Previous studies have demonstrated the importance of assessing biomechanical thoracic aorta properties for the prediction of adverse cardiovascular outcomes, inclusive of heart failure and all-cause and cardiovascular mortality [32–35]. Recently it has been demonstrated that vascular loading conditions may change dramatically with relief of valvular obstruction following TAVR, unmasking highly elevated aortic stiffness resulting in significant postprocedure hypertension [7]. Whether pre-procedure 3D thoracic aorta PPSA analysis incrementally improves prediction of similar adverse outcomes in this population requires further investigation. Our study found highly significant correlations between lower 3D thoracic aorta PPSA and worsening measures of AS severity. These findings suggest that the presence of severe AS has a

Table 3 Correlations between 3-dimensional peak principal strain amplitude calculations using ECG-gated CTA of the ascending aorta and global thoracic aorta and clinical, hemodynamic and echocardiographic variables using linear regression analysis

Parameter	Ascending Aorta		Global Thoracic Aorta	
	β	p-value	β	p-value
Clinical				
Age	-0.07	0.76	0.005	0.97
Gender	2.43	0.41	0.59	0.69
Height	-0.23	0.13	-0.09	0.2650
Weight	0.04	0.61	0.02	0.68
Body mass index	0.45	0.09	0.18	0.19
Body surface area	1.04	0.86	0.57	0.84
Hypertension	1.85	0.50	-0.001	1.00
Diabetes mellitus	-2.88	0.45	-2.20	0.24
Hyperlipidemia	0.43	0.87	0.31	0.82
Coronary artery disease	-0.56	0.84	-0.08	0.95
Prior myocardial infarction	0.86	0.77	0.65	0.66
Congestive heart failure	-1.14	0.68	0.04	0.97
Stroke	9.89	0.004	4.05	0.02
Hemodynamic				
Heart rate	0.009	0.94	-0.005	0.93
Systolic blood pressure	0.03	0.71	0.02	0.68
Diastolic blood pressure	-0.09	0.41	-0.06	0.28
Mean arterial pressure	-0.05	0.69	-0.03	0.59
Pulse pressure	0.11	0.25	0.07	0.16
Echocardiographic				
LV ejection fraction	0.07	0.50	0.02	0.67
LV end-diastolic volume index	0.001	0.99	0.03	0.41
LV end-systolic volume index	-0.002	0.98	0.03	0.49
AV annulus diameter	-0.08	0.85	0.17	0.43
AV area	15.41	0.0005	8.54	0.00004
AV mean pressure gradient	-0.38	0.0004	-0.19	0.0005
AV peak pressure gradient	-0.23	0.0003	-0.11	0.0005
Systemic vascular resistance	-0.0001	0.49	-0.001	0.30
Systemic arterial compliance	-2.29	0.55	-0.97	0.61
Systemic arterial elastance	-0.64	0.73	-0.61	0.51
Valvulo-arterial impedance	0.03	0.77	0.01	0.74

AV, aortic valve; LV, left ventricle

dominant influence on aortic deformation and remodeling that may significantly outweigh concurrent physiologic factors, a relationship that has also been described in prior reports [7, 12, 36].

Localized, 2D aortic distensibility has been previously evaluated using cardiovascular magnetic resonance imaging (CMR) by measuring the difference in maximal and minimal short-axis lumen area at different phases of the cardiac cycle [32]. Despite being a simple and therefore attractive approach, this technique is unable to account for changes in longitudinal or other directions of aortic deformation, and therefore may be less sensitive for detecting clinically important alterations in thoracic aortic function [37, 38]. Bell et al. measured proximal thoracic aorta strain using CMR in N=375 subjects by constructing a longitudinal centerline that follows the aortic curvature in a 2D plane, applying intersecting perpendicular chords to characterize changes in axial diameter throughout the cardiac cycle [37]. They found that proximal aortic stiffness was over-estimated when measured using circumferential strain calculations assessed from cross-sectional imaging due to the latent effects of longitudinal strain, and that incorporation of longitudinal strain into aortic biomechanical assessment may be an important component of cardiovascular risk assessment. Our technique derives 3D PPSA and therefore is not subject to the limitations of single-plane assessment, incorporating the 3D properties of aortic deformation without the need for further correction. Principal strain analysis has been previously used to characterize the complex fibre interactions occurring during ventricular contraction,[16] and this same approach may be beneficial for providing a more physiologic metric of thoracic aorta deformation in AS and other cardiovascular diseases.

Previous reports have investigated 2D speckle-tracking echocardiography-based strain calculations of the thoracic aorta, postulating that strain is an accurate marker of aortic stiffness [39, 40]. The association demonstrated between aortic strain and collagen content provides further support for its value as a surrogate marker of vascular stiffness [41]. Teixeira et al. reported 2D circumferential ascending aorta strain values corrected for blood pressure were highly correlated with stroke volume and valvulo-arterial impedance in AS patients, concluding that both vessel wall and flow properties influence strain values [39]. Despite being widely available, echocardiography remains subject to coverage limitations and acoustic artifact for thoracic aorta imaging, particularly for multi-planar or 3D acquisitions, which may present challenges for accuracy and reproducibility.

Expanding interest in the study of ECG-gated CTA for the evaluation of vascular deformation is related to its full anatomic coverage of the thoracic aorta coupled with its superior spatial resolution, providing a dynamic isotropic dataset appropriate for quantitative biomechanical assessments [12]. Previous studies have used CTA to calculate circumferential and longitudinal 2D thoracic aorta strain based upon differences in vessel caliber throughout the cardiac cycle [10, 11, 15, 37]. More recently, Mileto et al. demonstrated the feasibility of

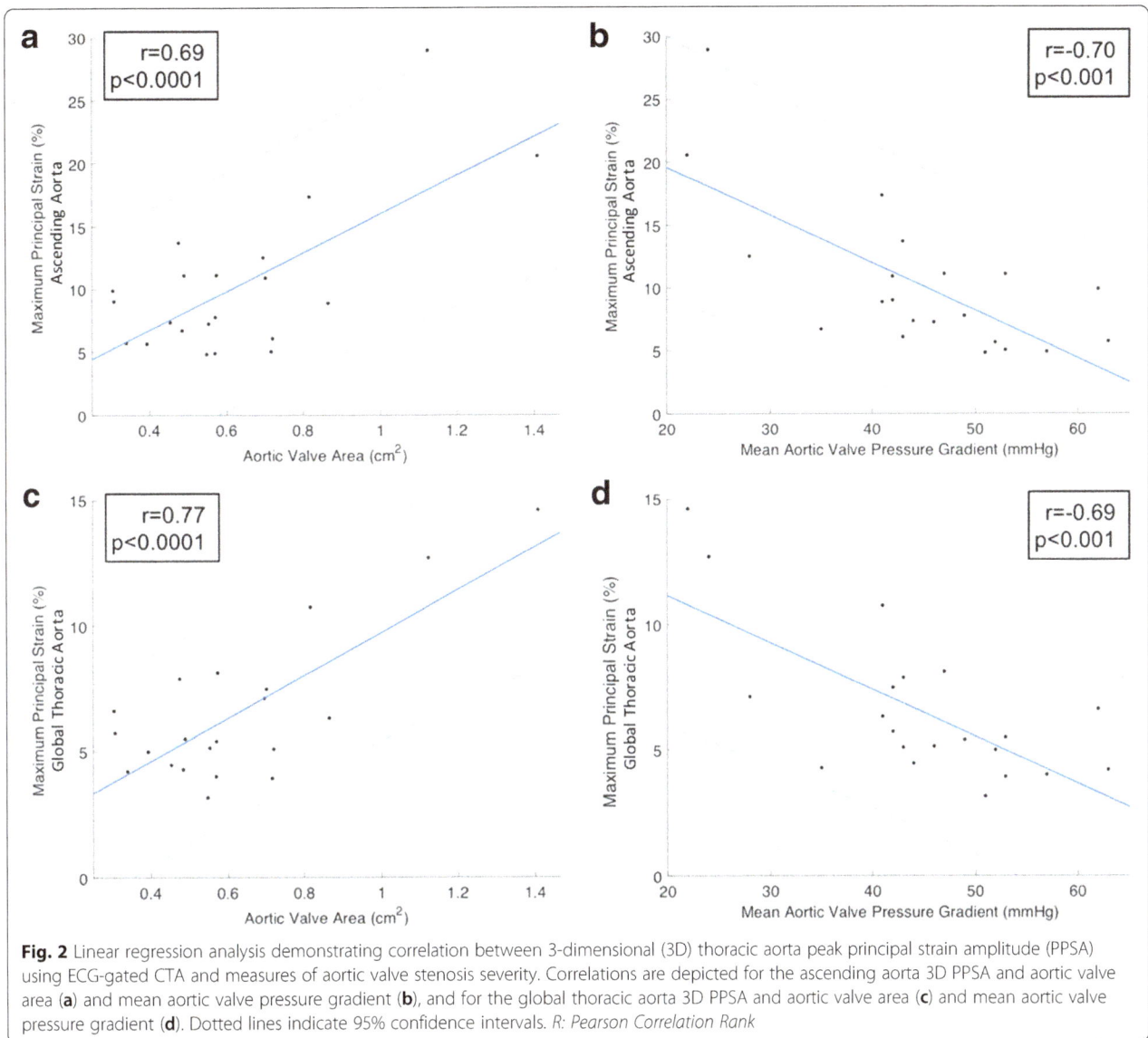

Fig. 2 Linear regression analysis demonstrating correlation between 3-dimensional (3D) thoracic aorta peak principal strain amplitude (PPSA) using ECG-gated CTA and measures of aortic valve stenosis severity. Correlations are depicted for the ascending aorta 3D PPSA and aortic valve area (**a**) and mean aortic valve pressure gradient (**b**), and for the global thoracic aorta 3D PPSA and aortic valve area (**c**) and mean aortic valve pressure gradient (**d**). Dotted lines indicate 95% confidence intervals. *R: Pearson Correlation Rank*

performing aortic strain calculation at seven discrete locations using a deformable, motion-coherent modelling approach based on ECG-gated CTA acquisitions in a large cohort of patients (N=250) undergoing AV replacement [12]. Our technique offers a complimentary approach to provide a contiguous 3D principal strain analysis along the thoracic aortic. This provides a comprehensive spatial evaluation of deformation that is independent of aortic shape and orientation. We have identified regions of increased aortic wall strain in the aortic root and proximal ascending aorta that we speculate is secondary to the high velocity aortic valve outflow jet present in this population with severe AS referred for TAVR. Additionally, we have located high-strain regions in correspondence of the vessel branches, which are regions where curvature changes rapidly and can be

concave. Our strain findings are consistent with previously described aortic regions of increased wall strain found in computer models [42, 43], ex-vivo optical strain measurements [44], and multi-segmentation based in-vivo strain analysis [14]. The need to quantify this inhomogeneity has been recently described [45]. Further, improved potential exists for inter-study registration given that a full volumetric evaluation is achieved, eliminating reliance on correct identification of specific anatomic landmarks [46].

Limitations
This study was a single-center feasibility study in a small number of subjects. Therefore, this technique requires validation in broader patient cohorts with a wider range of aortic disease. Due to the exposure to ionizing

Table 4 Independent correlates of 3-dimensional peak principal strain amplitude calculations using ECG-gated CTA for the ascending aorta and global thoracic aorta

Parameter	Ascending Aorta		Global Thoracic Aorta	
	β	p-value	β	p-value
Age	-0.02	0.91	0.05	0.61
Gender	3.05	0.15	0.89	0.37
Hypertension	0.08	0.97	-0.65	0.51
Stroke	**8.85**	**0.03**	**3.72**	**0.046**
Heart rate	-0.04	0.75	0.003	0.95
Pulse pressure	-0.03	0.75	0.009	0.86
Left ventricular ejection fraction	-0.06	0.47	-0.04	0.31
Aortic valve area	**14.41**	**0.008**	**3.73**	**0.003**
Valvulo-arterial impedance	0.02	0.80	-0.004	0.93
Model-adjusted r^2	0.58	0.015	0.608	0.012

The global r^2 of the model represents the amount of variance accounted for by these correlates

radiation and iodinated contrast dye required for this CTA-based technique, a control population was not recruited for comparison with the TAVR population in this analysis. Such comparison is an important consideration for future research into the clinical utility of this approach. However, future aims will include establishing reference values from broader registry data across a range of age, sex and comorbidity. Although such analyses were beyond the scope of this analysis, our approach was previously validated against ground-truth strain data obtained from a digital phantom [13]. Additionally, this study was not longitudinal, and therefore the prognostic value of

aortic 3D strain analysis is uncertain. Further research is needed to determine the correlation between 3D aortic PSSA and clinical outcomes. Finally, we were unable to perform CTA and echocardiography in the same imaging session, therefore we cannot exclude the potential for altered loading conditions that may confound comparison of results between these two modalities.

Conclusions

Three-dimensional aortic wall principal strain analysis from routine, ECG-gated CTA is clinically feasible and shows good reproducibility. In this cohort of patients

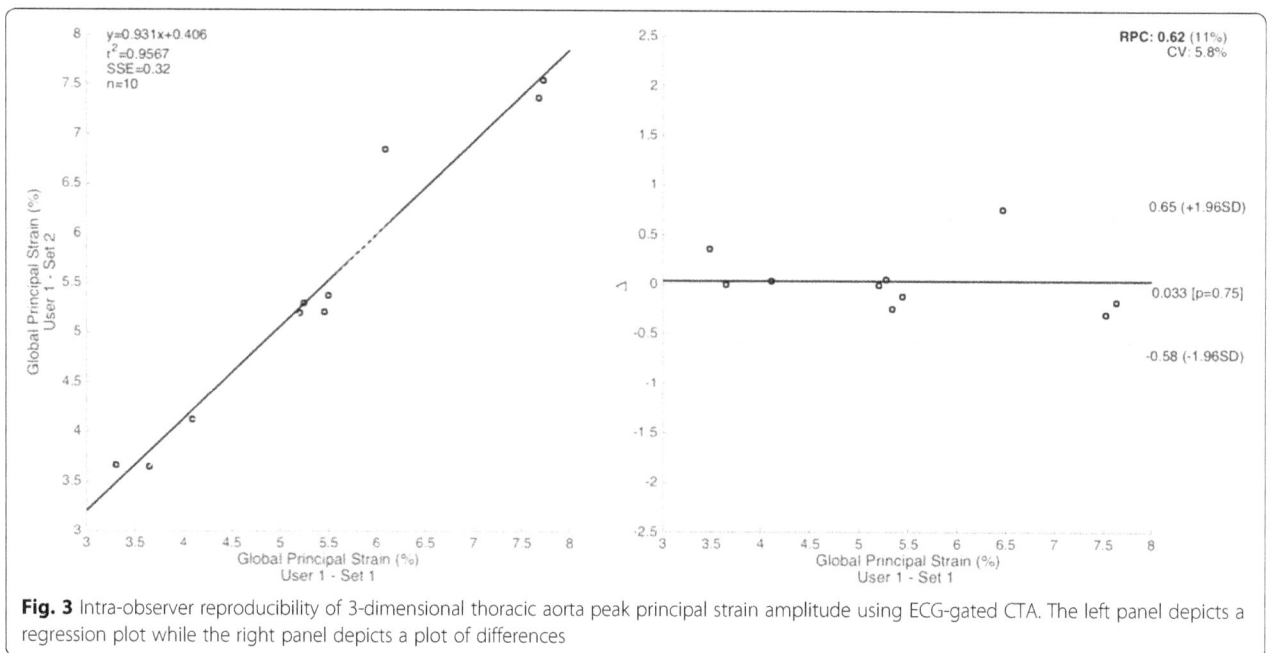

Fig. 3 Intra-observer reproducibility of 3-dimensional thoracic aorta peak principal strain amplitude using ECG-gated CTA. The left panel depicts a regression plot while the right panel depicts a plot of differences

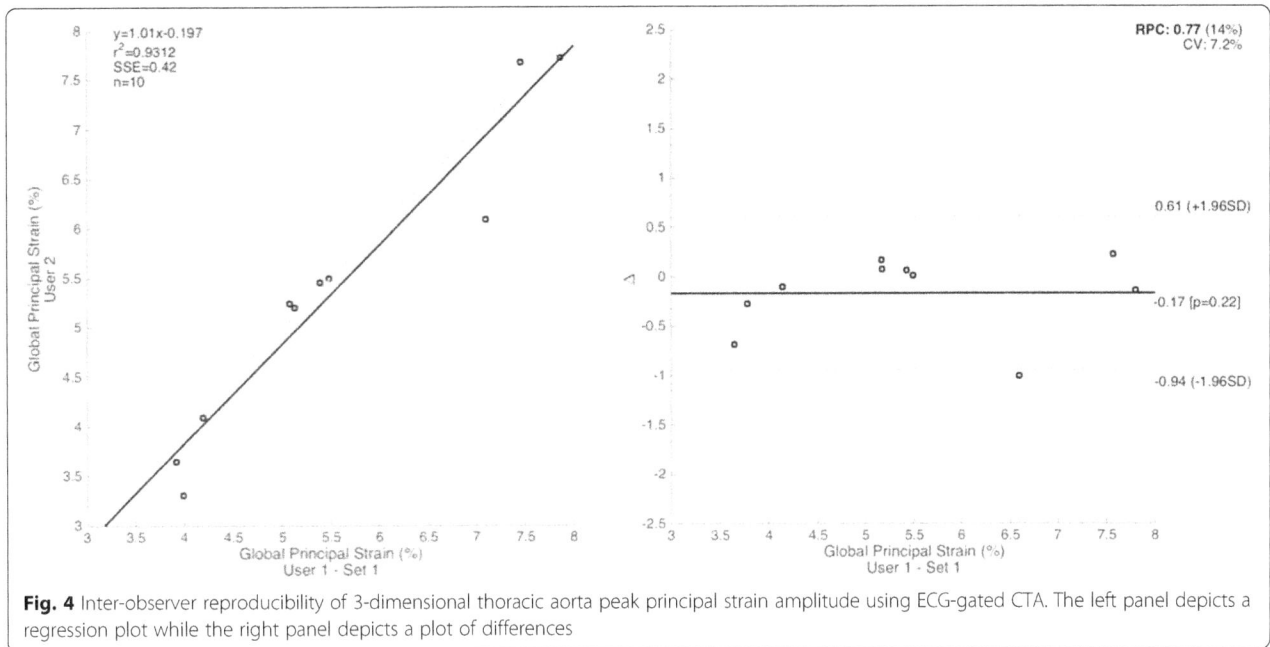

Fig. 4 Inter-observer reproducibility of 3-dimensional thoracic aorta peak principal strain amplitude using ECG-gated CTA. The left panel depicts a regression plot while the right panel depicts a plot of differences

with severe AS referred for TAVR, lower 3D PPSA values were appropriately identified in patients with greater hemodynamic severity of AS, as assessed by echocardiography. Future research is warranted to explore the value of this novel technique in other patient cohorts with aortic disease routinely imaged by ECG-gated CTA.

Abbreviations

2D: 2-dimensional; 3D: 3-dimensional; ANOVA: Analysis of variance; AR: Aortic valve regurgitation; AS: Aortic stenosis; AV: Aortic valve; AVA: Aortic valve area; BMI: Body mass index; BSA: Body surface area; CO: Cardiac output; CTA: Computerized tomography angiography; ECG: Electrocardiography; LV: Left ventricle; LVEF: Left ventricular ejection fraction; LVOT: Left ventricle outflow tract; MAP: Mean aortic pressure; MG: Mean gradient; PPSA: Peak principal strain amplitude; SD: Standard deviation; TAVR: Transcatheter aortic valve replacement; VTI: Velocity time integral

Funding

Dr. Satriano was funded by the Mitacs Elevate Postdoctoral Fellowship Program and by Medtronic of Canada, Ltd. Dr. White received research support from Circle Cardiovascular Inc. and is Chief Medical Officer of Cohesic Inc. Dr. White is supported by a Heart and Stroke Foundation of Alberta Early Investigator Award. This research was funded in part by the Calgary Health Trust.

Authors' contributions

Conception and design: AS, ZG, JAW, FAQ, CPL, and NMF; analysis and interpretation of the data: AS, ZG, ESDM, NM, JAW and NMF; drafting of the article: AS, ZG, JAW, and NMF; revising of the article: AS, ZG, JAW, CPL, NM, ESDM, FAQ, and NMF. All authors have read and approved the final manuscript.

Competing interests

The authors declare that they have no competing interests.

Author details

[1]Stephenson Cardiac Imaging Centre, University of Calgary, Calgary, Alberta, Canada. [2]Division of Cardiology, Department of Cardiac Sciences, Libin Cardiovascular Institute of Alberta, University of Calgary, South Health Campus, 4448 Front Street SE, Calgary, Alberta T3M 1M4, Canada. [3]Department of Diagnostic Imaging, Cummings School of Medicine, University of Calgary, Calgary, Alberta, Canada. [4]Department of Civil Engineering and Centre for Bioengineering Research and Education, University of Calgary, Calgary, Alberta, Canada.

References

1. Lee H-Y, Oh B-H. Aging and arterial stiffness. Circ J. 2010;74(11):2257–62.
2. Sun Z. Aging, arterial stiffness, and hypertension. Hypertension. 2015;65(2):252–6.
3. Laurent S, Cockcroft J, Van Bortel L, Boutouyrie P, Giannattasio C, Hayoz D, Pannier B, Vlachopoulos C, Wilkinson I, Struijker-Boudier H, et al. Expert consensus document on arterial stiffness: methodological issues and clinical applications. Eur Heart J. 2006;27(21):2588–605.
4. Mancia G, De Backer G, Dominiczak A, Cifkova R, Fagard R, Germano G, Grassi G, Heagerty AM, Kjeldsen SE, Laurent S, et al. 2007 Guidelines for the Management of Arterial Hypertension: The Task Force for the Management of Arterial Hypertension of the European Society of Hypertension (ESH) and of the European Society of Cardiology (ESC). J Hypertens. 2007;25(6):1105–87.
5. Veerasamy M, Ford GA, Neely D, Bagnall A, MacGowan G, Das R, Kunadian V. Association of aging, arterial stiffness, and cardiovascular disease: a review. Cardiol Rev. 2014;22(5):223–32.
6. Hachicha Z, Dumesnil JG, Pibarot P. Usefulness of the valvuloarterial impedance to predict adverse outcome in asymptomatic aortic stenosis. J. Am. Coll. Cardiol. 2009;54(11):1003–11.

7. Yotti R, Bermejo J, Gutierrez-Ibanes E, Perez del Villar C, Mombiela T, Elizaga J, Benito Y, Gonzalez-Mansilla A, Barrio A, Rodriguez-Perez D, et al. Systemic vascular load in calcific degenerative aortic valve stenosis: insight from percutaneous valve replacement. J. Am. Coll. Cardiol. 2015;65(5):423–33.

8. Briand M, Dumesnil JG, Kadem L, Tongue AG, Rieu R, Garcia D, Pibarot P. Reduced systemic arterial compliance impacts significantly on left ventricular afterload and function in aortic stenosis: implications for diagnosis and treatment. J. Am. Coll. Cardiol. 2005;46(2):291–8.

9. Rosca M, Magne J, Calin A, Popescu BA, Pierard LA, Lancellotti P. Impact of aortic stiffness on left ventricular function and B-type natriuretic peptide release in severe aortic stenosis. Eur J Echocardiogr. 2011;12(11):850–6.

10. Morrison TM, Choi G, Zarins CK, Taylor CA. Circumferential and longitudinal cyclic strain of the human thoracic aorta: age-related changes. J Vasc Surg. 2009;49(4):1029–36.

11. Martin C, Sun W, Primiano C, McKay R, Elefteriades J. Age-dependent ascending aorta mechanics assessed through multiphase CT. Ann Biomed Eng. 2013;41(12):2565–74.

12. Mileto A, Heye TJ, Makar RA, Hurwitz LM, Marin D, Boll DT. Regional Mapping of Aortic Wall Stress by Using Deformable, Motion-coherent Modeling based on Electrocardiography-gated Multidetector CT Angiography: Feasibility Study. Radiology. 2016;280(1):230–6.

13. Satriano A, Rivolo S, Martufi G, Finol EA, Di Martino ES. In vivo strain assessment of the abdominal aortic aneurysm. J Biomech. 2015;48(2):354–60.

14. Pasta S, Agnese V, Di Giuseppe M, Gentile G, Raffa GM, Bellavia D, Pilato M. In Vivo Strain Analysis of Dilated Ascending Thoracic Aorta by ECG-Gated CT Angiographic Imaging. Ann Biomed Eng. 2017;45(12):2911–20.

15. Wittek A, Karatolios K, Fritzen CP, Bereiter-Hahn J, Schieffer B, Moosdorf R, Vogt S, Blase C. Cyclic three-dimensional wall motion of the human ascending and abdominal aorta characterized by time-resolved three-dimensional ultrasound speckle tracking. Biomech Model Mechanobiol. 2016;15(5):1375–88.

16. Pedrizzetti G, Sengupta S, Caracciolo G, Park CS, Amaki M, Goliasch G, Narula J, Sengupta PP. Three-dimensional principal strain analysis for characterizing subclinical changes in left ventricular function. J Am Soc Echocardiogr. 2014;27(10):1041–50. e1041

17. Holmes DR Jr, Mack MJ, Kaul S, Agnihotri A, Alexander KP, Bailey SR, Calhoon JH, Carabello BA, Desai MY, Edwards FH, et al. 2012 ACCF/AATS/SCAI/STS expert consensus document on transcatheter aortic valve replacement. J. Am. Coll. Cardiol. 2012;59(13):1200–54.

18. Freeman M, Webb JG, Willson AB, Wheeler M, Blanke P, Moss RR, Thompson CR, Munt B, Norgaard BL, Yang TH, et al. Multidetector CT predictors of prosthesis-patient mismatch in transcatheter aortic valve replacement. J Cardiovasc Comput Tomogr. 2013;7(4):248–55.

19. Caselles V, Catté F, Coll T, Dibos F. A geometric model for active contours in image processing. Numerische mathematik. 1993;66(1):1–31.

20. Yushkevich PA, Piven J, Hazlett HC, Smith RG, Ho S, Gee JC, Gerig G. User-guided 3D active contour segmentation of anatomical structures: significantly improved efficiency and reliability. Neuroimage. 2006;31(3):1116–28.

21. Taubin G. A signal processing approach to fair surface design. In: Proc 22nd Annu Conf Comput Graph Interact Tech: 1995; 1995. p. 351–8.

22. Cignoni P, Callieri M, Corsini M, Dellepiane M, Ganovelli G, Ranzuglia G. Meshlab: an open-source mesh processing tool. In: Eurographics Italian Chapter Conference; 2008. p. 129–36.

23. Goldstein SA, Evangelista A, Abbara S, Arai A, Asch FM, Badano LP, Bolen MA, Connolly HM, Cuellar-Calabria H, Czerny M, et al. Multimodality imaging of diseases of the thoracic aorta in adults: from the American Society of Echocardiography and the European Association of Cardiovascular Imaging: endorsed by the Society of Cardiovascular Computed Tomography and Society for Cardiovascular Magnetic Resonance. Journal of the American Society of Echocardiography : official publication of the American Society of Echocardiography. 2015;28(2):119–82.

24. Baumgartner H, Hung J, Bermejo J, Chambers JB, Evangelista A, Griffin BP, Iung B, Otto CM, Pellikka PA, Quinones M, et al. Echocardiographic assessment of valve stenosis: EAE/ASE recommendations for clinical practice. Journal of the American Society of Echocardiography : official publication of the American Society of Echocardiography. 2009;22(1):1 23. quiz 101-102

25. Lang RM, Badano LP, Mor-Avi V, Afilalo J, Armstrong A, Ernande L, Flachskampf FA, Foster E, Goldstein SA, Kuznetsova T, et al.

Recommendations for cardiac chamber quantification by echocardiography in adults: an update from the American Society of Echocardiography and the European Association of Cardiovascular Imaging. J Am Soc Echocardiogr. 2015;28(1):1–39. e14

26. Zoghbi WA, Enriquez-Sarano M, Foster E, Grayburn PA, Kraft CD, Levine RA, Nihoyannopoulos P, Otto CM, Quinones MA, Rakowski H, et al. Recommendations for evaluation of the severity of native valvular regurgitation with two-dimensional and Doppler echocardiography. Journal of the American Society of Echocardiography : official publication of the American Society of Echocardiography. 2003;16(7):777–802.

27. Kadem L, Dumesnil JG, Rieu R, Durand LG, Garcia D, Pibarot P. Impact of systemic hypertension on the assessment of aortic stenosis. Heart. 2005;91(3):354–61.

28. Hachicha Z, Dumesnil JG, Bogaty P, Pibarot P. Paradoxical low-flow, low-gradient severe aortic stenosis despite preserved ejection fraction is associated with higher afterload and reduced survival. Circulation. 2007; 115(22):2856–64.

29. Beller CJ, Labrosse MR, Thubrikar MJ, Robicsek F. Role of aortic root motion in the pathogenesis of aortic dissection. Circulation. 2004;109(6):763–9.

30. Allison MA, Cheung P, Criqui MH, Langer RD, Wright CM. Mitral and aortic annular calcification are highly associated with systemic calcified atherosclerosis. Circulation. 2006;113(6):861–6.

31. Ohyama Y, Ambale-Venkatesh B, Noda C, Chugh AR, Teixido-Tura G, Kim JY, Donekal S, Yoneyama K, Gjesdal O, Redheuil A, et al. Association of Aortic Stiffness With Left Ventricular Remodeling and Reduced Left Ventricular Function Measured by Magnetic Resonance Imaging: The Multi-Ethnic Study of Atherosclerosis. Circ. Cardiovasc. Imaging. 2016;9(7)

32. Redheuil A, Wu CO, Kachenoura N, Ohyama Y, Yan RT, Bertoni AG, Hundley GW, Duprez DA, Jacobs DR Jr, Daniels LB, et al. Proximal aortic distensibility is an independent predictor of all-cause mortality and incident CV events: the MESA study. J. Am. Coll. Cardiol. 2014;64(24):2619–29.

33. Redfield MM, Jacobsen SJ, Borlaug BA, Rodeheffer RJ, Kass DA. Age- and gender-related ventricular-vascular stiffening: a community-based study. Circulation. 2005;112(15):2254–62.

34. Hundley WG, Kitzman DW, Morgan TM, Hamilton CA, Darty SN, Stewart KP, Herrington DM, Link KM, Little WC. Cardiac cycle-dependent changes in aortic area and distensibility are reduced in older patients with isolated diastolic heart failure and correlate with exercise intolerance. J. Am. Coll. Cardiol. 2001;38(3):796–802.

35. Mitchell GF, Hwang SJ, Vasan RS, Larson MG, Pencina MJ, Hamburg NM, Vita JA, Levy D, Benjamin EJ. Arterial stiffness and cardiovascular events: the Framingham Heart Study. Circulation. 2010;121(4):505–11.

36. Harbaoui B, Courand PY, Girerd N, Lantelme P. Aortic Stiffness: Complex Evaluation But Major Prognostic Significance Before TAVR. J. Am. Coll. Cardiol. 2015;66(13):1521–2.

37. Bell V, Mitchell WA, Sigurethsson S, Westenberg JJ, Gotal JD, Torjesen AA, Aspelund T, Launer LJ, de Roos A, Gudnason V, et al. Longitudinal and circumferential strain of the proximal aorta. J. Am. Heart Assoc. 2014;3(6):e001536.

38. Weber TF, Muller T, Biesdorf A, Worz S, Rengier F, Heye T, Holland-Letz T, Rohr K, Kauczor HU, von Tengg-Kobligk H. True four-dimensional analysis of thoracic aortic displacement and distension using model-based segmentation of computed tomography angiography. Int J Cardiovasc Imaging. 2014;30(1):185–94.

39. Teixeira R, Moreira N, Baptista R, Barbosa A, Martins R, Castro G, Providencia L. Circumferential ascending aortic strain and aortic stenosis. Eur Heart J Cardiovasc Imaging. 2013;14(7):631–41.

40. Kim KH, Park JC, Yoon HJ, Yoon NS, Hong YJ, Park HW, Kim JH, Ahn Y, Jeong MH, Cho JG, et al. Usefulness of aortic strain analysis by velocity vector imaging as a new echocardiographic measure of arterial stiffness. Journal of the American Society of Echocardiography : official publication of the American Society of Echocardiography. 2009;22(12):1382–8.

41. Kim SA, Lee KH, Won HY, Park S, Chung JH, Jang Y, Ha JW. Quantitative assessment of aortic elasticity with aging using velocity-vector imaging and its histologic correlation. Arterioscler Thromb Vasc Biol. 2013;33(6):1306–12.

42. Pasta S, Rinaudo A, Luca A, Pilato M, Scardulla C, Gleason TG, Vorp DA. Difference in hemodynamic and wall stress of ascending thoracic aortic aneurysms with bicuspid and tricuspid aortic valve. J Biomech. 2013;46(10): 1729–38.

43. Liang L, Liu M, Martin C, Sun W. A deep learning approach to estimate stress distribution: a fast and accurate surrogate of finite-element analysis. R Soc Interface. 2018;15(138)
44. Genovese K, Humphrey JD. Multimodal optical measurement in vitro of surface deformations and wall thickness of the pressurized aortic arch. J Biomed Opt. 2015;20(4):046005.
45. Ferraro M, Trachet B, Aslanidou L, Fehervary H, Segers P, Stergiopulos N. Should We Ignore What We Cannot Measure? How Non-Uniform Stretch, Non-Uniform Wall Thickness and Minor Side Branches Affect Computational Aortic Biomechanics in Mice. Ann Biomed Eng. 2018;46(1):159–70.
46. Csobay-Novak C, Fontanini DM, Szilagyi BR, Szeberin Z, Szilveszter BA, Maurovich-Horvat P, Huttl K, Sotonyi P. Thoracic aortic strain can affect endograft sizing in young patients. J Vasc Surg. 2015;62(6):1479–84.

23

Cardiac autotransplantation and ex vivo surgical repair of giant left atrium

Zan Mitrev[*†] ⓘ, Milka Klincheva, Tanja Anguseva, Igor Zdravkovski and Rodney Alexander Rosalia[†]

Abstract

Background: Chronic Mitral Valve disease is strongly associated with Left atrial enlargement; the condition has a high mortality risk. Clinical manifestations include atrial fibrillation, pulmonary hypertension, thromboembolic events, and in cases of Giant Left Atrium (GLA) and a distorted cardiac silhouette. Full sternotomy, conventional open-heart surgery, reductive atrioplasty and atrioventricular valve repair are required to resolve symptoms. However, these procedures can be complicated due to the posterior location of the GLA and concomitant right lateral protrusion.

Cardiac autotransplantation is superior under these conditions; it provides improved visual access to the posterior atrial wall and mitral valve, hence, facilitates corrective surgical procedures.

We aimed to assess the clinical outcome of patients undergoing cardiac autotransplantation as the primary treatment modality to resolve GLA. Moreover, we evaluated the procedural safety profile and technical feasibility.

Case presentation: Four patients, mean EuroSCORE II of 23.7% ± 7.7%, presented with heart failure, atrial fibrillation, left atrial diameter > 6.5 cm and a severe distorted cardiac silhouette; X-ray showed prominent right lateral protrusion. We performed cardiac autotransplantation using continuous retrograde perfusion with warm blood supplemented with glucose followed by atrioplasty, atrial plication, valve annuloplasty and valve repair on the explanted beating heart. The surgical approach reduced the left atrial area, mean reduction was − 90.71 cm^2 [CI95% -153.3 cm^2 to − 28.8 cm^2, $p = 0.02$], and normalized pulmonary arterial pressure, mean decrease − 11.25 mmHg [CI95% -15.23 mmHg to − 7.272 mmHg, $p = 0.003$]. 3 out of 4 patients experienced an uneventful postoperative course; 2 out of 4 patients experienced a transient return to sinus rhythm following surgery. One was operated on in 2017 and is still in good condition; two other patients survived for more than 10 years; Kaplan-Meier determined median survival is 10.5 years.

Conclusions: Cardiac autotransplantation is an elegant surgical procedure that facilitates the surgical remodelling of Giant Left Atrium. Surgical repair on the ex vivo beating heart, under continuous warm blood perfusion, is a safe procedure applicable also to high-risk patients.

Keywords: Giant left atrium, Warm blood perfusion, Atrial fibrillation, Cardiac autotransplantation

Background

Chronic mitral valve diseases are considered the primary trigger for pathological Left Atrial Enlargement (LAE) [1–3]. LAE is predictive for adverse outcomes and is independently related to cardiovascular morbidity and mortality [4, 5].

Untreated chronic mitral valve disease predisposes the patients to secondary illnesses such as pulmonary hypertension [6, 7], respiratory complications [8] thromboembolic events [9] and atrial fibrillation (AF); the degree of the left atrium morphological and functional abnormalities determine the severity of AF [10–12].

In rare cases, with an estimated 0.3–0.6% incidence rate, patients present with Giant Left Atrium (GLA), characterised by an LA diameter > 6.5 cm or an LA area > 40 cm^2 [2, 5, 13]. Patients with GLA frequently present with a severely distorted cardiac silhouette and

---
* Correspondence: zan@zmc.mk
†Zan Mitrev and Rodney Rosalia contributed equally to this work.
Zan Mitrev Clinic, Bledski Dogovor 8, Skopje 1000, Republic of Macedonia

abnormal cardiothoracic ratio. LA protrusion into the right chest cavity may be observed via X-ray. Moreover, these patients often suffer from chronic AF [12]. Circumferential corrective surgery of GLA would ideally require complete cardiac explantation, ex vivo surgical remodelling and autotransplantation.

Cardiac autotransplantation is mostly reserved to debulk cardiac tumours [14–16]. However, it offers distinct advantages to achieve efficient surgical remodelling; cardiac autotransplantation is highly suitable for reductive (left) atrioplasty as the ex vivo handling of the heart allows full access to the posterior left atrial wall and complete visualisation of the mitral valve.

This paper describes our experience with cardiac autotransplantation, and concomitant cardiac corrections, in the treatment of four patients who presented with cardiac and pulmonary complications because of chronic mitral valve disease. All patients presented with NYHA IV and GLA.

Our observations point to a substantial clinical benefit, emphasised by a decrease in symptom severity, successful cardiac remodelling, restoration of left atrial morphology, normalisation of pulmonary hypertension and a median survival time of 10.5 years in the absence of postoperative complications.

Surgical technique
Patients (Table 1) were operated using general cardiac anaesthesia. We access the heart via a median sternotomy. Surgery was performed under cardiopulmonary bypass (CPB), without cardiac arrest under normothermic conditions (> 34 °C) applying bicaval venous cannulation, coronary sinus (CS) cannulation and continuous retrograde warm blood perfusion - beating heart methodology. We controlled the mean systemic arterial pressure at 65 mmHg and used a blood auto-reinfusion system (auto trans®) in all cases.

Cardiac autotransplantation (Fig. 1) is initiated via a bicaval cannulation of the superior and inferior vena cava. A catheter is placed in the CS ostium using a purse-string suture for retrograde perfusion; we continuously perfuse the heart with warm blood supplemented with 50% Glucose – flow rate is maintained at 200 ml/min, and the in-vessel-pressure set at 40–50 mmHg.

Next, the aorta is cross-clamped followed by the transverse cut of the aorta and the pulmonary trunk. At this stage, we perform a longitudinal cut in the posterior wall of the LA. We preserve the vena cava and perform the incision in the interatrial septum followed by a cut along the crista terminalis of the right atrium (RA). In summary, our cardiac autotransplantation method allows the explantation of the cannulated heart while preserving the major veins.

Surgical cardiac remodelling was performed combining atrial reconstruction, reductive atrioplasty - rough debulking of excess atrial tissue - and left atrial appendage excision and concomitant Cox-Maze procedure [17]. Following surgical remodelling and autotransplantation of the heart, we reconnect the LA to its base, the anastomosis of the aorta and pulmonary artery are performed, and the RA sutured and closed. The aorta, pulmonary

Table 1 Patient characteristics, diagnosis, echocardiography parameters and overview of surgical procedures

Patient/Case #	1●	2✳	3▲	4◻
Age	42	64	65	64
Gender	M	M	F	F
Date of Hospitalisation	29/11/2001	30/03/2003	15/03/2004	28/09/2017
Weight (Kg)	48	61	50	63
Height (m)	1.86	1.58	1.49	1.6
BMI (kg/m2)	13.9	24.4	22.5	24.6
BSA (m2)	1.57	1.64	1.44	1.67
EuroSCORE II (%)	16.4	18.3	28.9	31.9
Aetiology	Congenital	Degenerative	Rheumatic	Degenerative
Performed cardiac corrections & Surgical Remodelling				
Reductive Left Atrioplasty	Yes	Yes	Yes	Yes
Reductive Right Atrioplasty	No	Yes	No	Yes
Mitral Annuloplasty	Yes	Yes	No	No
Mitral Valve Replacement	No	No	Yes	Yes
Tricuspid annuloplasty	Yes	Yes	No	Yes

BMI Body mass index
BSA Body Surface Index
EuroSCORE II European System for Cardiac Operative Risk Evaluation (II)
Symbols adjacent to the patient case # correspond to the symbols used in Fig. 2 to facilitate individual analysis

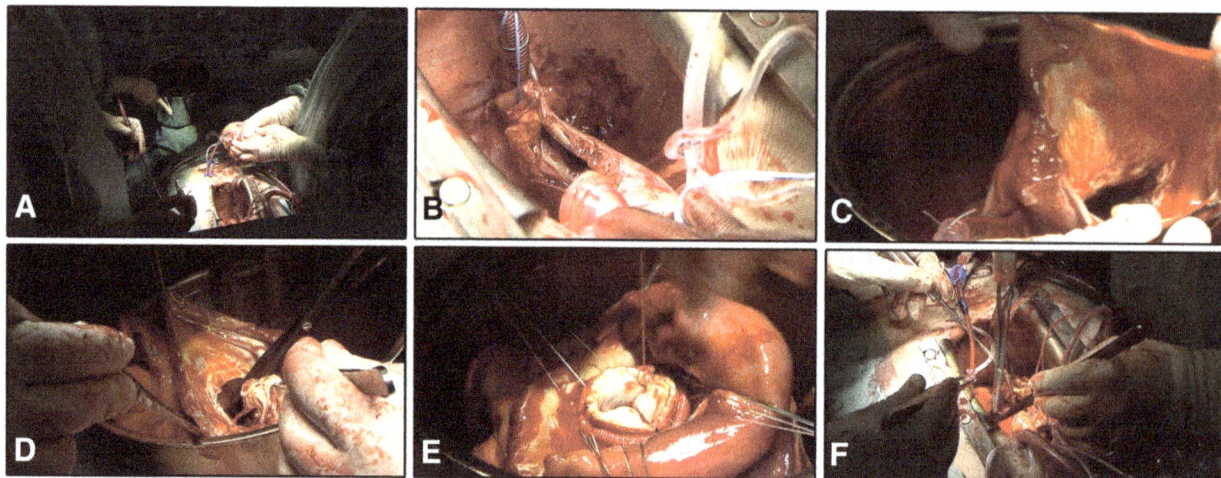

Fig. 1 Intraoperative images of the cardiac autotransplantation procedure. **a** Explanted and ex vivo handling of the enlarged heart. **b** Preserved, cannulated vena cava and residual Right Atrial wall tissue. **c** The open left Atria with the diseased mitral valve. **d** The full excision of the diseased mitral valve. **e** Implantation biological valve prosthesis. **f** depicts the sternum with the re-implanted, surgically corrected heart

artery and both caval veins are unclamped and weaning from CPB is initiated.

Table 2 describes the total surgery duration, cardiopulmonary bypass time, aortic cross-clamp time and duration of perioperative respiratory support.

Case series summary

Four patients with left atrial cardiomegaly and concomitant atrial fibrillation were treated at our clinic in 2001, 2003, 2004 and 2017. Table 1. describes the basic patient characteristics and the corrective surgical procedures and Table 2. presents a summary of the perioperative echocardiography examinations and duration of care.

Primary symptoms reported were dyspnoea and angina. All patients presented with NYHA class IV. Three patients presented with syncope; we observed peripheral oedema in 2 patients. Echocardiography showed a reduced left ventricular contractility, LVEF 43.3 ± 5.4%, with no distinct outliers among patients. All patients presented with severe mitral valve disease, we observed 3 cases of grade 4 regurgitation and one case of severe MV stenosis.

Surgical corrections performed were atrioplasty, valve annuloplasty or replacement (Table 1). Three out of four patients experienced a swift and uneventful recovery. The procedure successfully reduced left atrial area, mean difference 90.71 cm^2 [CI95% 153.3 cm^2 to 28.8 cm^2], $p = 0.02$ (Fig. 2a), stabilised LVEF (Fig. 2b) and reduced the pulmonary hypertension by (mean) 11.25 mmHg [CI95% 15.23 mmHg to 7.272 mmHg], $p = 0.003$ (Fig. 2c).

In these three patients, we could control the minor decrease in renal and liver function without artificial support (Fig. 2d–g). Two out of four patients experienced transient relief from AF, of which one patient

converted to and remained in sinus rhythm for nearly 1 year after surgery (Table 2). The median survival was 10.5 years in the absence of MACCE (Fig. 2h).

Long-term follow up confirms a sustained atrial reverse remodelling after 10 and 13 years, respectively.

Patient 1

A 42-year-old male patient with a 21-year cardiac medical history presented at our emergency department in 2001. His symptoms worsened in the days preceding the surgical intervention. Upon examination, he was heavily dyspneic, with severe palpitations, worsening chest discomfort, coughing and haemoptysis.

Since 1983, on numerous occasions he was advised to undergo cardiac surgery to alleviate his symptoms; however, the patient was unable to decide on surgery.

Transthoracic echocardiography (TTE) revealed a Giant Left Atrium (GLA), dilated cardiomyopathy, prominent right atrial protrusion, and hemodynamically significant mitral and tricuspid regurgitation (Table 2). Computed tomography showed mid-oesophageal and bilateral pulmonary compression from the left atrium combined with congenital bilateral bullous emphysema – specific for congenital lung cystic emphysema. Cardiac autotransplantation and surgical remodelling were successful (Table 1).

Nevertheless, the patient experienced several respiratory complications related to the underlying congenital disease. Also, he experienced thrombocytopenia and excessive bleeding during the postoperative course.

Severe bacterial pneumonia and recurrent pneumothorax further complicated the clinical condition. The patient required prolonged ventilation support and surgical tracheostomy.

Table 2 Preoperative, Intraoperative and postoperative patient characteristics

Patient/Case #	1●	2✱	3▲	4☐
Preoperative data				
MV regurgitation (grade)	Severe	Severe	No	Severe
MV Stenosis (grade)	No	No	Severe	No
MV annulus (cm)	5.5	4.4	4.0	4.6
TV regurgitation (grade)	Severe	Severe	Moderate	Moderate
TV annulus (cm)	4.1	3.8	2.7	3.7
LA diameter (cm) (Fig. 2)	13	17	9.2	9
LA area (cm^2)	143	221	120	81
IVSd (cm)	12	12	10	11
LVPWD(cm)	12	12	10	11
LVEDd (cm)	6.8	6.0	6.2	5.1
LVEDs (cm)	3.5	3.5	3.8	3.4
LVEF (%) (Fig. 2)	40	40	35	45
SPAP (mmHg) (Fig. 2)	> 40	> 40	> 35	> 30
NYHA classification	IV	IV	IV	IV
Coronary angiography	Normal	Normal	Normal	normal
Perioperative data				
Cardiopulmonary bypass (min)	87	135	253	135
Aorta cross-clamp time (min)	48	73	177	82
Total operation duration (min)	215	250	338	195
Mechanical ventilation (hours)	96	46	96	24
ICU LOS (hours)	202	3	7	14
Total Hospitalisation (days)	202	19	15	20
Postoperative analysis				
MV annulus (cm)	3.2	3.0	3.1	2.7
MV regurgitation (grade)	No	No	No	No
MV stenosis (grade)	No	No	No	No
TV (grade)	No	No	No	mild
LA diameter (cm)	6.5	5.6	3.5	4.7
LA area (cm^2) (Fig. 2)	42.5	36	16.8	29.8
LVEF (%) (Fig. 2)	50	40	40	50
Complications	Fever	No	Mild fever	No
SPAP (mmHg) (Fig. 2)	30	30	20	20
NYHA classificaton	–	II	I	I
Follow up (days)	214	3816	4855	249
Postoperative Sinus rhythm duration (days)	0	364	0	5
Intrahospital mortality (days)	214	No	No	No
Cause of death	Mesenteric ischemia	Sepsis	Malignancy	–

MV Mitral Valve
TV Tricuspid Valve
LA Left Atrium
IVSd Interventricular Septal Thickness at Diastole
LVPWD Left ventricular posterior wall dimension
LVEDd Left ventricular diastolic diameter
LVESd Left ventricular systolic diameter
LVEF Left Ventricular Ejection Fraction
SPAP Systolic Pulmonary Arterial Pressure
NYHA New York Heart Association
SPAP is measured via a *Swan-Ganz catheter*
Symbols adjacent to the patient case # correspond to the symbols used in Fig. 2 to facilitate individual analysisv

His condition further deteriorated in the following months. Our examinations revealed severe mesenteric ischemia with the involvement of the ileum at day 190; This complication was finale fatal after 202 days.

Patient 2

We hospitalised a 65-years-old man, in 2003, complaining of fatigue, dyspnoea, heart palpitations, hepatomegaly and peripheral oedema. TTE revealed severe mitral and tricuspid regurgitation resulting from myxomatous degeneration of both valves, with significant atrial cardiomegaly (Table 2).

The postoperative course was uneventful. Due to progressive rheumatic disease, 4 years after the surgical procedure the patient developed high-grade atrioventricular block for which a single chamber pacemaker was implanted; no other cardiac abnormalities were detected since then.

The patient succumbed to an acute septic shock, as a consequence of a neglected right lateral incarcerated inguinoscrotal hernia, after 10 years and 5 months.

Patient 3

A 65-years-old woman was referred to our hospital, in 2004, with severe mitral valve stenosis that manifested with severe chest pain, fatigue, dyspnoea, hepatomegaly and peripheral oedema. Her symptoms started 8 years before her hospitalisation.

She had an episode of rheumatic fever when she was 10 years old and had undergone a left nephrectomy.

TTE indicated severe mitral stenosis with severely enlarged left atrium (Table 2). Mitral valve replacement, reconstruction of the tricuspid valve and surgical remodelling of the left atrium was performed on the explanted heart. The patient recovered swiftly in the absence of postoperative complications.

The patient experienced a symptom-free postoperative course until 2016 when she complained about significant chest pain. Magnetic resonance imaging detected bone metastasis; the patient refused further medical care and passed away, presumably from cancer, mid-2017.

Patient 4

We hospitalised a 64-year-old woman due to palpitations, fatigue, dyspnoea, and giddiness. TTE revealed severe mitral and tricuspid regurgitation (Table 2) - due to myxomatous degeneration - with bi-atrial enlargement. X-ray analysis indicated a significantly enlarged left atrium. Subsequent confirmed the case of GLA, indicated by a distorted cardiac silhouette and a cardiothoracic ratio of 0.8 (Fig. 2a). Given the high degree of right lateral protrusion and LA dimensions, we opted for cardiac autotransplantation (Fig. 1) in order to perform mitral valve replacement, tricuspid valvuloplasty and

reductive atrioplasty. The Intrahospital postoperative course was uneventful. Several check-ups at our outpatient clinic during the first postoperative year confirmed her improved clinical condition, improving cardiac silhouette, a better cardiothoracic ratio of 0.6 (Fig. 3) and a normalised left atrial area of $23\,cm^2$ (Fig. 2a). We noted only low-grade residual mitral insufficiency and AF that is successfully managed using anti-coagulation medication and conventional medical treatment.

Discussion and conclusions

Mitral Valve diseases are associated with high morbidity and mortality [1–3]. Mitral valve dysfunction, but also other congenital disorders such as Atrioventricular (AV) Septal Defect (AVSD), result in an increased intra-atrial pressure leading to constant strain and dilation of the left atrial chamber. Consequently, these diseases trigger progressive pathophysiological changes to the left atrial structure and mechanical function.

Chronic disease can lead to severe LA dilatation; Giant left atrium (GLA), characterised by a left atrial diameter exceeding 6.5 cm [5]. Left atrial dilatation is strongly associated with the onset of AF [11].

Oral anticoagulants and minimally invasive ablation techniques have improved the care of AF patients; these treatments can directly or indirectly trigger LA reverse remodelling and thus normalise left atrium dimensions [18–23]. Nevertheless, in some instances, treatment failure results in persistent pathogenic LA remodelling and consequently, GLA.

Corrective surgery is indicated as the primary approach to resolving severe mitral valve dysfunction and GLA [5, 24, 25].

Several surgical techniques have been described for the treatment of GLA. Conventional cardiac surgery [5], partial autotransplantation [26–28] and orthotopic heart transplantation [29] have been performed to resolve GLA and mitral valve disease with varying success [5].

Complete cardiac explantation was initially devised to excise malignant tissues posterior located in the left heart [30, 31], difficult to reach through standard open-heart surgery. Caution is warranted because of the high morbidity and mortality rates associated with the procedure; especially when GLA corrective surgery is accompanied by mitral valve corrections [32–34]. Consequently, not many surgeons attempt cardiac autotransplantation.

One successful case of cardiac autotransplantation was previously reported [29] with a 30-day follow up; few studies have evaluated cardiac autotransplantation as a treatment modality for mitral valve diseases with concomitant GLA.

Nevertheless, we show that cardiac autotransplantation is reasonably safe and offers substantial clinical

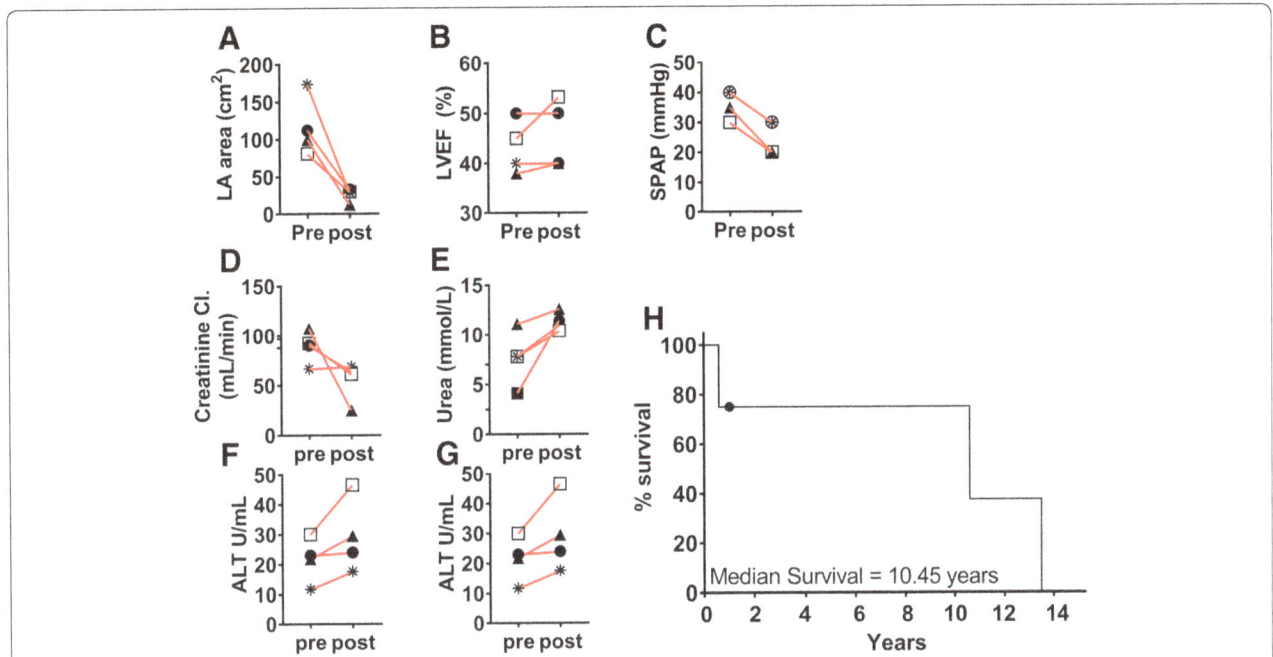

Fig. 2 Perioperative Echocardiography, Laboratory analysis results and Survival. Panels depict the paired pre- and postoperative measurements for Left Atrium area (**a**), Left Ventricular Ejection Fraction (**b**) and Pulmonary Arterial Pressure (**c**). Panels show the paired pre- and postoperative creatine clearance (**d**), blood Urea levels (**e**), the liver enzyme Alanine transaminase (**f**) and Aspartate transaminase (**g**) levels. The estimated median survival following cardiac autotransplantation to perform atrial corrective surgery and atrioventricular valve reconstruction or replacement, censored subject (patient #4) is indicated, (**h**). Symbols in graphs correspond to the patient case # described in Tables 1 and 2

benefits – it allows efficient cardiac surgical remodelling and resolves symptom severity. 3 out of 4 patients recovered well postoperatively and experienced a generally good quality of life. One patient suffered a postoperative aggravation related to his congenital lung disease which proved fatal. Despite the unfortunate outcome, the surgery was technically successful and did relief the patient from his cardiac complications and related clinical symptoms.

As mentioned previously, left atrial dilatation is a risk factor for AF [11, 35]. Surgical management, reductive atrioplasty and concomitant Cox maze procedures [17] have been shown to efficiently restore sinus rhythm in a select patient population [5, 36]. For example, attaining postoperative normal atrial size was critical in restoring sinus rhythm [5]. Despite several negative predictive factors, namely long-term episodes of AF, two out of four patients experienced a transient return to sinus rhythm.

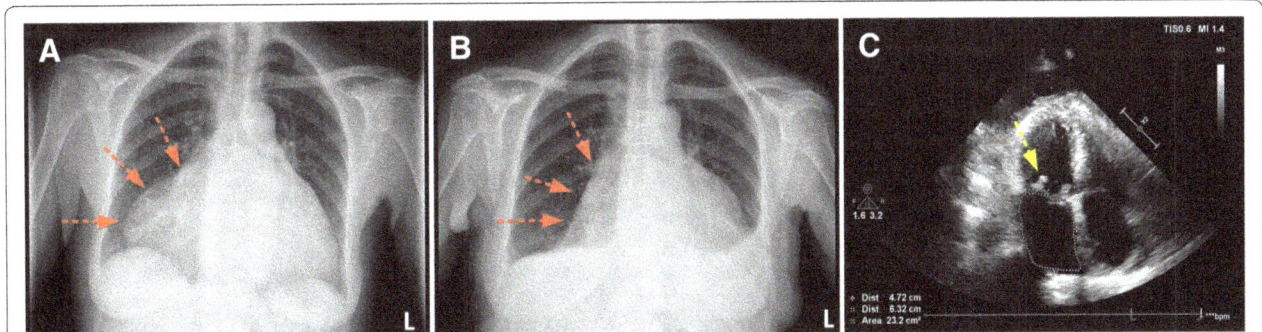

Fig. 3 The Radiological examinations of a patient with GLA and right lateral protrusion. Pre- (**a**) and postoperative (**b**) AP X-ray images of the cardiac silhouette of a 65-year-old woman with severe mitral regurgitation, pulmonary hypertension, tricuspid regurgitation and dilation of the left atrium (LA area, 81 cm^2 and a cardiothoracic ratio of 0.8). Red arrows point to the right heart border (**a** and **b**). Heart auto-transplantation was performed to replace the mitral valve with a biological prosthesis (yellow arrow) (St. Jude Medical, 27 mm). Excess atrial tissue was surgically removed followed by LA atrioplasty. Red arrows point to the right-lateral lining of the cardiac silhouette (**a** and **b**). The procedure successfully restored normal concave left heart border (**b**), (LA area, 23 cm^2 and a cardiothoracic ratio of 0.6). Postoperative echocardiogram displayed a normalised left atrium area (indicated by the dotted line) and other chambers without significant morphological distortions (**c**)

Although all patients relapsed, we could effectively manage AF through medication and regular clinical examinations.

Our cardiac autotransplantation technique mirrors the methods initially described by Cooley et al.,1985 [31] and, more recently, by Reardon et al., 2010 [37]. We adapted these elegant surgical methods by 1) preserving both caval veins and performing the cut along the crista terminalis of the RA, and 2) by using continuous retrograde perfusion using warm blood supplemented with 50% Glucose, and 3) completing all cardiac corrections on the beating heart.

At our clinic, most conventional open-heart valve repair/replacement surgeries and CABG procedures are performed on the beating heart; our approach to cardiac protection, *on-pump/continuous perfusion of the beating heart with warm blood supplemented with glucose*, leads to shorter reperfusion times after aortic unclamping and faster postoperative recovery.

A technical limitation of our study is the use of 2D-measurements to diagnose and follow-up our patients. Volumetric approaches offer higher sensitivity to asses LA abnormalities than LA diameter-based measurements. Nonetheless, the four patients described here presented with such severe GLA that both analytical methods would suffice to diagnose their condition. Furthermore, the X-ray and CT examinations complemented our 2D-echocardiography measurements. To this end, our multi-modal diagnostic approach successfully identified GLA and allowed us to set up a successful surgical treatment modality based on cardiac autotransplantation [11, 38].

We are particularly interested in determining whether our surgical corrections promote long-term post-operative structural and functional atrial reverse remodelling [39]. The longitudinal evaluation of the LA area revealed a stable diameter. (patient #1 was excluded from the longitudinal analysis due to Intrahospital death). In patients #2 and #3, the LA area remained stable as assessed at 10.5 and 13.4 years, respectively. Interestingly, in patient 4, our most recent case, a further reduction in the LA area to 15.2 cm^2 was observed after 172 days, from 29.8 cm^2 Long-term follow up of this patient will offer insights to the continuity of the left atrial reverse remodelling. To the best of our knowledge, this case series, albeit based on a small cohort, for the first time describes the long-term clinical outcome of patients who underwent cardiac autotransplantation.

It is plausible that the continuous perfusion of the explanted beating heart with glucose-supplemented warm blood, during the corrective surgical procedures, helps cardiac reverse remodelling by supporting the foetal gene and metabolic programs of the damaged myocardium, hence promote recovery [40, 41].

The clinical management of GLA requires an individual approach tailored to the specific cardiac abnormalities. Few cases on the successful treatment of GLA have been reported in the literature with limited follow-up period. Data sharing among other clinical centres and evaluation of new patients might identify an optimal method to treat GLA; nevertheless, based on the long-term assessment of the patients described here, cardiac autotransplantation seems promising.

In conclusion, cardiac auto-transplantation is a safe approach to address GLA and underlying atrioventricular valve diseases surgically. Size reduction proved to be stable in the long run.

Abbreviations

AF: Atrial Fibrillation; GLA: Giant Left Heart; LA: Left Atrium; LV: Left Ventricle; RA: Right Atrium; SVC: Superior Vena Cava

Acknowledgements

The authors are grateful to Dr. Nikola Gjorgov for critical reviewing earlier versions of this manuscript and providing valuable suggestions and comments. The authors are thankful for the digital imaging assistance provided by Daniel Veljanoski,

Funding

Not applicable Internal hospital funds supported this work.

Authors' contributions

ZM performed the surgeries; TA and MK were responsible for the perioperative patient care. IZ, RR, TA and MK were responsible for clinical data management, T.A. and M.K. did the risk evaluation and assessed causes of death. R.R. performed the data statistics and wrote the manuscript with the assistance of MK and ZM. All authors approved of the manuscript submission.

Competing interests

Dr. Zan Mitrev is the hospital director at the Zan Mitrev Clinic. The authors of scientific publications receive financial incentives, as a function of the scientific impact of the journal, awarded by the ZMC board.
The ZMC chief scientific officer, R.A. Rosalia, is exempt from any financial incentive system and attests that all clinical and patient data described in this manuscript is devoid of any deliberate falsification or other fraudulent practices. The authors declare no other competing interests.

References

1. Ray R, Chambers J. Mitral valve disease. Int J Clin Pract. 2014;68(10):1216–20.
2. El Maghraby A, Hajar R. Giant left atrium: a review. Heart views : the official journal of the Gulf Heart Association. 2012;13(2):46–52.
3. Di Eusanio G, Gregorini R, Mazzola A, Clementi G, Procaccini B, Cavarra F, Taraschi F, Esposito G, Di Nardo W, Di Luzio V. Giant left atrium and mitral valve replacement: risk factor analysis. Eur J Cardiothoracic Surg : official journal of the European Association for Cardio-thoracic Surgery. 1988;2(3):151–9.
4. Hoit BD. Left atrial size and function: role in prognosis. J Am Coll Cardiol. 2014;63(6):493–505.
5. Apostolakis E, Shuhaiber JH. The surgical management of giant left atrium. Eur J Cardiothoracic Surg : official journal of the European Association for Cardio-thoracic Surgery. 2008;33(2):182–90.
6. Schwammenthal E, Vered Z, Agranat O, Kaplinsky E, Rabinowitz B, Feinberg MS. Impact of atrioventricular compliance on pulmonary artery pressure in mitral stenosis: an exercise echocardiographic study. Circulation. 2000; 102(19):2378–84.
7. Nunes MC, Hung J, Barbosa MM, Esteves WA, Carvalho VT, Lodi-Junqueira L,

Fonseca Neto CP, Tan TC, Levine RA. Impact of net atrioventricular compliance on clinical outcome in mitral stenosis. Circ Cardiovasc Imaging. 2013;6(6):1001–8.

8. Tamura Y, Nagasaka S, Abe T, Taniguchi S. Reasonable and effective volume reduction of a giant left atrium associated with mitral valve disease. Ann Thorac Cardiovasc Surg : official journal of the Association of Thoracic and Cardiovascular Surgeons of Asia. 2008;14(4):252–5.

9. Darwazah AK, El Sayed H. Giant left atrium associated with massive thrombus formation. Thromb J. 2013;11(1):5.

10. Gupta DK, Shah AM, Giugliano RP, Ruff CT, Antman EM, Grip LT, Deenadayalu N, Hoffman E, Patel I, Shi M, et al. Left atrial structure and function in atrial fibrillation: ENGAGE AF-TIMI 48. Eur Heart J. 2014;35(22): 1457–65.

11. Delgado V, Di Biase L, Leung M, Romero J, Tops LF, Casadei B, Marrouche N, Bax JJ. Structure and function of the left atrium and left atrial appendage: AF and Stroke Implications. J Am Coll Cardiol. 2017;70(25):3157–72.

12. Mitrev Z, Hristov N. Cardiac silhouette following a mitral valve replacement, tricuspid annuloplasty and atrioplasty of both atria. Eur J Cardiothoracic Surg : official journal of the European Association for Cardio-thoracic Surgery. 2008;34(4):905.

13. Oh JK. Echocardiographic evaluation of morphological and hemodynamic significance of giant left atrium. An important lesson. Circulation. 1992;86(1): 328–30.

14. Park HO, Yang JH, Kim SH, Moon SH, Byun JH, Choi JY, Lee CE, Yang JW, Kim JW. Autotransplantation of the heart for recurrent inflammatory Myofibroblastic tumor. J Korean Med Sci. 2017;32(9):1548–51.

15. Andrushchuk U, Ostrovsky Y, Zharkov V, Amelchanka S, Krutau V, Yudina O, Ilyina T, Grinchuk I. Surgery for massive malignant tumors of the left atrium - one center's experience. Kardiochir Torakochirurgia Pol. 2016;13(3):229–35.

16. Conklin LD, Reardon MJ. Autotransplantation of the heart for primary cardiac malignancy: development and surgical technique. Tex Heart Inst J. 2002;29(2):105–8 discussion 108.

17. Sueda T. History and development of surgical procedures for atrial fibrillation. Surg Today. 2015;45(12):1475–80.

18. Lang RM, Bierig M, Devereux RB, Flachskampf FA, Foster E, Pellikka PA, Picard MH, Roman MJ, Seward J, Shanewise JS, et al. Recommendations for chamber quantification: a report from the American Society of Echocardiography's guidelines and standards committee and the chamber quantification writing group, developed in conjunction with the European Association of Echocardiography, a branch of the European Society of Cardiology. J Am Soc Echocardiogr. 2005;18(12):1440–63.

19. Pritchett AM, Jacobsen SJ, Mahoney DW, Rodeheffer RJ, Bailey KR, Redfield MM. Left atrial volume as an index of left atrial size: a population-based study. J Am Coll Cardiol. 2003;41(6):1036–43.

20. Solomon SD, Foster E, Bourgoun M, Shah A, Viloria E, Brown MW, Hall WJ, Pfeffer MA, Moss AJ, Investigators M-C. Effect of cardiac resynchronization therapy on reverse remodeling and relation to outcome: multicenter automatic defibrillator implantation trial: cardiac resynchronization therapy. Circulation. 2010;122(10):985–92.

21. Dogliotti A, Paolasso E, Giugliano RP. Novel oral anticoagulants in atrial fibrillation: a meta-analysis of large, randomized, controlled trials vs warfarin. Clin Cardiol. 2013;36(2):61–7.

22. Stulak JM, Dearani JA, Sundt TM 3rd, Daly RC, Schaff HV. Ablation of atrial fibrillation: comparison of catheter-based techniques and the cox-maze III operation. Ann Thorac Surg. 2011;91(6):1882–8 discussion 1888-1889.

23. Kearney K, Stephenson R, Phan K, Chan WY, Huang MY, Yan TD. A systematic review of surgical ablation versus catheter ablation for atrial fibrillation. Ann Cardiothorac Surg. 2014;3(1):15–29.

24. Garcia-Villarreal OA, Gouveia AB, Gonzalez R, Arguero R. Left atrial reduction. A new concept in surgery for chronic atrial fibrillation. Rev Esp Cardiol. 2002;55(5):499–504.

25. Kang DH, Heo R, Lee S, Baek S, Kim DH, Song JM, Song JK, Lee JW. Initial surgery versus conservative management of symptomatic severe mitral regurgitation in the elderly. Heart. 2018;104(10):849-54.

26. Pan J, Li QG, Li J, Wang DJ. Partial cardiac autotransplantation with a concomitant mitral valve, aortic valve replacement and tricuspid plasty. Interact Cardiovasc Thorac Surg. 2013;17(5):906–7.

27. Erdogan HB, Kirali K, Omeroglu SN, Goksedef D, Isik O, Yakut C. Partial cardiac autotransplantation for reduction of the left atrium. Asian Cardiovasc Thorac Ann. 2004;12(2):111–4.

28. Garcia-Villarreal OA. eComment. Mini-partial heart autotransplantation for atrial fibrillation and mitral valve surgery. Interact Cardiovasc Thorac Surg. 2013;17(5):907–8.

29. Boldyrev SY, Lepshokov MK, Yakuba II, Barbukhatty KO, Porhanov VA. A patient with giant left atrium undergoes orthotopic heart transplantation. Tex Heart Inst J. 2014;41(1):87–90.

30. Ramlawi B, Al-Jabbari O, Blau LN, Davies MG, Bruckner BA, Blackmon SH, Ravi V, Benjamin R, Rodriguez L, Shapira OM, et al. Autotransplantation for the resection of complex left heart tumors. Ann Thorac Surg. 2014;98(3):863–8.

31. Cooley DA, Reardon MJ, Frazier OH, Angelini P. Human cardiac explantation and autotransplantation: application in a patient with a large cardiac pheochromocytoma. Tex Heart Inst J. 1985;12(2):171–6.

32. Novitzky D, Perry R, Ndaba D, Bowen T. Cardiac autotransplantation for mitral valve replacement. The heart surgery forum. 2003;6(5):424–8.

33. Piccoli GP, Massini C, Di Eusanio G, Ballerini L, Iacobone G, Soro A, Palminiello A. Giant left atrium and mitral valve disease: early and late results of surgical treatment in 40 cases. J Cardiovasc Surg. 1984;25(4):328–36.

34. Badhwar V, Rankin JS, Jacobs JP, Shahian DM, Habib RH, D'Agostino RS, Thourani VH, Suri RM, Prager RL, Edwards FH. The Society of Thoracic Surgeons adult cardiac surgery database: 2016 update on research. Ann Thorac Surg. 2016;102(1):7–13.

35. Terpenning S, Ketai LH, Teague SD, Rissing SM. Prevalence of left atrial abnormalities in atrial fibrillation versus normal sinus patients. Acta Radiol Open. 2016;5(6):2058460116651899.

36. Kawaguchi AT, Kosakai Y, Isobe F, Sasako Y, Eishi K, Nakano K, Kobayashi J, Kawashima Y. Surgical stratification of patients with atrial fibrillation secondary to organic cardiac lesions. Eur J Cardiothorac Surg. 1996;10(11): 983–9 discussion 989-990.

37. Blackmon SH, Reardon MJ. Cardiac Autotransplantation. Oper Tech Thorac Cardiovasc Surg. 2010;15(2):147–61.

38. Vyas H, Jackson K, Chenzbraun A. Switching to volumetric left atrial measurements: impact on routine echocardiographic practice. Eur J Echocardiogr. 2011;12(2):107–11.

39. Thomas L, Abhayaratna WP. Left atrial reverse remodeling: mechanisms, evaluation, And Clinical Significance. JACC Cardiovasc Imaging. 2017;10(1): 65–77.

40. Baskin KK, Taegtmeyer H. Taking pressure off the heart: the ins and outs of atrophic remodelling. Cardiovasc Res. 2011;90(2):243–50.

41. Kim GH, Uriel N, Burkhoff D. Reverse remodelling and myocardial recovery in heart failure. Nat Rev Cardiol. 2017;15:83.

Permissions

The contributors of this book come from diverse backgrounds, making this book a truly international effort. This book will bring forth new frontiers with its revolutionizing research information and detailed analysis of the nascent developments around the world.

We would like to thank all the contributing authors for lending their expertise to make the book truly unique. They have played a crucial role in the development of this book. Without their invaluable contributions this book wouldn't have been possible. They have made vital efforts to compile up to date information on the varied aspects of this subject to make this book a valuable addition to the collection of many professionals and students.

This book was conceptualized with the vision of imparting up-to-date information and advanced data in this field. To ensure the same, a matchless editorial board was set up. Every individual on the board went through rigorous rounds of assessment to prove their worth. After which they invested a large part of their time researching and compiling the most relevant data for our readers.

The editorial board has been involved in producing this book since its inception. They have spent rigorous hours researching and exploring the diverse topics which have resulted in the successful publishing of this book. They have passed on their knowledge of decades through this book. To expedite this challenging task, the publisher supported the team at every step. A small team of assistant editors was also appointed to further simplify the editing procedure and attain best results for the readers.

Apart from the editorial board, the designing team has also invested a significant amount of their time in understanding the subject and creating the most relevant covers. They scrutinized every image to scout for the most suitable representation of the subject and create an appropriate cover for the book.

The publishing team has been an ardent support to the editorial, designing and production team. Their endless efforts to recruit the best for this project, has resulted in the accomplishment of this book. They are a veteran in the field of academics and their pool of knowledge is as vast as their experience in printing. Their expertise and guidance has proved useful at every step. Their uncompromising quality standards have made this book an exceptional effort. Their encouragement from time to time has been an inspiration for everyone.

The publisher and the editorial board hope that this book will prove to be a valuable piece of knowledge for researchers, students, practitioners and scholars across the globe.

List of Contributors

Anna Marcinkiewicz, Ryszard Jaszewski and Radosław Zwoliński
Cardiac Surgery Clinic, Chair of Cardiology and Cardiac Surgery, Military Medical Academy University Teaching Hospital - Central Veterans' Hospital in Lodz, Sterling 1/3 St, Lodz 91-425, Poland

Katarzyna Piestrzeniewicz
Department of Cardiology, Chair of Cardiology and Cardiac Surgery, Military Medical Academy University Teaching Hospital - Central Veterans' Hospital in Lodz, Lodz, Poland

Mahdieh Abbasalizad Farhangi
Drug Applied Research Center, Nutrition Research Center, Faculty of Nutrition, Tabriz University of Medical Sciences, Tabriz, Iran

Mahdi Najafi
Department of Research, Tehran Heart Center, Tehran University of Medical Sciences, North Karegar Street, Tehran 1411713138, Iran

Mohammad Asghari Jafarabadi
Road Traffic Injury Research Center, Tabriz University of Medical Sciences, Tabriz, Iran

Leila Jahangiry
Tabriz Health Services Managment Research Center, Tabriz University of Medical Sciences, Tabriz, Iran

Rickard P. F. Lindblom, Camilla Sandström, Nadjira Ligata, Beata Larsson and Christine Leo Swenne
Department of Cardiothoracic Surgery and Anesthesia, Uppsala University Hospital, 751 85 Uppsala, Sweden

Birgitta Lytsy and Ulrika Ransjö
Department of Medical Sciences, Unit for Clinical Microbiology and Infectious Medicine, Uppsala University, Uppsala, Sweden

Christine Leo Swenne
Department of Public Health and Caring Sciences, Uppsala University, Uppsala, Sweden

Hang Wang and Ke-Yin Cai
Cadre Ward Two, Wuhan General Hospital of Guangzhou Military Command, Wuhan 430070, China

Yang-Guang Yin
Intensive Care Unit, The sixth people's hospital of Chongqing, Nan'an District, Chongqing 400060, China

Hao Huang
Clinic center, Shenzhen Hornetcorn Biotechnology Company, Ltd, Shenzhen 518400, China

Xiao-Hui Zhao, Jie Yu, Qiang Wang and Wei Li
Institute of Cardiovascular Science, Xinqiao Hospital, Third Military Medical University, Chongqing 400037, China

Shi-Fang Ding
Institute of Cardiovascular Science, Wuhan General Hospital of Guangzhou Military Command, Wuhan 430070, China

H. Kirov, M. Schwarzer, G. Faerber, M. Diab and T. Doenst
Department of Cardiothoracic Surgery, Friedrich Schiller University Jena, University Hospital, Am Klinikum 1, 07747 Jena, Germany

M. Diab
Department of Cardiothoracic Surgery, Cairo University, Cairo, Egypt

S. Neugebauer
Department of Clinical Chemistry and Laboratory Medicine, Friedrich-Schiller-University Jena, University Hospital, Jena, Germany
Integrated Research and Treatment Center, Center for Sepsis Control and Care (CSCC), Jena, Germany

Arn Migowski, Vitor Manuel Pereira Azevedo, Rogério Brant Martins Chaves and Regina Maria de Aquino Xavier
Instituto Nacional de Cardiologia - INC (National Institute of Cardiology, Ministry of Health), Coordenação de Ensino e Pesquisa, Divisão de Saúde Coletiva, rua das Laranjeiras 374, Laranjeiras, Rio de Janeiro, RJ, Brazil

Antonio Luiz Ribeiro
University Hospital and School of Medicine, Federal University of Minas Gerais (UFMG), Minas Gerais, Brazil

Marilia Sá Carvalho
Oswaldo Cruz Foundation (FIOCRUZ), Rio de Janeiro, Brazil

Lucas de Aquino Hashimoto and Carolina de Aquino Xavier
School of Medicine, Federal University of Rio de Janeiro (UFRJ), Rio de Janeiro, Brazil

Marco Barbanti and Corrado Tamburino
Catania Division of Cardiology, Ferrarotto Hospital, University of Catania, Via Salvatore Citelli 6, Catania, Italy

Jan Baan, Marije Vis and Martijn S. van Mourik
Department of Cardiology, Academic Medical Center, Amsterdam, The Netherlands

Mark S. Spence
Cardiology Department, Royal Victoria Hospital, Belfast, UK

Fortunato Iacovelli
Interventional Cardiology Service, "Montevergine" Clinic, Mercogliano, Italy
Division of Cardiology, Department of Advanced Biomedical Sciences, University of Naples "Federico II", Naples, Italy

Gian Luca Martinelli
Novara Department of Cardiac Surgery, Clinica San Gaudenzio, Novara, Italy

Francesco Saia
Cardiovascular and Thoracic Department, S. Orsola-Malpighi University Hospital, Bologna, Italy

Alessandro Santo Bortone
Department of Interventional Cardiology, University of Bari "Aldo Moro", Bari, Italy

Frank van der Kley
Department of Cardiology, Leiden University Medical Center, Leiden, The Netherlands

Douglas F. Muir
Cardiothoracic Division, The James Cook University Hospital, Middlesbrough, UK

Cameron G. Densem
Department of Interventional Cardiology, Papworth Hospital, Cambridge, UK

Lenka Seilerova
Edwards Lifesciences, Prague, Czech Republic

Claudia M. Lüske and Peter Bramlage
Institute for Pharmacology and Preventive Medicine, Cloppenburg, Germany

Paolo Cotogni
Department of Anesthesia and Intensive Care, S. Giovanni Battista Hospital, University of Turin, Via Giovanni Giolitti 9, 10123 Turin, Italy

Cristina Barbero and Mauro Rinaldi
Department of Cardiovascular Surgery, S. Giovanni Battista Hospital, University of Turin, Turin, Italy

Roberto Passera
Nuclear Medicine Unit, S. Giovanni Battista Hospital, University of Turin, Turin, Italy

Lucina Fossati
Microbiology and Virology Laboratory, S. Giovanni Battista Hospital, University of Turin, Turin, Italy

Giorgio Olivero
Department of Surgical Sciences, S. Giovanni Battista Hospital, University of Turin, Turin, Italy

Jessica G. Y. Luc, Colleen M. Norris, Sadek Al Shouli, Yugmel S. Nijjar and Steven R. Meyer
Division of Cardiac Surgery, Department of Surgery, Faculty of Medicine and Dentistry, University of Alberta, Edmonton, Canada

Michelle M. Graham, Colleen M. Norris, Sadek Al Shouli and Steven R. Meyer
Mazankowski Alberta Heart Institute, Edmonton, Canada

Michelle M. Graham and Colleen M. Norris
Division of Cardiology, Department of Medicine, Faculty of Medicine and Dentistry, University of Alberta, Edmonton, Canada

Yunpeng Ling
Department of Cardiac Surgery, Peking University Third Hospital, Beijing, China

Liming Bao
Department of Cardiac Surgery, Aero Space Center Hospital, Beijing, China

Wei Yang, Yu Chen and Qing Gao
Department of Cardiac Surgery, Peking University People's Hospital, Beijing, China

Troels Thim, Gro Egholm Chisholm, Anne Kaltoft, Leif Thuesen, Steen Dalby Kristensen, Lars Romer Krusell, Jens Flensted Lassen and Michael Maeng
Department of Cardiology, Aarhus University Hospital, Aarhus, Denmark

Henrik Toft Sørensen, Martin Berg Johansen, Morten Schmidt and Hans Erik Bøtker
Department of Clinical Epidemiology, Aarhus University Hospital, Brendstrupgaardsvej 100, Aarhus, N 8200, Denmark

Per Thayssen and Lisette Okkels Jensen
Department of Cardiology, Odense University Hospital, Odense, Denmark

Hans-Henrik Tilsted
Department of Cardiology, Aalborg University Hospital, Aalborg, Denmark

Jaehuk Choi
Division of Cardiology, Hangang Sacred Heart Hospital, Hallym University Medical Center, Seoul, South Korea

Min-Kyung Kang, Chaehoon Han, Sang Muk Hwang, Sung Gu Jung, Han-Kyul Kim, Kwang Jin Chun, Seonghoon Choi, Jung Rae Cho and Namho Lee
Cardiology Division, Kangnam Sacred Heart Hospital, Hallym University Medical Center, Seoul, South Korea

Kwang Jin Chun
Division of Cardiology, Department of Medicine, College of Medicine, Kangwon National University, Chuncheon, South Korea

Tomoko S. Kato, Hiroshi Nakamura, Mai Murata, Kishio Kuroda, Yasutaka Yokoyama, Akie Shimada, Satoshi Matsushita, Taira Yamamoto and Atsushi Amano
Department of Cardiovascular Surgery, Heart Center, Juntendo University, 2-1-1, Hongo, Bunkyo-ku, Tokyo 113-8421, Japan

Hitoshi Suzuki
Division of Nephrology,Department of Internal Medicine, Juntendo University School of Medicine, Bunkyo-ku, Tokyo, Japan

Mehmet Oezkur, Jens Holger Krannich, Christoph Schimmer and Rainer Leyh
Department of Cardiovascular Surgery, University Hospital Würzburg, Würzburg, Germany

Martin Wagner, Christoph Riegler, Victoria Rücker and Peter U. Heuschmann
Institute of Clinical Epidemiology and Biometry, University of Würzburg, Würzburg, Germany

Martin Wagner, Dirk Weismann and Peter U. Heuschmann
Comprehensive Heart Failure Center, University of Würzburg, Würzburg, Germany

Martin Wagner
Department of Internal Medicine I, Division of Nephrology, University Hospital Würzburg, Würzburg, Germany

Dirk Weismann
Department of Internal Medicine I, Endocrine and Diabetes Unit, University Hospital Würzburg, Würzburg, Germany

Peter U. Heuschmann
Clinical Trial Center Würzburg, University Hospital Würzburg, Würzburg, Germany

Anna Wysocka, Andrzej Wysokiński and Tomasz Zapolski
Cardiology Department, Medical University of Lublin, ul. Jaczewskiego 8, 20– 954 Lublin, Poland

Anna Wysocka and Jadwiga Daniluk
Internal Medicine in Nursing Department, Medical University of Lublin, ul. Jaczewskiego 8, 20–954 Lublin, Poland

Marek Cybulski and Henryk Berbeć
Biochemistry and Molecular Biology Department, Medical University of Lublin, ul. Chodźki 1, 20-093 Lublin, Poland

Janusz Stążka
Cardiosurgery Department, Medical University of Lublin, ul. Jaczewskiego 8, 20–954 Lublin, Poland

Lei Zheng, Qing-Ming Fan and Zhen-Yu Wei
Department of Cardiovascular Surgery, Yantai Yuhuangding Hospital, No.20 Yuhuangding East Road, Yantai 264000, P. R. China

Andrea Ungar, Giulio Mannarino and Gennaro Santoro
Geriatric Intensive Care Unit, Department of Geriatrics and Medicine, Careggi Hospital and University of Florence, Florence, Italy

Nathalie van der Velde and Sofie Jansen
Internal Medicine, Section of Geriatric Medicine, Academic Medical Center, Amsterdam, Netherlands

Jan Baan and Martijn van Mourik
Cardiology, Academic Medical Center, Amsterdam, Netherlands

Marie-Pierre Thibodeau and Jean-Bernard Masson
Centre Hospitalier de l'Université de Montréal, Montréal, Canada

Cornelia Deutsch and Peter Bramlage
Institute for Pharmacology und Preventive Medicine, Cloppenburg, Germany

Jana Kurucova and Martin Thoenes
Edwards Lifesciences, Nyon, Switzerland

Stefania Maggi
CNR–Institute of Neuroscience, Aging Branch, Padua, Italy

Andreas W. Schoenenberger
Department of Geriatrics, Inselspital, Bern University Hospital, University of Bern, Bern, Switzerland

Jenny Bjerre, Anne Mielke Christensen, Gunnar Gislason and Anne-Christine Ruwald
Department of Cardiology, Cardiovascular Research, Copenhagen University Hospital Herlev-Gentofte, Kildegaardsvej 28, 2900 Hellerup, Denmark

Simone Hofman Rosenkranz
Research and Test Center for Health Technologies, Copenhagen University Hospital, Rigshospitalet-Glostrup, Valdemar Hansens Vej 1-23, 2600 Glostrup, Denmark

Morten Schou and Christian Jøns
Department of Cardiology, Copenhagen University Hospital Rigshospitalet-Glostrup, Blegdamsvej 9, 2100 Copenhagen Ø, Denmark

Anne-Christine Ruwald
Department of Medicine, Zealand University Hospital, Sygehusvej 10, 4000 Roskilde, Denmark

Grzegorz Bielicki, Kinga Kosiorowska, Jacek Jakubaszko, Rafal Nowicki and Marek Jasinski
Department of Cardiac Surgery, Wroclaw Medical University, Wroclaw, Poland

Marceli Lukaszewski and Marek Jasinski
Department of Anaesthesiology and Intensive Therapy, Wroclaw Medical University, Borowska 213, 50-556 Wroclaw, Wroclaw, Poland

Wen Ge
Department of Cardiothoracic Surgery, Shuguang Hospital, affiliated to Shanghai University of TCM, Shanghai 200021, China

Chang Gus
Department of Thoracic Surgery, Shanghai Chest Hospital, Shanghai Jiao Tong University, Shanghai 200030, China

Chao Chen, Wangwang Chen, Zhengqiang Cang and Chennan Shi
The First Clinical Medical College of Nanjing Medical University, Nanjing 210029, China

Yuliang Wang
Department of Hygiene Analysis and Detection School of Public Health Nanjing Medical University, Nanjing 210029, China

Yangyang Zhang
Department of Cardiovascular Surgery, East Hospital, Tongji University School of Medicine, 150 Jimo Road, Shanghai 200120, China
Key Laboratory of Arrhythmias of the Ministry of Education of China, East Hospital, Tongji University School of Medicine, Shanghai 200120, China

Ping Zhu, Xin Zhou, Chenliang Zhang, Huakang Li, Zhihui Zhang and Zhiyuan Song
Department of Cardiology, Southwest Hospital, Third Military Medical University (Army Medical University), Chongqing, China

Alessandro Satriano, Zachary Guenther, James A. White, Naeem Merchant and Carmen P. Lydell
Stephenson Cardiac Imaging Centre, University of Calgary, Calgary, Alberta, Canada

Alessandro Satriano, James A. White, Faisal Al-Qoofi and Nowell M. Fine
Division of Cardiology, Department of Cardiac Sciences, Libin Cardiovascular Institute of Alberta, University of Calgary, South Health Campus, 4448 Front Street SE, Calgary, Alberta T3M 1M4, Canada

Zachary Guenther, Naeem Merchant and Carmen P. Lydell
Department of Diagnostic Imaging, Cummings School of Medicine, University of Calgary, Calgary, Alberta, Canada

Elena S. Di Martino
Department of Civil Engineering and Centre for Bioengineering Research and Education, University of Calgary, Calgary, Alberta, Canada

Zan Mitrev, Milka Klincheva, Tanja Anguseva, Igor Zdravkovski and Rodney Alexander Rosalia
Zan Mitrev and Rodney Rosalia contributed equally to this work. Zan Mitrev Clinic, Bledski Dogovor 8, Skopje 1000, Republic of Macedonia

Index